SEDATION AND ANALGESIA FOR DIAGNOSTIC AND THERAPEUTIC PROCEDURES

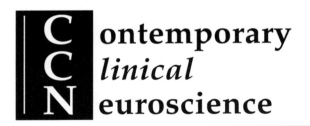

C
C ontemporary
C linical
N euroscience

Series Editors:
Ralph Lydic and
Helen A. Baghdoyan

Contemporary Clinical Neuroscience

SEDATION AND ANALGESIA FOR DIAGNOSTIC AND THERAPEUTIC PROCEDURES

Edited by

SHOBHA MALVIYA, MD,
NORAH N. NAUGHTON, MD,

and

KEVIN K. TREMPER, MD, PhD

*Department of Anesthesiology,
University of Michigan Health System,
Ann Arbor, MI*

Humana Press ✳ Totowa, New Jersey

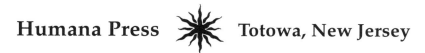

© 2003 Humana Press Inc.
999 Riverview Drive, Suite 208
Totowa, New Jersey 07512

humanapress.com

Production Editor: Kim Hoather-Potter.

Cover design by Patricia F. Cleary.

For additional copies, pricing for bulk purchases, and/or information about other Humana titles, contact Humana at the above address or at any of the following numbers: Tel.: 973-256-1699; Fax: 973-256-8341; E-mail: humana@humanapr.com or visit our website at www.humanapress.com

The opinions expressed herein are the views of the authors and may not necessarily reflect the official policy of the National Institute on Drug Abuse or any other parts of the US Department of Health and Human Services. The US Government does not endorse or favor any specific commercial product or company. Trade, proprietary, or company names appearing in this publication are used only because they are considered essential in the context of the studies reported herein.

This publication is printed on acid-free paper. ⊚
ANSI Z39.48-1984 (American National Standards Institute) Permanence of Paper for Printed Library Materials.

Printed in the United States of America. 10 9 8 7 6 5 4 3 2 1

Library of Congress Cataloging-in-Publication Data

Sedation and analgesia for diagnostic and therapeutic procedures / [edited by] Shobha Malviya, Norah N. Naughton and Kevin K. Tremper.
        p. ; cm.-- (Contemporary clinical neuroscience)
    Includes bibliographical references and index.
    ISBN 0-89603-863-7 (alk. paper)
    E-ISBN 1-59259-295-3
        1. Anesthesia. 2. Analgesia. I. Malviya, Shobha. II. Naughton, Norah N. III. Tremper, Kevin K. IV. Series.
        [DNLM: 1. Anesthesia. 2. Analgesia. 3. Diagnostic Techniques and Procedures. WO 200 S4466 2003]
    RD81 .S39 2003
617.9'6--dc21   2002032817

DEDICATION

In memory of my parents Mr. Laxmi Narain Goel and Mrs. Janak Dulari Goel who gave me the privilege of learning. To my husband Vinay, and our children Samir and Sanjana with whom I continue to learn.

Shobha Malviya, MD

To Bridget, Julie, Michael, and Pat: your presence makes my dreams possible.

Norah N. Naughton, MD

PREFACE

Pharmacologically induced sedation has become pervasive throughout medical practice to accomplish diagnostic and minor therapeutic procedures effectively and humanely. As diagnostic techniques and technical procedures become more complex, the need for sedation in patients with varied co-morbid conditions, in diverse settings produces a series of questions regarding safety and effectiveness. The administration of sedation and analgesia for diagnostic and therapeutic procedures has therefore evolved into a unique discipline that is practiced by clinicians with varying skills and training. Disparities in sedation practices have led regulatory agencies to mandate that patients receive the same standard of care regardless of the location in which the care is provided within an institution. To ensure that the standard of care is of high quality, institutions are required to develop guidelines for the practice of sedation, ensure that these guidelines are followed, and provide quality data and outcome measures. In addition, practitioners who administer sedatives and analgesics specifically for a diagnostic and/or a therapeutic procedure require specific credentials for this practice.

It is the intent of *Sedation and Analgesia for Diagnostic and Therapeutic Procedures* to review sedation and analgesia from a wide variety of perspectives starting with the basic neurobiology and physiology of the sedated state, proceeding through clinical guidelines and practices, and concluding with a section on quality-outcome measures and processes. The practical aspects of this book have been further emphasized by incorporating a series of tables and figures in each chapter that highlight protocols, regulatory requirements, recommended dosages of pharmacologic agents, monitoring requirements, and quality assurance tools. The target audience for this text spans multiple disciplines that range from investigators, physicians, and nurses to hospital administrators.

The editors are indebted to all the authors for contributing their knowledge, time, and effort. Special thanks are due to Dr. Ralph Lydic who conceived this project and to Ms. Terri Voepel-Lewis, MSN, RN for her invaluable assistance throughout the development of this text. Finally, we thank Mrs. Colleen Rauch and Mrs. Melissa Bowles for their administrative assistance.

Shobha Malviya, MD
Norah Naughton, MD
Kevin K. Tremper, MD, PhD

vii

CONTENTS

CONTRIBUTORS

HELEN A. BAGHDOYAN, PhD • *Department of Anesthesiology, University of Michigan Medical School, Ann Arbor, MI*

JEFFREY L. BLUMER, MD, PhD • *Department of Pediatrics, Rainbow Babies and Children's Hospital, Case Western Reserve University School of Medicine, Cleveland, OH*

LOREE A. COLLETT, BSN, RN • *Pediatric PACU, C. S. Mott Children's Hospital, University of Michigan Health System, Ann Arbor, MI*

SABINE KOST-BYERLY, MD • *Department of Anesthesiology/Critical Care Medicine, The Johns Hopkins University, Baltimore, MD*

LIA H. LOWRIE, MD • *Department of Pediatrics, Rainbow Babies and Children's Hospital, Case Western Reserve University School of Medicine, Cleveland, OH*

RALPH LYDIC, PhD • *Department of Anesthesiology, University of Michigan Medical School, Ann Arbor, MI*

SHOBHA MALVIYA, MD • *Department of Anesthesiology, University of Michigan Health System, Ann Arbor, MI*

LYNNE G. MAXWELL, MD • *Department of Anesthesiology, The Children's Hospital of Philadelphia, Philadelphia, PA*

JACINTA MCGINLEY, MB, FFARCSI • *Department of Anesthesia and Intensive Care, Our Lady's Hospital for Sick Children, Dublin, Ireland*

NORAH N. NAUGHTON, MD • *Director of Obstetric Anesthesiology, Department of Anesthesiology, University of Michigan Health System, Ann Arbor, MI*

J. ELIZABETH OTHMAN, MS, RN • *Department of Anesthesiology, University of Michigan Health System, Ann Arbor, MI*

DAVID M. POLANER, MD, FAAP • *Department of Anesthesia, The Children's Hospital, and University of Colorado School of Medicine, Denver, CO*

RANDOLPH STEADMAN, MD • *Vice Chairman, Department of Anesthesiology, UCLA School of Medicine, Center for Health Sciences, Los Angeles, CA*

JOSEPH D. TOBIAS, MD • *Vice Chairman, Department of Anesthesiology, Chief, Division of Pediatric Anesthesia/Critical Care, University of Missouri Health Sciences Center, Columbia, MO*

KEVIN K. TREMPER, MD, PhD • *Department of Anesthesiology, University of Michigan Health System, Ann Arbor, MI*

SHEILA A. TROUTEN, BSN, RN • *Pediatric PACU, C. S. Mott Children's Hospital, University of Michigan Health System, Ann Arbor, MI*

TERRI VOEPEL-LEWIS, MSN, RN • *Department of Anesthesiology, C. S. Mott Children's Hospital, University of Michigan Health System, Ann Arbor, MI*

MYRON YASTER, MD • *Departments of Anesthesiology/Critical Care Medicine and Pediatrics, The Johns Hopkins Hospital, Baltimore, MD*

STEVE YUN, MD • *UCLA School of Medicine, Center for Health Sciences, Los Angeles, CA*

Opioids, Sedation, and Sleep

Different States, Similar Traits,
and the Search for Common Mechanisms

Ralph Lydic, PhD, Helen A. Baghdoyan, PhD, and Jacinta McGinley, MB, FFARCSI

1. INTRODUCTION

Sedation is an area of active research motivated by the clinical need for safe and reliable techniques. An understanding of the cellular and molecular physiology of sedation will contribute to the rational development of sedating drugs. These important goals are hampered, however, by the complexity of sedation as an altered state of arousal and by the diversity of sedating drugs. The purpose of this chapter is to selectively review data in support of a working hypothesis that conceptually unifies efforts to understand the neurochemical basis of sedation.

We hypothesize that brain mechanisms that evolved to generate naturally occurring states of sleep *(1)* generate the traits that define levels of sedation *(2)* and various states of general anesthesia *(3–5)*. Our hypothesis offers several key advantages. First, it is simpler and more direct than the alternate hypothesis, which requires a cartography of cellular changes that are unique to each disparate drug and associated co-variates such as dose, route of delivery, and pharmacokinetics. Even a decade ago, this alternate hypothesis would have required evaluation of more than 80 different drugs and drug combinations used to produce sedation *(6)*. Second, our hypothesis encourages characterization of alterations in traits such as the electroencephalogram (EEG), respiration, or muscle tone, which are characteristic of sedation. Third, the hypothesis offers a standardized control condition (normal wakefulness) to which drug-induced trait and state changes can be compared. Finally, the hypothesis is empowered by the fact that natural sleep is the most thoroughly characterized arousal state at the cellular level *(1,7,8)*. Thus, sleep neurobiology offers a conceptual framework for unifying the diverse collection of descriptive data that now characterize sedation.

From: *Contemporary Clinical Neuroscience: Sedation and Analgesia for Diagnostic and Therapeutic Procedures*
Edited by: S. Malviya, N. N. Naughton, and K. K. Tremper © Humana Press Inc., Totowa, NJ

During sedation, the effects of pharmacological agents are superimposed on a patient's emotional state and level of arousal. A patient's endogenous behavioral state is particularly relevant for the practitioners who use sedation to enhance patient comfort. One study of 76 children aged 18–61 mo noted that parental perception of a child being tired was related to poor sedation *(9)*. It has been noted that "the declaration of any given state may be incomplete and that states can oscillate rapidly, resulting in bizarre and important clinical syndromes" *(10)*. Narcolepsy provides one example during which physiological and behavioral traits characteristic of rapid eye movement (REM) sleep intrude upon and disrupt wakefulness *(11)*. A better understanding of the endogenously generated traits outlined in this chapter is likely to advance understanding of the mechanisms that actively generate states of sedation.

2. SEDATION DOES NOT PUT PATIENTS TO SLEEP

There are compelling questions concerning the development of accurate and medically sophisticated definitions of sedation. For example, is it disingenuous to advise a patient that they will be "put to sleep"? In both research and purely clinical environments, patients are routinely told they will be "put to sleep." Examples from human drug research refer to "wake-sleep transitions" displayed by patients receiving hypnotic infusion *(12)* and refer to children who are "asleep but rousable" following doses of ketamine/ midazolam *(13)*. Clinical sedation has been described as "light sleep" *(14)*, and textbooks note that "the terms sleep, hypnosis, and unconsciousness are used interchangeably in anesthesia literature to refer to the state of artificially induced (i.e., drug-induced) sleep" *(15)*. Is it any wonder that so much thoughtful attention has been directed toward operationally defining "procedural sedation" *(16)*, "monitored anesthesia care" *(17)*, "conscious versus deep sedation" *(18)*, and "sedation/analgesia" *(2)*? Practice guidelines recommend monitoring the level of consciousness during sedation *(2,19)*. Therefore, a clear understanding of the similarities and differences between sedation and natural sleep are directly relevant to any objective assessment of arousal level. Aldrich provides an example from the neurology of akinetic mutism reflecting frontal lobe lesion or diffuse cortical injury resulting in a state of silent immobility that resembles sleep *(11)*. A clear distinction between natural sleep and sedation is likely to prove important from a medical-legal perspective.

All arousal states are manifest on a continuum that is operationally defined by physiological and behavioral traits (Fig. 1). The component traits are generated by anatomically distributed neuronal networks *(1,20)*. The traits

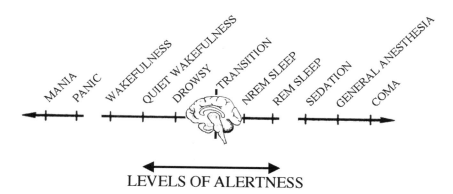

MANIA PANIC WAKEFULNESS QUIET WAKEFULNESS DROWSY TRANSITION NREM SLEEP REM SLEEP SEDATION GENERAL ANESTHESIA COMA

LEVELS OF ALERTNESS

Fig. 1. Schematic illustrating dynamic changes in levels of alertness displayed by the brain. The figure conveys continuity between states of naturally occurring sleep and wakefulness. The individual states, such as wakefulness, are defined using a constellation of physiological and behavioral traits generated by the brain. Pharmacologically induced states of sedation and general anesthesia are characterized by some of the same traits observed during naturally occurring sleep/waking states. The broken lines between REM sleep and sedation and between wakefulness and manic states indicate a discontinuity in the state transitions.

(e.g., activated EEG, motor tone, and orientation to person, place, and time) are clustered into groups that define a particular arousal state, such as wakefulness. In many cases, central pattern-generating neurons are known to orchestrate the constellation of traits *(21)* from which states are assembled as an emergent process *(22)*. It is clear that sleep is not a passive process resulting from the loss of waking consciousness. Rather, sleep is actively generated by the brain, and considerable progress in sleep neurobiology has identified many of the neuronal and molecular mechanisms regulating sleep *(1)*. These basic data provide a knowledge base for the rational development of a clinical sub-specialty referred to as sleep disorders medicine *(7,11,23)*. Cogent arguments for empiric definitions of traits and states have been presented elsewhere *(10,24,25)*.

Many lines of evidence demonstrate that pharmacologic sedation is not physiologic sleep. The remainder of this paragraph illustrates this point through five examples of specific differences in sleep and sedation. First, the duration of sedation is a function of drug, dose, and a host of patient variables. In contrast, the duration and temporal organization of the sleep cycle, like the cardiac cycle, are homeostatically regulated. Just as cardiovascular health requires a normal cardiac cycle, restorative sleep that enhances daytime performance requires a normal sleep cycle. Throughout the night,

Table 1
States are Defined by a Constellation of Traits

Traits defining NREM/REM sleep	Traits defining sedation	Traits defining general anesthesia
• Hypotonia/atonia • Slow/fast eye movements • Regular/irregular breathing, heart rate, blood pressure • EEG slow, deactivated/ fast, activated	• Analgesia • Amnesia • Obtundation of waking • Anxiolysis	• Analgesia • Amnesia • Unconsciousness • Muscle relaxation • Reduced autonomic responses

the distinct phases of REM and non-rapid eye movement (NREM) sleep occur periodically about every 90 min. This actively generated NREM/REM cycle has particular relevance for patients who are sedated during periods of the night that would normally comprise the sleep phase of their sleep/wake cycle (for example, patients sedated in the intensive care unit). A second difference is that sleep is reversible with sensory stimulation, whereas one goal of sedation is to depress sensory processing in the face of noxious physical and/or aversive psychological stimulation. Third, nausea and vomiting are not associated with sleep, but can be positively correlated with sedation level (26). Fourth, a characteristic trait of REM sleep is postural muscle atonia that is actively generated by the brainstem (27,28). Virtually all humans experience this motor blockade each night, yet are unaware of the process. In contrast, motor blockade is not observed or induced during sedation. Finally, sedation analgesia is a dissociated state comprised of some traits characteristic of wakefulness (ability to follow verbal commands) and some traits characteristic of natural sleep (diminished sensory processing, memory impairment, and autonomic depression). Table 1 illustrates some of the traits used to define states of sleep, sedation, and general anesthesia. The presence of dissociated traits satisfies the diagnostic criteria for sleep disorders when waking traits occur during natural sleep (7,10) and disorders of arousal when sleep traits intrude upon wakefulness (11).

For more than 30 years, it has been known that opioids administered acutely obtund wakefulness but disrupt the normal sleep cycle and inhibit the REM phase of sleep (29). This finding from the substance abuse literature is directly relevant for sedation analgesia. Opioids administered to intensive care unit (ICU) patients have been shown to contribute to the sleep deprivation and delirium that characterize ICU syndrome (30).

Despite these differences between sleep and sedation, the two states share remarkable similarities. For example, NREM sleep is characterized by slow eye movements and REM sleep was named (arbitrarily) for the "rapid," saccadic eye movements. Stereotypic eye movements can be observed in sedated patients, and these eye movements may vary as a function of dose and drug *(12)*. Mammalian temperature regulation is disrupted during the REM phase of sleep (reviewed in ref. *31*), and sedation can alter the relationship between body temperature and energy expenditure *(32)*. Compared to wakefulness, mentation during both sleep and sedation can be bizarre and hallucinoid. For each of the foregoing examples, however, there are qualitative differences between the traits characterizing states of sleep and states of sedation. The remainder of this chapter highlights data consistent with the working hypothesis that the similarities between sedation and natural sleep are mediated by common neurobiological mechanisms.

3. SEDATION AND SLEEP INHIBIT MEMORY AND ALTER EEG FREQUENCY

A distinctive feature of both natural sleep and drug-induced sedation is the blunting or elimination of normal waking consciousness. The diminution in arousal associated with both sedation and sleep has profound and complex effects on recall and memory. The amnesic properties of sedating drugs are widely regarded as a positive feature for preventing the recall of unpleasant, frightening, or painful procedures. A caveat is that sedating drugs also are known to disrupt natural sleep. This disruption can contribute to the negative features of impaired alertness and delirium *(30,33)*, resulting in delayed discharge time from the hospital or clinic. Dose-dependent impairment of memory by ketamine and propofol has been demonstrated repeatedly, and the most reliable anterograde amnesia is produced by benzodiazepines *(34)*. This conclusion is supported by studies emphasizing that benzodiazepines more potently impair implicit memory (word stem completion) than explicit memory (cued recall) *(35,36)*. Papper's insights into the potential contributions anesthesiology can make to the formal study of consciousness *(37)* also apply to sedation as a unique tool for understanding learning and memory *(38)*.

A large body of research has established a reliable and complex relationship between natural sleep and memory. As reviewed elsewhere *(39–41)*, memory can be impaired by sleep onset and by sleep deprivation. Selective deprivation of REM sleep impairs recall. Intense learning of new materials significantly increases REM sleep. During NREM (slow wave) sleep, the EEG is comprised of low-frequency, high-amplitude waves often referred to as "sleep spindles" (Fig. 2). During waking and REM sleep, brainstem systems that project to the thalamus and cortex produce an activated EEG

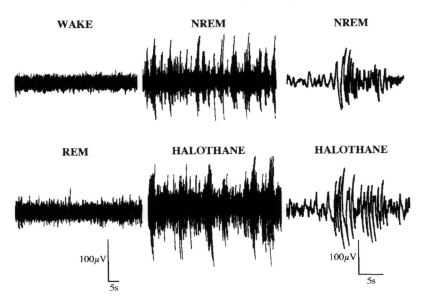

Fig. 2. Electroencephalographic recording from the cortex of the cat during wakefulness, NREM sleep, REM sleep, and halothane anesthesia. The left-most column illustrates that REM sleep is an activated brain state. Note that the EEG during REM sleep is similar to the EEG of wakefulness. The middle portion of the figure shows that the EEG spindles characteristic of halothane anesthesia are similar to the EEG spindles generated during NREM sleep. The right column shows the EEG spindles recorded at a faster sweep speed; note that these spindles are comprised of waves with frequencies of 8–14 Hz. (Reprinted with permission from ref. *[92]*, Lippincott Williams & Wilkins, 1996).

containing high-frequency waves of 30–40 Hz known as gamma oscillations *(42)*. These state-dependent changes in EEG are consistent with data suggesting that sleep may play a key role in the cortical reorganization of memories *(43)*. The ability of sleep to modulate recall and memory may involve state-dependent modulation of thalamocortical plasticity *(44)*. Cellular and electrographic studies of learning have found that patterns of neuronal discharge in the rat hippocampus during NREM sleep contain traces of neuronal activity patterns associated with behaviors that occurred during previous waking experience *(45)*. This finding implies that normal sleep offers a period during which the brain replays the neuronal correlates of some daily experience. The degree to which sedating drugs alter such neuronal discharge patterns has not yet been reported.

Many studies have examined the relationship between EEG power, memory, and level of sedation. Many of these studies aim to derive an EEG index for the quantitative assessment of arousal level or as a marker of amnesia. There is good agreement for slowing of EEG frequency into the Beta range (Beta$_1 \cong$ 15–20 Hz; Beta$_2 \cong$ 20.5–30 Hz) caused by midazolam *(46)* and propofol *(47–49)*, and for EEG slowing caused by dexmedetomidine *(50)*. Few studies have systematically compared sedating drugs from different chemical families, but comparison of a benzodiazepine (midazolam), an alkylphenol (propofol), and a barbiturate (thiopental) also revealed increasing EEG beta-power resulting from all three drugs *(51)*.

Historically, studies of EEG in relation to sedation employed spectral analyses to identify a dominant frequency among a complex collection of waveforms and frequencies *(52)*. The complexities of EEG signal processing and the time required for raw EEG interpretation have stimulated efforts to obtain a processed EEG signal (i.e., a single number) that can be interpreted in near-real time. One such processed EEG signal for which there has been enthusiasm in the context of anesthesia and/or sedation is referred to as the bispectral index (BIS) *(53)*. The BIS uses a scale of 0 to 100 to quantify the degree of coherence among the different EEG components *(54)*. In general, quiet wakefulness is associated with high BIS values *(53–55)*. A preliminary study of five normal, non-drugged subjects reported mean BIS levels during quiet wakefulness = 92, light sleep = 81, slow-wave sleep = 59, and REM sleep = 83 *(55)*. This initial study of the BIS as a measure of natural sleep acknowledged three limitations. First, the BIS values have not been validated against a full 12–16-channel polysomnographic recording. Second, some periods of REM sleep and waking may have been mixed. Third, NREM sleep was not divided into its four known stages: I–IV *(55)*. Even with these caveats, it is interesting to compare the BIS sleep data to previous BIS values of <50 produced by propofol doses needed to inhibit movement in response to surgical stimulation *(56)*. The finding that the transition from waking to sleep produces BIS values *(55)*, similar to the transition to unconsciousness produced by sedation, is consistent with our working hypothesis that sleep and sedation are mediated by some of the same neuronal mechanisms.

BIS monitoring may prove useful for patients in intensive care, where assessments of the depth of sedation are difficult *(57)*. Data obtained from 14 sedated volunteers revealed a linear relationship between BIS value and propofol blood concentration *(58)*. BIS values also have been shown to be a good predictor for the conscious processing of information during propofol sedation and hypnosis *(59)*. In a study of 72 healthy volunteers, the developers of BIS measured: i) blood concentrations of propofol, midazolam, and alfentanil, and end tidal concentrations of isoflurane; ii) sedation level, and iii) recall *(60)*. None of the subjects in this study who received alfentanil lost consciousness, and none had a change in their BIS values. For propofol, midazolam, and isoflurane, BIS values were significantly correlated with level of consciousness and with recall. The BIS values at which 50% and 95% of volunteers were unconscious were 67 and 50, respectively. Thus, this study showed that BIS values were a reliable predictor of sedation level for all drugs tested. Practitioners who are interested in BIS monitoring as an adjunct to oximetry and capnometry should be aware of the limitation that the ability to predict hypoxia or airway obstruction using the BIS index is confounded by co-administration of hypnotics and muscle relaxants *(61)*.

Evoked potentials are a measurement of the electrical responses to nervous system activation by sensory, electrical, magnetic, or cognitive stimulation. Measurement of auditory-evoked potentials (AEPs) may be used to evaluate wakefulness. Most tests of awareness require subjects who can respond to verbal commands *(62–64)*. Providing a standardized click to the auditory canal produces AEPs. The click generates three distinct wave complexes, brainstem (BAEP, 0–20 ms), midlatency (MLAEP, 20–80 ms) and long latency (LLAEP, 80–100 ms). These responses correspond to transmission of the sound (BAEP), knowledge that one has heard the sound (MLAEP), and understanding the meaning of the sound (LLAEP). It is assumed that if the primary auditory cortex (MLAEP) is no longer receiving input (i.e., no waveform) one is unaware. The general evoked potential response to propofol is a dose-dependent decrease in amplitude and an increase in latency *(65,66)*. Studies that have compared MLAEP-derived information with BIS measures agree that MLAEP derivatives more sharply define and predict the transition between conscious and unconscious states *(67–69)*.

Traditionally, the depth of anesthesia is correlated with the response to painful stimuli during intravenous (i.v.) anesthetic drug administration or minimum alveolar concentration (MAC). To assess the level of sedation, one uses the MAC_{awake} or the drug concentration for which the subject arouses to sound (a command) or touch. The Observer's Assessment of Alertness/Sedation Scale (OAA/S) was developed to measure the response during MAC_{awake} *(70)* and is reviewed in detail in Chapter 9.

4. BRAINSTEM CHOLINERGIC NEURONS MODULATE EEG SPINDLE GENERATION

More than 50 years ago, the neurotransmitter acetylcholine (ACh) was shown to activate the EEG *(71)*. EEG activation was next demonstrated to be produced by a reticular system in the brainstem that sends ascending projections to the thalamus and cerebral cortex *(72)*. The discovery in 1953 of the REM phase of human sleep *(73)* further stimulated efforts to under-

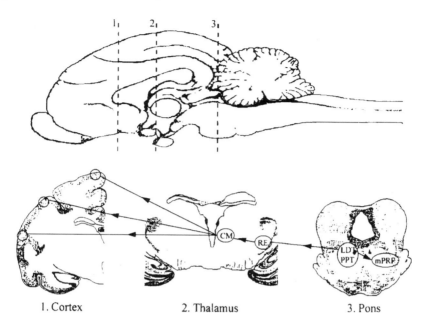

1. Cortex   2. Thalamus   3. Pons

Fig. 3. Schematic drawing of brain regions regulating cortical ACh release and EEG. The top view shows a lateral section of brain with dotted lines at the level of the cortex, thalamus, and pons. The lower portion shows these three brain regions in coronal section. The point of the figure is to illustrate how discreet nuclei localized to the pontine brainstem can modulate thalamocortical circuits generating EEG spindles. The laterodorsal (LDT) and pedunculopontine (PPT) tegmental nuclei in the pons project rostrally to the thalamus and caudally to medial pontine reticular formation (mPRF) regions known to regulate arousal. (Reprinted with permission from ref. *[92]*, Lippincott Williams & Wilkins, 1996).

stand the cellular and molecular basis of arousal-state control. Data demonstrating the active generation of sleep by the pontine brainstem is described in a now classic monograph *(74)*.

EEG spindles, one of the EEG traits characteristic of both sedation and sleep, are regulated by pontine cholinergic neurons. These brainstem neurons modulate the ability of specific thalamic nuclei to generate cortical EEG spindles (Fig. 3). Within the thalamus, the centromedian nucleus and nucleus reticularis generate cortical EEG spindles *(75)*. Spindles occur when diminished cholinergic input to the thalamus decreases cholinergic inhibition of nucleus reticularis, enabling the centromedian reticularis circuit to generate cortical EEG spindles *(76)*. Basic studies also have shown that muscarinic cholinergic receptors of the M2 subtype within the medial pontine reticular formation (mPRF) modulate the amount of REM sleep *(77)*. This is relevant for the ability of opioids to inhibit REM sleep because the synthetic opioid fentanyl binds to and antagonizes muscarinic cholinergic receptors and can produce negative side effects similar to central anticholinergic syndrome *(78)*. Microdialysis delivery of morphine sulfate or fentanyl to mPRF regions regulating REM sleep significantly decreases ACh release (Fig. 4).

The dorsal pons contains neurons that produce ACh and provide cholinergic input caudally to pontine reticular formation activating systems *(79,80)* and rostrally to thalamic nuclei regulating the EEG *(81,82)*. These cholinergic neurons descriptively named for their location are referred to as laterodorsal (LDT) and pedunculopontine (PPT) tegmental nuclei (reviewed in refs. *1,8*). Functional data from studies in which the electrical activity of LDT/PPT neurons recorded from intact, sleeping animals demonstrate a decreased discharge rate during NREM sleep relative to waking *(83)*. LDT/PPT neurons exhibit an increased discharge that begins 60 s before—and persists throughout—the EEG activation of REM sleep *(84)*. Opioids also decrease ACh release within the LDT/PPT nuclei, and this finding helps to elucidate one mechanism by which opioids inhibit the REM phase of sleep *(5)*.

Microdialysis data have quantified ACh release from LDT/PPT projections caudally into the mPRF and from LDT/PPT projections rostrally into the thalamus. Microdialysis of the mPRF showed that electrical stimulation of the LDT/PPT significantly increased ACh release *(85)*. These ACh measures were obtained from the same regions of the mPRF where EEG activation is evoked by direct application of cholinergic agonists and acetylcholinesterase inhibitors (reviewed in ref. *86*). Microinjection of the acetylcholinesterase inhibitor neostigmine into the mPRF causes a REM sleep-like state *(87)*. In humans, physostigmine administration during NREM sleep reduces the latency to REM sleep onset and increases REM sleep *(88)*. The finding that propofol-induced unconsciousness can be reversed with physostigmine *(89)* is consistent with data indicating cholinergic activation of EEG. Electrical stimulation of the LDT/PPT regions of the cat brain also produces the EEG activation of REM sleep *(90)*. Within the thalamus, microdialysis revealed that ACh levels originating from LDT/PPT neurons are high in association with EEG activation of waking and REM sleep, and significantly decreased during NREM sleep when EEG spindles are present *(91)*. This anatomical, electrophysiological, and neurochemical data are consistent with decreased LDT/PPT discharge causing decreased acetylcholine release associated with a synchronized EEG and sleep spindles. This is important in understanding the neurobiology of sedation analgesia because opioids have been shown to decrease ACh release within the LDT/PPT nuclei *(5)*.

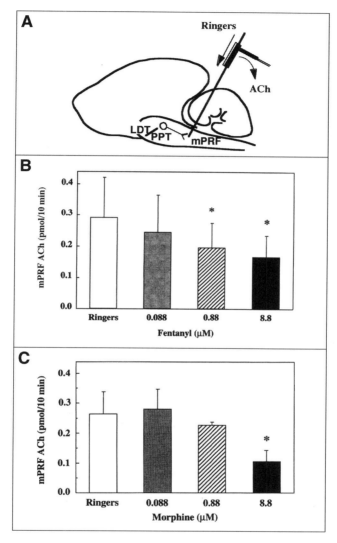

Fig. 4. Opioids inhibit ACh release in brain regions known to regulate EEG and behavioral arousal. (**A**) Illustrates a microdialysis probe aimed for the mPRF. These probes make it possible to measure neurotransmitter release during dialysis delivery of artificial cerebrospinal fluid (CSF) (Ringers). The schematic also shows cholinergic LDT/PPT neurons projecting ACh-containing terminals to the mPRF. (**B**) Shows that mPRF dialysis delivery of the opioid fentanyl caused a dose-dependent decrease in mPRF ACh release (mean + s.d.). (**C**) Shows that morphine sulfate also decreased mPRF ACh release. Data such as these help identify the neural circuits and neurotransmitters altered by sedating drugs. (Modified with permission from ref. *[5]*, Lippincott Williams & Wilkins, 1999).

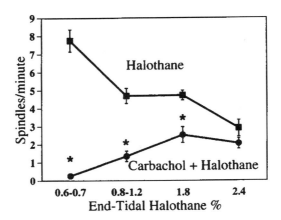

Fig. 5. Cholinergic neurotransmission modulates EEG arousal. The top curve shows that the number of EEG spindles of the type illustrated in Fig. 2 is increased by low concentrations of halothane (0.6–1.2%) and suppressed by higher concentrations of halothane (2.4%). The bottom curve shows that the cholinergic agonist carbachol decreases the ability of halothane to produce EEG spindles. Carbachol was delivered into the pontine mPRF region illustrated in Fig. 3. These data imply that the EEG spindles produced by halothane are regulated by cholinergic and cholinoceptive pontine neurons. (Reprinted with permission from ref. *[92]*, Lippincott Williams & Wilkins, 1996).

Two additional lines of evidence provide direct support for our hypothesis that the EEG spindles of sleep and anesthesia are regulated by the same cholinergic LDT/PPT neurons. First, halothane anesthesia causes both EEG spindle generation and significantly decreased acetylcholine release from LDT/PPT cholinergic terminals in the mPRF *(92)*. Since some LDT/PPT neurons also project to the thalamus *(82)*, the decreased pontine ACh release data are consistent with halothane also causing decreased thalamic acetylcholine release. As described previously, decreased thalamic acetylcholine release disinhibits thalamic neurons known to produce EEG spindle generation *(75)*. Second, microinjection of the cholinergic agonist carbachol into the mPRF decreased halothane-induced EEG spindles *(92)*. This finding indicates that enhancing brainstem cholinergic neurotransmission can activate the cortical EEG (Fig. 5).

Considered together, these results are consistent with the hypothesis that the EEG spindles of both sleep and halothane anesthesia are caused by brainstem cholinergic neurons localized to the LDT/PPT nuclei. Although opioids have been shown to cause decreased ACh release in pontine networks regulating EEG and behavioral arousal *(93)*, the extent to which other sedating drugs decrease pontine cholinergic neurotransmission has not yet been studied. It will also be important to extend microdialysis studies to additional brain regions such as the basal forebrain and cortex. Basal forebrain cholinergic neurons contribute to the regulation of wakefulness and normal mentation. In sleeping animals, ACh release in the basal forebrain is significantly decreased during NREM sleep over waking levels, and further increased during the cortical activation of REM sleep *(94)*. In mice anesthetized with isoflurane, muscarinic autoreceptors modulate ACh in the prefrontal cortex *(95)*.

5. GAMMA-AMINOBUTYRIC ACID A (GABA$_A$) RECEPTORS AND AROUSAL

GABA is the major inhibitory neurotransmitter in the nervous system, and GABA is estimated to be present in 20–50% of all synapses *(96)*. Agonist activation of the GABA$_A$ receptor enhances chloride ion (Cl$^-$) conductance. Barbiturates, benzodiazepines, and neuroactive steroids all alter GABA$_A$ receptor function, leading to increased neuronal inhibition *(96)*. Data reviewed in this section support the conclusion that sedation and natural sleep occur, in part, as a result of enhanced GABAergic neurotransmission.

Chloral hydrate administered orally is one of the most widely used sedatives in children undergoing magnetic resonance imaging (MRI) *(97)* and dental procedures *(98)*. Chloral hydrate is a sedative-hypnotic drug that produces little or no analgesia. Hepatic alcohol dehydrogenase rapidly converts chloral hydrate to the active metabolite trichloroethanol, which causes sedation. Similar to barbiturates, steroids, and halogenated volatile anesthetics, trichloroethanol potentiates synaptic transmission at the GABA$_A$ receptor *(99)*. In vitro studies have shown that trichloroethanol prolongs inhibitory postsynaptic currents resulting from Cl$^-$ *(99)*. This finding is consistent with the interpretation that chloral hydrate produces sedation by enhancing inhibitory synaptic transmission mediated by the GABA$_A$ receptor.

The time-course for sedation produced by chloral hydrate is a function of dose, patient age, and health. One study of 596 pediatric patients noted that following oral chloral hydrate (68 mg/kg), effective sedation for MRI was achieved in 26 min without respiratory depression *(100)*. Studies of chloral hydrate metabolism following a single 50 mg/kg oral dose in critically ill children 57–708 wk old found the half-life for trichloroethanol to be 9.7 h *(101)*. Another metabolite of chloral hydrate—trichloroacetic acid—failed to decline within 6 d after the single oral dose *(101)*. The effect of these metabolites on breathing is not clear. There is agreement in the available literature that with careful medical screening, monitoring, and patient management chloral hydrate provides effective sedation without respiratory depression. Animal data indicating that chloral hydrate causes chromosome changes has raised the question of long-term effects. Chloral hydrate is a reactive metabolite of the known carcinogen trichloroethylene, and oral administration of chloral hydrate to mice was found to be carcinogenic following a single dose lower than that typically used to produce sedation in children *(102)*. Although chloral hydrate came into use in the early 1900s, its short-term actions and interaction with GABAergic neurotransmission are not yet fully understood. The mechanisms by which chloral hydrate causes the adverse reaction of paradoxical excitement are also unclear. These questions represent important opportunities for sedation research.

Benzodiazepines remain the most frequently prescribed hypnotics. Oral administration of benzodiazepines shortens NREM sleep-onset latency and increases the duration of NREM sleep *(96)*. The sedative and sleep-enhancing actions of benzodiazepines are blocked by the benzodiazepine-receptor antagonist flumazenil *(103,104)*. Midazolam has become the benzodiazepine of choice for procedural sedation. Midazolam can be administered by a variety of routes (oral, intranasal, rectal, intramuscular, and i.v.) but the i.v. route is used most commonly. Benzodiazepines increase the Cl^- current generated by $GABA_A$-receptor activation, potentiating GABAergic inhibition and calming the patient, relaxing skeletal muscles, and producing loss of consciousness in high doses *(105)*. There have been some concerns about the possibility of direct neurotoxicity of nasally administered drugs, which may travel along the olfactory nerves to the central nervous system (CNS). High blood levels of midazolam (160 ng/mL at 10 min) were reported in an infant who received 0.2 mg/kg intranasally and developed apnea *(106)*.

Paradoxical excitement has been reported in up to 10% of patients after oral, i.v., and rectal administration of midazolam, and may appear in the recovery phase *(107)* or even after discharge. This complication is disturbing for family members and healthcare personnel because the excitement phase can be quite violent. The mechanism underlying this paradoxical excitement is unknown.

There is a large body of evidence showing that the actions of GABAergic neurotransmission on arousal level vary as a function of brain region. Direct administration of bicuculline ($GABA_A$ antagonist) and muscimol ($GABA_A$ agonist) into the pontine reticular formation alters cycles of sleep and wakefulness in both the rat *(108)* and cat *(109)*. The REM phase of sleep has also been shown to be enhanced following administration of muscimol into the ventrolateral periaqueductal gray *(110)*. Nociception and arousal vary together, and in the periaqueductal gray of the rat the analgesic effect of nitrous oxide is mediated by opiate receptors *(111)*.

Microdialysis studies measuring the release of endogenous GABA across the sleep cycle have revealed results consistent with a role for GABA in the regulation of arousal. Nuclei in the pons, such as the locus coeruleus and the dorsal raphe nucleus, exhibit cellular discharge rates that are positively correlated with wakefulness and inversely correlated with REM sleep (reviewed in ref. *1*). These findings have led to the suggestion that cessation of discharge by cells in these regions is somehow permissive for REM sleep onset. This interpretation is also consistent with an active modulation of arousal by monoamine-containing neurons. The dorsal raphe nucleus contains a high concentration of serotonin. Microdialysis of cat dorsal raphe reveals increased GABA release during REM sleep, and microinjection of the GABA agonist muscimol into the dorsal raphe increased REM sleep *(112)*. GABA levels in the locus coeruleus also increase during REM sleep *(113)*, and locus coeruleus administration of $GABA_A$ antagonist decreases REM sleep *(114)*. During sleep, noradrenergic neurons in the locus coeruleus are also tonically inhibited by GABA *(115)*, a finding consistent with monoaminergic modulation of arousal. In rostral brain regions such as the posterior hypothalamus, known to be important for maintaining wakefulness, an increase in GABA release occurs during non-REM sleep *(116)*. The emerging data suggest that GABAergic transmission contributes to sleep and sedation by inhibiting neurons and neurotransmitters that promote wakefulness. Further illustrating the complexity of pharmacological interaction is the finding that opiates administered into the locus coeruleus enhance non-REM sleep via mu opioid receptors *(117)*. Additional effects of GABA on sleep and wakefulness are reviewed in detail elsewhere *(118)*.

6. SEDATION AND SLEEP ALTER RESPIRATORY CONTROL

Drug-induced respiratory depression is the primary cause of morbidity associated with sedation analgesia *(2)*. This follows from the repeated observation that sedation produced by different classes of drugs depresses the ability to generate an appropriate ventilatory response to hypercapnic and/or hypoxic stimuli. For example, halothane depresses the ventilatory response to isocapnic hypoxia and hyperoxic hypercapnia *(119)*. Isoflurane causes dose-dependent reductions in the ability to respond to hypoxic and hypercapnic stimuli *(120)*. Comparative data show that the loss of consciousness produced by isoflurane, sevoflurane, and desflurane was associated with respiratory depression *(121)*. Nitrous oxide sedation also enhanced apneic episodes (respiratory pauses of ≥20 s) following hyperventilation, and led to oxygen desaturation averaging 75% *(122)*. Sedation produced by combinations of midazolam and opioids causes apnea and hypoxemia *(123)*, and sedation produced by intrathecal morphine sulfate causes dose-related respiratory depression *(124)*. One important concern regarding sedation produced by opioids is that the respiratory rate and level of sedation did not reliably predict hypoxemia *(124,125)*. Propofol infused at sub-anesthetic doses can cause oxygen desaturation to 70% and a depressed response to hypoxia *(126)*. Opioids also increase apneas when injected into areas of the brainstem that regulate the REM phase of sleep (Fig. 6).

As reviewed elsewhere *(4)*, anesthesiologists have long appreciated the respiratory-facilitatory effect of behavioral arousal as a "wakefulness stimulus for breathing." The safety of sedation analgesia will be greatly improved by advances in understanding the cellular and molecular mechanisms comprising the wakefulness stimulus for breathing. However, it is now clear that cholinergic neurotransmission in pontine regions known to regulate arousal can significantly alter breathing *(4)*. Basic studies have shown that pontine administration of cholinergic agonists and acetylcholinesterase inhibitors significantly diminishes upper-airway muscle tone, afferent responsiveness to hypercapnic stimuli, and respiratory rhythm generation (reviewed in ref. *127*). Of relevance for mechanistic studies of sedation is the finding that this cholinergic respiratory depression was produced from regions of the mPRF that contain no pre- or upper motor respiratory neurons *(4,127)*. Thus, cholinergic mechanisms known to regulate levels of behavioral arousal can significantly alter respiratory control (Fig. 7).

Cholinergic modulation of arousal and breathing can be direct, indirect via interactions with other neurotransmitters and neuromodulators, or through a mixture of direct and indirect actions. By 1987, existing data made it possible to predict that "a leading candidate for neurons that mediate the stimulating effect of wakefulness on respiration includes serotonin-containing cells in the brainstem raphe nuclei" *(128)*. Subsequent studies have demonstrated an excitatory serotoninergic drive to hypoglossal motoneurons *(129)* and microdialysis measurement of serotonin in hypoglossal nucleus reveals significant decrements in serotonin caused by pontine administration of carbachol *(130)*. Sleep and sedation depress upper-airway muscle function, and the foregoing data are consistent with the possibility that tongue muscle hypotonia can contribute to upper-airway obstruction. Such obstructions comprise one of the mechanisms by which deaths have occurred in children receiving chloral hydrate *(131)*.

Studies designed to foster an understanding of how sedatives alter neurotransmitters and brain regions regulating arousal and breathing must also contend with the complexity of non-uniform drug effects. Although anesthetics hyperpolarize vertebrate neurons, thereby decreasing neuronal excitability *(132)*, drug actions vary as a function of brain region, route of

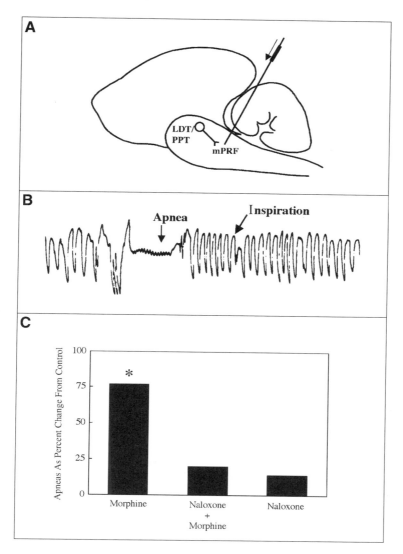

Fig. 6. The effect of pontine opioid administration on respiratory pauses (apneas). **(A)** Schematizes a sagittal brain section and a microinjection of morphine made directly into the mPRF. Since the brain contains no pain receptors, these injections can be made in intact, unanesthetized animals. **(B)** Shows a respiratory trace recorded from a thermistor placed at the nose. **(C)** Shows that the number of apneas was significantly increased by mPRF administration of morphine sulfate, and that the morphine-induced increase in respiratory apneas was blocked by naloxone. Thus the mPRF, a region of the brain that contains no respiratory neurons but does regulate arousal, can significantly alter breathing. (Reprinted with permission from ref. *[167]*, Lippincott Williams & Wilkins, 1992).

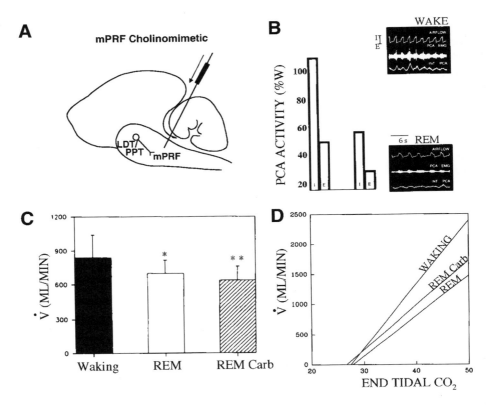

Fig. 7. Cholinergic neurotransmission in the medial pontine reticular formation significantly alters respiratory control. **(A)** Shows that cholinergic drugs can be delivered directly into the mPRF. **(B)** Shows that the posterior cricoarytenoid (PCA) muscle activity in the upper airway is decreased following carbachol injections producing a REM sleep-like state. The PCA activity during inspiration (I) and expiration (E) is shown as a percent of waking discharge and the muscle EMG is shown on the inserts labeled "WAKE" and "REM." (Reprinted with permission from ref. *[168], FASEB Journal,* 1989). **(C)** Shows minute ventilation during wakefulness, REM sleep, and the REM sleep-like state produced by mPRF administration of carbachol. Note that cholinergic compounds injected into the mPRF depressed minute ventilation. (Reprinted with permission from ref. *[169],* Elsevier Science, 1989). **(D)** Shows that the ability to respond to CO_2 is diminished during both natural REM sleep and during the REM sleep-like state produced by carbachol. (Reprinted with permission from ref. *[170],* The American Physiological Society, 1991). Thus, enhanced cholinergic neurotransmission in areas of the brain known to regulate arousal states **(A)** depresses efferent upper airway motor output **(B)**, central respiratory pattern generation **(C)**, and ability to respond to CO_2 **(D)**.

administration, and transmitter system studied. For example, ACh release in brain regions regulating arousal and breathing is diminished by opioids *(5)*, volatile anesthetics *(92)*, and ketamine *(133)*. Propofol can alter both serotoninergic *(134)* and cholinergic *(135)* neurotransmission, although one mechanism of propofol action occurs via receptor systems for the inhibitory amino acids glycine and GABA *(136)*. As we have demonstrated for the antinociceptive actions of morphine *(137)*, the effects of propofol on ACh release vary depending on the brain region examined *(138)*.

Efforts to elucidate the mechanisms by which sedation alters breathing are further complicated by the complexity of interacting autonomic control systems. Generation of the normal respiratory rhythm *(139)* and gasping *(140)* arise from the medullary brainstem. Paralleling the effects of systemically administered opioids, NREM sleep is enhanced, whereas waking and REM sleep are inhibited by delivering a mu opioid agonist directly into the medullary nucleus of the solitary tract *(141)*. The rostral ventrolateral medulla (RVLM) is the most potent pressor region in the brain *(142)*. The ability of propofol to produce hypotension remains poorly understood, but available data suggest that propofol can disrupt vasomotor control via the RVLM *(143)*. The specific mechanisms by which propofol causes hypotension are not yet clear, but may be partially caused by central cholinergic neurotransmission, since the RVLM is known to contain a high number of muscarinic cholinergic receptors *(144)*. Opioids inhibit cholinergic neurotransmission in many areas of the brain, and in humans the acetylcholinesterase inhibitor physostigmine antagonizes the ability of morphine to cause respiratory depression *(145)*.

Alpha-2 agonist-induced analgesia and sedation are likely to involve brain regions that are known to regulate naturally occurring states of arousal. As noted previously, the locus coeruleus contributes to the maintenance of wakefulness, and also modulates the ability of the α-2 agonist dexmedetomidine to produce antinociception *(146)*. The sedative action of dexmedetomidine is altered by serotonergic *(147)* but not by cholinergic *(148)* neurotransmission.

Central respiratory control is modulated by an interaction between adrenergic and cholinergic neurotransmission *(149)*. Activation of α-2 adrenoreceptors by norepinephrine and by clonidine inhibits medullary respiratory neurons *(150)*. The sedative and analgesic actions of epidural clonidine, mediated in part by α-2 adrenoreceptors, are accompanied by respiratory depression *(151)* and a diminished respiratory response to hypercapnia *(152)*. Hypotonia of oral-pharyngeal muscles such as the genioglossus likely contributes to state-dependent airway obstruction *(153)*, and clonidine hyperpolarizes hypoglossal motoneurons *(154)*. Recent studies show that dilator muscles of the upper airway are tonically activated by clonidine, resulting in airway obstruction *(155)* and disrupted respiratory rhythm generation *(156)*. Thus, sedatives with mechanisms of action involving central α-2 adrenoreceptors may be anticipated to have a negative impact on chemosensitivity, maintenance of upper-airway patency, and respiratory rhythm generation.

7. CONCLUSION: RESEARCH WILL ENHANCE PATIENT SAFETY DURING SEDATION

In November 1999, the U.S. Institute of Medicine (IOM) released data showing that medical errors are a leading cause of death and injury. This report indicated that more people in the U.S. die from medical mistakes each year than from highway accidents, breast cancer, or AIDS *(157)*. During the past 50 years, there have been tremendous advances in patient safety for anesthesia delivered in the operating room environment. In 1952, the potential for harm resulting from anesthesia was several times greater than the odds of death from polio *(158)*. Presently, deaths from anesthesia in the operating room environment are estimated at 1:250,000 cases *(159)*. Current data of the same scope as the Beecher and Todd study are unavailable on morbidity and mortality associated with sedation and anesthesia outside the operating room. Data showing high morbidity and mortality rates from cardiorespiratory complications during diagnostic endoscopy have been presented *(160)*. Economic factors have made it routine to discharge ambulatory patients as soon as possible following even prolonged anesthesia or sedation *(161)*. *The New York Times* reported a study by the New York State Senate Committee indicating that patients who undergo surgery in locations remote from a hospital are protected by few regulations *(162)*. Non-hospital venues for sedation have also been identified as an independent factor associated with permanent neurological injury or death following sedation analgesia *(163)*. Office-based elective surgeries such as liposuction are expected to rise from 6% in 1999 to 20% in 2001. Recent data suggest liposuction-related death rates of 1 in 5224 *(164)*. These death rates are 50 times higher than current anesthesia-related deaths anticipated by the American Society of Anesthesiologists (ASA) *(165)*. This chapter has summarized data illustrating gaps in existing knowledge concerning the cellular and molecular mechanisms that cause sedation. Improved anesthetic drugs are a key factor contributing to enhanced anesthetic safety *(166)*. Therefore, basic and clinical sedation research are essential for continued advances in patient safety and comfort.

ACKNOWLEDGEMENT

Supported by NIH grants HL57120, MH45361, HL40881, HL65272, and the Department of Anesthesiology. We gratefully acknowledge help by C.A. Lapham, A. English, and M. A. Norat.

REFERENCES

1. Lydic, R. and Baghdoyan, H. A. (eds). (1999) *Handbook of Behavioral State Control: Cellular and Molecular Mechanisms,* CRC Press, Boca Raton, FL.
2. Gross, J. B., Bailey, P. L., Caplan, R. A., Connis, R. T., Coté, C. J., Davis, F. G., et al. (1996) Practice guidelines for sedation and analgesia by non-anesthesiologists. *Anesthesiology* **84,** 459–471.
3. Lydic, R. and Biebuyck, J. F. (1994) Sleep neurobiology: relevance for mechanistic studies of anesthesia. *Br. J. Anaesth.* **72,** 506–508.
4. Lydic, R. (1996) Reticular modulation of breathing during sleep and anesthesia. *Curr. Opin. Pulm. Med.* **2,** 474–481.
5. Mortazavi, S., Thompson, J., Baghdoyan, H. A., and and Lydic, R. (1999) Fentanyl and morphine, but not remifentanil, inhibit acetylcholine release in pontine regions modulating arousal. *Anesthesiology* **90,** 1070–1077.
6. Jastak, J. T. and Peskin, R. M. (1991) Major morbidity or mortality from office anesthetic procedures: A closed-claim analysis of 13 cases. *Anesth. Prog.* **38,** 39–44.
7. Kryger, M. H., Roth, T., and Dement, W. C. (eds). (1994) *Principles and Practice of Sleep Medicine,* 2nd ed., W. B. Saunders, Philadelphia, PA.
8. Steriade, M., and McCarley, R. W. (1990) *Brainstem Control of Wakefulness and Sleep.* Plenum Press, New York, NY.
9. Sanders, B. J. and Avery, D. R. (1997) The effect of sleep on conscious sedation: A follow-up study. *J. Clin. Pediatr. Dent.* **21,** 131–134.
10. Mahowald, M. W. and Schenck, C. H. (1992) Dissociated states of wakefulness and sleep. *Neurology* **42,** 44–52.
11. Aldrich, M. S. (1999) *Sleep Medicine,* Oxford University Press, New York, NY.
12. Van Steveninck, A. L., Mandema, J. W., Tuk, B., Van Dijk, J. G., Schoemaker, H. C., Danhof, M., et al. (1993) A comparison of the concentration-effect relationships for midazolam for EEG-derived parameters and saccadic peak velocity. *Br. J. Clin. Pharmacol.* **36,** 109–115.
13. Roelofse, J. A., Louw, L. R., and Roelofse, P. G. (1998) A double blind randomized comparison of oral trimeprazine-methadone and ketamine-midazolam for sedation of pediatric dental patients for oral surgical procedures. *Anesth. Prog.* **45,** 3–11.
14. Ramsay MAE, Savege, T. M., Simpson, B. R. J., and Goodwin, R. (1974) Controlled sedation with alphaxalone-alphadolone. *Br. Med. J.* **2,** 656–659.
15. Fragen, R. J., Avram, M. J. (1992) Nonopioid intravenous anesthetics, in *Clinical Anesthesia,* 2nd ed. (Barash, P. G., Cullen, B. F., and Stoelting, R. K., eds.), J. B. Lippincott, Philadelphia, PA.

16. Jagoda, A. S., Campbell, M., Karas, S., Mariani, P. J., and Shepherd, S. M. (1998) Clinical policy for procedural sedation and analgesia in the emergency department. *Ann. Emerg. Med.* **31,** 663–677.

17. Novak, C. I. (1998) ASA updates its position on monitored anesthesia care. *Am. Soc. Anes. News* **62,** 22–23.

18. Coté, C. J. (1994) Sedation for the pediatric patient. *Paediatr. Anaesth.* **41,** 31–53.

19. Holzman, R. S., Cullen, D. J., Eichhorn, J. H., and Philips, J. H. (1994) Guidelines for sedation by nonanesthesiologists during diagnostic and therapeutic procedures. *J. Clin. Anesth.* **6,** 265–275.

20. Baghdoyan, H. A., Rodrigo-Angulo, M. L., McCarley, R. W., and Hobson, J. A. (1984) Site-specific enhancement and suppression of desynchronized sleep signs following cholinergic stimulation of three brain stem regions. *Brain Res.* **306,** 39–52.

21. Lydic, R. (1989) Central pattern-generating neurons and the search for general principles. *FASEB J.* **3,** 2457–2478.

22. Churchland, P. S. (1986) *Neurophilosophy: Toward a Unified Science of the Mind-Brain.* A Bradford Book, The MIT Press, Cambridge, MA.

23. Chokroverty, S. (ed). (1999) *Sleep Disorders Medicine: Basic Science, Technical Considerations, and Clinical Aspects.* Butterworth-Heinmann, Boston, MA.

24. Folstein, M. F., Folstein, S. E., and McHugh, P. R. (1975) Mini-mental state. A practical method for grading the cognitive state of patients for the clinician. *J. Psychiatr. Res.* **12,** 189–198.

25. Kraemer, H. C., Gullion, C. M., Rush, A. J., Frank, E., and Kupfer, D. J. (1994) Can state and trait variables be disentangled? A methodological framework for psychiatric disorders. *Psychiatry Res.* **52,** 55–69.

26. Avramov, M. N., Smith, I., and White, P. F. (1996) Interactions between midazolam and remifentanil during monitored anesthesia care. *Anesthesiology* **85,** 1283–1289.

27. Fung, S. J., Boxer, P., Morales, F. R., and Chase, M. (1982) Hyperpolarizing membrane responses induced in lumbar motoneurons by stimulation of the nucleus reticularis pontis oralis during active sleep. *Brain Res.* **248,** 267–273.

28. Morales, F. R., Boxer, P., and Chase, M. H. (1987) Behavioral state-specific inhibitory postsynaptic potentials impinge on cat lumbar motoneurons during active sleep. *Exp. Neurol.* **98,** 418–435.

29. Kay, D. C., Eisenstein, R. B., and Jasinski, D. R. (1969) Morphine effects on human REM state, waking state, and NREM sleep. *Psychopharmacologia* **14,** 404–416.

30. Krachman, S. L., D'Alonzo, G. E., and Criner, G. J. (1995) Sleep in the intensive care unit. *Chest* **107,** 1713–1720.

31. Lydic, R. and Biebuyck, J. F. (eds). (1988) *The Clinical Physiology of Sleep.* The American Physiological Society, Bethesda, MD.

32. Bruder, N., Raynal, M., Pellissier, D., Courtinat, C., and Francois, G. (1998) Influence of body temperature, with or without sedation, on energy expenditure in severe head-injured patients. *Crit. Care Med.* **26,** 568–572.

33. Parikh, S. and Chung, F. (1995) Postoperative delirium in the elderly. *Anesth. Analg.* **80,** 1223–1232.
34. Wagner, B. K., O'Hara, D. A., and Hammond, J. S. (1997) Drugs for amnesia in the ICU. *Am. J. Crit. Care* **6,** 192–201.
35. Buffett-Jerrott, S. E., Stewart, S. H., Bird, S., and Teehan, M. D. (1998) An examination of differences in the time course of oxazepam's effects on implicit vs explicit memory. *J. Psychopharm.* **12,** 338–347.
36. Buffett-Jerrott, S. E., Stewart, S. H., and Teehan, M. D. (1998) A further examination of the time-dependent effects of oxazepam and lorazepam on implicit and explicit memory. *Psychopharmacologia* **138,** 344–353.
37. Papper, E. M. (1987) The state of consciousness: some humanistic considerations, in *Consciousness, Awareness and Pain in General Anaesthesia.* (Rosen, M., and Lunn, J. N., eds.), Butterworths, London, pp. 10–11.
38. Andrade, J. (1996) Investigations of hypesthesia: using anesthetics to explore relationships between consciousness, learning, and memory. *Conscious Cogn.* **54,** 562–580.
39. Bloch, V., Hennevin, E., Leconte P. (1979) Relationship between paradoxical sleep and memory processes, in *Brain Mechanisms in Memory and Learning: From the Single Neuron to Man,* (Brazier, M. A. B., ed.), Raven Press, New York, NY, pp. 329–343.
40. Hennevin, E., Hars, B., and Bloch, E. (1989) Improvement of learning by mesencephalic reticular stimulation during postlearning paradoxical sleep. *Behav. Neural. Biol.* **51,** 291–306.
41. Smith, C. (1996) Sleep states, memory processes and synaptic plasticity. *Behav. Brain Res.* **78,** 49–56.
42. Steriade, M. (1996) Awakening the brain. *Nature* **383,** 24–25.
43. Sejnowski, T. J. (1995) Sleep and memory. *Curr. Biol.* **5,** 832–834.
44. Castro-Alamancos, M. A. and Connors, B. W. (1996) Short-term plasticity of a thalamocortical pathway dynamically modulated by behavioral state. *Science* **272,** 274–276.
45. Kudrimoti, H. S., Barnes, C. A., and McNaughton, B. L. (1999) Reactivation of hippocampal cell assemblies: Effects of behavioral state, experience, and EEG dynamics. *J. Neurosci.* **19,** 4090–4101.
46. Engelhardt, W., Friess, K., Hartung, E., Sold, M., and Dierks, T. (1992) EEG and auditory evoked potential P300 compared with psychometric tests in assessing vigilance after benzodiazepine sedation and antagonism. *Br. J. Anaesth.* **69,** 75–80.
47. Veselis, R. A., Reinse, R. A., Wronski, M., Marino, P., Tong, W. P., and Bedford, R. F. (1992) EEG and memory effects of low-dose infusions of propofol. *Br. J. Anaesth.* **69,** 246–254.
48. Seifert, H. A., Blouin, R. T., Conrad, P. F., and Gross, J. B. (1993) Sedative doses of propofol increase beta activity in the processed electroencephalogram. *Anesth. Analg.* **76,** 976–978.
49. Kishimoto, T., Kadoya, C., Sneyd, R., Samra, S. K., and Domino, E. F. (1995) Topographic electroencephalogram of propofol-induced conscious sedation. *Clin. Pharmacol. Ther.* **58,** 666–774.

50. Dowlatshahi, P. and Yaksh, T. L. (1997) Differential effects of two intraventricularly injected alpha 2 agonists ST-91 and dexmedetomidine on electroencephalogram, feeding and electromyogram. *Anesth. Analg.* **84,** 133–138.

51. Feshchenko, V. A., Veselis, R. A., and Reinsel, R. A. (1997) Comparison of the EEG effects of midazolam, thiopental, and propofol: the role of underlying oscillatory systems. *Neuropsychobiology* **35,** 211–220.

52. Rampil, I. J. (1998) A primer for EEG signal processing in anesthesia. *Anesthesiology* **89,** 980–1002.

53. Vernon, J. M., Long, E., Sebel, P. S., and Manberg, P. (1995) Prediction of movement using bispectral electroencephalographic analysis during propofol/alfentanil or isoflurane/alfentanil anesthesia. *Anesth. Analg.* **80,** 780–785.

54. Sigl, J. C. and Chamoun, N. C. (1994) An introduction to bispectral analysis for the electroencephalogram. *J. Clin. Monit.* **10,** 392–404.

55. Sleigh, J. W., Andrzejowski, J., Steyn-Ross, A., and Steyn-Ross, M. (1999) The bispectral index: A measure of depth of sleep? *Anesth. Analg.* **88,** 659–661.

56. Leslie, K., Sessler, D. I., Smith, W. D., Larson, M. D., Ozaki, M., Blanchard, D., and Crankshaw, D. P. (1996) Prediction of movement during propofol/nitrous oxide anesthesia. *Anesthesiology* **84,** 52–63.

57. De Deyne, C., Struys, M., Decruyenaere, J., Creupelandt, J., Hoste, E., and Colardyne, F. (1998) Use of continuous bispectral EEG monitoring to assess depth of sedation in ICU patients. *Intensive Care Med.* **24,** 1294–1298.

58. Leslie, K., Sessler, D. I., Schroeder, M., and Walters, K. (1995) Propofol blood concentration and the bispectral index predict suppression of learning during propofol/epidural anesthesia in volunteers. *Anesth. Analg.* **81,** 1269–1274.

59. Kearse, L. A., Rosow, C., Zaslavsky, A., Connors, P., Dershwitz, M., and Denman, W. (1998) Bispectral analysis of the electroencephalogram predicts conscious processing of information during propofol sedation and hypnosis. *Anesthesiology* **88,** 25–34.

60. Glass, P. S., Bloom, M., Kearse, L., Roscow, C., Sebel, P., and Manberg, P. (1997) Bispectral analysis measures sedation and memory effects of propofol, midazolam, isoflorane and alfentanil in healthy volunteers. *Anesthesiology* **86,** 836–847.

61. Singh, H. (1999) Bispectral index (BIS) monitoring during propofol-induced sedation and anaesthesia. *Eur. J. Anaesthesiol.* **16,** 31–36.

62. Ghoneim, M. M. and Block, R. I. (1992) Learning and consciousness during general anesthesia. *Anesthesiology* **76,** 279–305.

63. Ghoneim, M. M. and Block, R. I. (1997) Learning and memory during general anesthesia: an update. *Anesthesiology* **87,** 387–410.

64. McLeskey, C. H. (1999) Awareness during anaesthesia. *Can. J. Anaesth.* **46,** R80–R83.

65. Schwender, D., Daunderer, M., Schnatmann, N., Klasing, S., Finister, U., and Peter, K. (1997) Midlatency auditory evoked potentials and motor signs of wakefulness during anaesthesia and midazolam. *Br. J. Anaesth.* **79,** 53–58.

66. Tooley, M. A., Greenslade, G. L., and Prys-Roberts, C. (1996) Concentration-related effects of propofol on the auditory evoked response. *Br. J. Anaesth.* **77,** 720–726.

67. Doi, M., Gajraj, R. J., Mantzardis, H., and Kenny, G. N. (1997) Relationship between calculated blood concentrations of propofol and electrophysiological variables during emergence from anaesthesia: comparison of bispectral index, spectral edge frequency, median frequency and auditory evoked potential index. *Br. J. Anaesth.* **78**, 180–184.

68. Gajraj, R. J., Doi, M., Mantzardis, H., and Kenny, G. N. (1998) Analysis of the EEG bispectrum, auditory evoked potentials and the EEG power spectrum during repeated transitions from consciousness to unconsciousness. *Br. J. Anaesth.* **80**, 46–52.

69. Schraag, S., Bothner, U., Gajraj, R., Kenny, G., and Georgieff, M. (1999) The performance of electroencephalogram bispectral index and auditory evoked potential index to predict loss of consciousness during propofol infusion. *Anesth. Analg.* **89**, 1311–1315.

70. Rampil, I. J., Kim, J., Lenhard, T., Neigishi, C., and Sessler, D. I. (1998) Bispectral EEG index during nitrous oxide administration. *Anesthesiology* **89**, 671–677.

71. Wescoe, W. C., Green, R. E., McNamara, B. P., and Krop, S. (1948) The influence of atropine and scopolamine on the central effects of DFP. *J. Pharmacol. Exp. Ther.* **92**, 63–72.

72. Moruzzi, G. and Magoun, H. W. (1949) Brain stem reticular formation and activation of the EEG. *Electroencephalogr. Clin. Neurophysiol.* **1**, 455–473.

73. Aserinsky, E. and Kleitman, N. (1953) Regularly occurring periods of eye motility, and concomitant phenomena, during sleep. *Science* **118**, 273–274.

74. Jouvet, M. (1972) The role of monoamines and acetylcholine containing neurons in the regulation of the sleep waking cycle. *Ergeb. Physiol.* **64**, 116–307.

75. Steriade, M., Contreras, D., Curro' Dossi, R., and Nunez, A. (1993) The slow (<1 Hz) oscillation in reticular thalamic and thalamocortical neurons: scenario of sleep rhythm generation in interacting thalamic and neocortical networks. *J. Neurosci.* **13**, 3284–3299.

76. Steriade, M. (1993) Cholinergic blockage of network- and intrinsically-generated slow oscillations promotes waking and REM sleep activity patterns in thalamic and cortical neurons. Prog *Brain Res.* **98**, 345–355.

77. Baghdoyan, H. A. and Lydic, R. (1999) M2 muscarinic receptor subtype in the feline medial pontine reticular formation modulates the amount of rapid eye movement sleep. *Sleep* **22**, 835–847.

78. Hustveit, O. (1994) Binding of fentanyl and pethidine to muscarinic receptors in rat brain. *Jpn. J. Pharmacol.* **64**, 57–59.

79. Shiromani, P. J., Armstrong, D. M., and Gillin, J. C. (1988) Cholinergic neurons from the dorsolateral pons project to the medial pons: a WGA-HRP and choline acetyltransferase immunohistochemical study. *Neurosci. Lett.* **95**, 19–23.

80. Mitani, A., Ito, K., Hallanger, A. H., Wainer, B. H., Kataoka, K., and McCarley, R. W. (1988) Cholinergic projections from the laterodorsal and pedunculopontine tegmental nuclei to the pontine gigantocellular tegmental field in the cat. *Brain Res.* **451**, 397–402.

81. Honda, T. and Semba, K. (1995) An ultrastructural study of cholinergic and non-cholinergic neurons in the laterodorsal and pedunculopontine nuclei in the rat. *Neuroscience* **68**, 837–853.

82. Semba, K., Reiner, P. B., and Fibiger, H. C. (1990) Single cholinergic mesopontine tegmental neurons project to both the pontine reticular formation and the thalamus in the rat. *Neuroscience* **38,** 643–654.

83. El Mansari, M., Sakai, K., and Jouvet, M. (1989) Unitary characteristics of presumptive cholinergic tegmental neurons during the sleep-waking cycle in freely moving cats. *Exp. Brain Res.* **76,** 519–529.

84. El Mansari, M., Sakai, K., and Jouvet, M. (1990) Responses of presumed cholinergic mesopontine tegmental neurons to carbachol microinjections in freely moving cats. *Exp. Brain Res.* **83,** 115–123.

85. Lydic, R. and Baghdoyan, H. A. (1993) Pedunculopontine stimulation alters respiration and increases ACh release in the pontine reticular formation. *Am. J. Physiol.* **264,** R544–R554.

86. Baghdoyan, H. A. (1997) Cholinergic mechanisms regulating REM sleep, in *Sleep Science: Integrating Basic Research and Clinical Practice Monographs in Clinical Neuroscience,* Vol. 15. (Schwartz, W. J., ed.), Karger, Basel, pp. 88–116.

87. Baghdoyan, H. A., Monaco, A. P., Rodrigo-Angulo, M. L., Assens, F., McCarley, R. W., and Hobson, J. A. (1984) Microinjection of neostigmine into the pontine reticular formation of cats enhances desynchronized sleep signs. *J. Pharmacol. Exp. Ther.* **231,** 173–180.

88. Sitaram, N., Wyatt, R. J., Dawson, S., and Gillin, J. C. (1976) REM sleep induction by physostigmine infusion during sleep. *Science* **191,** 1281–1283.

89. Meuret, P., Backman, S. B., Bonhomme, V., Plourde, G., and Fiset, P. (2000) Physostigmine reverses propofol-induced unconsciousness and attenuation of the auditory steady state response in bispectral index in human volunteers. *Anesthesiology* **93,** 708–717.

90. Thakkar, M., Portas, C., and McCarley, R. W. (1996) Chronic low-amplitude electrical stimulation of the laterodorsal tegmental nucleus of freely moving cats increases REM sleep. *Brain Res.* **723,** 223–227.

91. Williams, J. A., Comisarow, J., Day, J., Fibiger, H. C., and Reiner, P. B. (1994) State-dependent release of acetylcholine in rat thalamus measured by in vivo microdialysis. *J. Neurosci.* **14,** 5236–5242.

92. Keifer, J. C., Baghdoyan, H. A., and Lydic, R. (1996) Pontine cholinergic mechanisms modulate the cortical EEG spindles of halothane anesthesia. *Anesthesiology* **84,** 945–954.

93. Lydic, R., Keifer, J. C., Baghdoyan, H. A., and Becker, L. (1993) Microdialysis of the pontine reticular formation reveals inhibition of acetylcholine release by morphine. *Anesthesiology* **79,** 1003–1012.

94. Vazquez, J. and Baghdoyan, H. A. (2001) Basal forebrain acetylcholine release during REM sleep is significantly greater than during waking. *Am. J. Physiol.* **280,** R598–R601.

95. Douglas, C. L., Baghdoyan, H. A., and Lydic, R. (2001) Muscarinic autoreceptors modulate release of ACh in frontal association cortex of C57BL/6J mouse. *J. Pharmacol. Exp. Ther.* **299,** 960–966.

96. Lancel, M. (1999) Role of GABAA receptors in the regulation of sleep: Initial sleep responses to peripherally administered modulators and agonists. *Sleep* **22,** 33–42.

97. Marti-Bonmati, L., Ronchera-Oms, C. L., Casillas, C., Poyatos, C., Torrijo, C., and Jimenez, N. V. (1995) Randomized double-blind clinical trial of intermediate versus high dose chloral hydrate for neuroimaging of children. *Neuroradiology* **37**, 687–691.

98. Needleman, H. L., Joshi, A., and Griffith, D. G. (1995) Conscious sedation of pediatric dental patients using chloral hydrate, hydroxyzine, and nitrous oxide—a retrospective study of 382 sedations. *Pediatr. Dent.* **17**, 424–431.

99. Lovinger, D. M., Zimmerman, S. A., Levitin, M., Jones, M. V., and Harrison, N. L. (1993) Trichloroentanol potentiates synaptic transmission mediated by gamma-aminobutyric acid A receptors in hippocampal neurons. *J. Pharmacol. Exp. Ther.* **264**, 1097–1103.

100. Ronchera-Oms, C. L., Casillas, C., Marti-Bonmati, L., Poyatos, C., Tomas, J., Sobejano, A., and et al. (1994) Oral chloral hydrate provides effective and safe sedation in paediatric magnetic resonance imaging. *J. Clin. Pharm. Ther.* **19**, 239–243.

101. Mayers, D. J., Hindmarsh, K. W., Sankaran, K., Gorecki, D. K., and Kasian, G. F. (1991) Chloral hydrate disposition following single-single dose administration to critically ill neonates and children. *Dev. Pharmacol. Ther.* **16**, 71–77.

102. Salmon, A. G., Kizer, K. W., Zwise, L., Jackson, R. J., and Smith, M. T. (1995) Potential carcinogenicity of chloral hydrate - a review. *J. Toxicol. Clin. Toxicol.* **33**, 115–121.

103. Mendelson, W. B. Cain, M., Cook, J. M., Paul, S. M., and Skolnick, P. (1983) A benzodiazepine receptor antagonist decreases sleep and reverses the hypnotic actions of flurazepam. *Science* **219**, 414–416.

104. Mendelson, W. B. and Martin, J. V. (1992) Characterization of the hypnotic effects of triazolam microinjections into the medial preoptic area. *Life Sci.* **50**, 1117–1128.

105. Reves, J. G., Fragen, R. J., Vinik, H. R., and Greenblatt, D. J. (1985) Midazolam: pharmacology and uses. *Anesthesiology* **63**, 310–324.

106. Malinovsky, J. M., Populaire, C., Cozian, A., Lepage, J. Y., Lejus, C., and Pinard, M. (1995) Premedication with midazolam in children effects of intranasal, rectal and oral routes on plasma midazolam concentrations. *Anaesthesia* **50**, 351–354.

107. Doyle, W. L. and Perrin, L. (1994) Emergence delirium in a child given oral midazolam for conscious sedation. *Ann. Emerg. Med.* **24**, 1173–1175.

108. Comacho-Arroyo, I., Alvarado, R., Manjarrez, J., and Tapia, R. (1991) Microinjections of muscimol and bicuculline into the pontine reticular formation modify the sleep-waking cycle in the rat. *Neurosci. Lett.* **129**, 95–97.

109. Xi M-C, Morales, F. R., and Chase, M. H. (1999) Evidence that wakefulness and REM sleep are controlled by a GABAergic pontine mechanism. *J. Neurophysiol.* **82**, 2015–2019.

110. Sastre, J. P., Buda, C., Kitahama, K., and Jouvet, M. (1996) Importance of the ventrolateral region of the periaqueductal gray and adjacent tegmentum in the control of paradoxical sleep as studied by muscimol microinjections in the cat. *Neuroscience* **74**, 415–426.

111. Fang, F., Guo, T. Z., Davies, M. F., and Maze, M. (1997) Opiate receptors in the periaqueductal gray mediate the analgesic effect of nitrous oxide in rats. *Eur. J. Pharmacol.* **336,** 137–141.

112. Nitz, D. and Siegel, J. (1997) GABA release in the dorsal raphe nucleus: role in the control of REM sleep. *Am. J. Physiol.* **273,** R451–R455.

113. Nitz, D. and Siegel, J. (1997) GABA release in the locus coeruleus as a function of sleep/wake state. *Neuroscience* **78,** 795–801.

114. Kaur, S., Saxena, R. N., and Mallick, B. N. (1997) GABA in locus coeruleus regulates spontaneous rapid eye movement sleep by acting on GABAA receptors in freely moving rat. *Neurosci. Lett.* **223,** 105–108.

115. Gervasoni, D., Darracq, L., Fort, P., Souliere, F., Chouvet, G., and Luppi, P. H. (1998) Electrophysiological evidence that noradrenergic neurons of the rat locus coeruleus are tonically inhibited by GABA during sleep. *Eur. J. Neurosci.* **10,** 964–970.

116. Nitz, D. and Siegel, J. M. (1996) GABA release in posterior hypothalamus across the sleep-wake cycle. *Am. J. Physiol.* **271,** R1707–R1712.

117. Garzon, M., Tejero, S., Beneitez, A. M., and de Andres, I. (1995) Opiate microinjections in the locus coeruleus area of the cat enhance slow wave sleep. *Neuropeptides* **29,** 229–239.

118. Baghdoyan, H. A. and Lydic R. (2002) Neurotransmitters and neuromodulators regulating sleep, in *Sleep and Epilepsy: The Clinical Spectrum.* (Bazil, C., Malow, B., and Sammaritano, M., eds.), Elsevier Science, New York, NY, pp. 17–44.

119. Knill, R. L. and Gelb, A. W. (1978) Ventilatory responses to hypoxia and hypercapnia during halothane sedation in man. *Anesthesiology* **49,** 244–251.

120. Soellevi, A. and Lindahl, S. G. (1995) Hypoxic and hypercapnic ventilatory responses during isoflurane sedation and anaesthesia in women. *Acta Anaesthesiol. Scand.* **39,** 931–938.

121. van der Elsen, M., Sarton, E., Teppema, L., Berkenbosch, A., and Dahan, A. (1998) Influence of 0.1 minimum alveolar concentration of sevoflurane, desflurane, and isoflurane on dynamic ventilatory response to hypercapnia in humans. *Br. J. Anaesth.* **80,** 174–182.

122. Northwood, D., Sapsford, D. J., Jones, J. G., Griffiths, D., and Wilkins, C. (1991) Nitrous oxide sedation causes post-hyperventilation apnoea. *Br. J. Anaesth.* **67,** 7–12.

123. Bailey, P. L., Pace, N. L., Ashburn, M. A., Moll, J. W., East, K. A., and Stanley, T. H. (1990) Frequent hypoxemia and apnea after sedation with midazolam and fentanyl. *Anesthesiology* **73,** 826–830.

124. Bailey, P. L., Rhondeau, S., Schafer, P. G., Lu, J. K., Timmins, B. S., Foster, W., et al. (1993) Dose-response pharmacology of intrathecal morphine in human volunteers. *Anesthesiology* **79,** 49–59.

125. Lu, J. K., Schafer, P. G., Gardner TL, Pace, N. L., Zhang, J., Niu, S., et al. (1997) The dose-response pharmacology of intrathecal sufentanil in female volunteers. *Anesth. Analg.* **85,** 372–379.

126. Blouin, R. T., Seifert, H. A., Babenco, H. D., Conrad, P. F., and Gross, J. B. (1993) Propofol depresses the hypoxic ventilatory response during conscious sedation and isohypercapnia. *Anesthesiology* **79,** 1177–1182.

127. Lydic, R. (1997) Respiratory modulation by nonrespiratory neurons, in *Sleep Science: Integrating Basic Research and Clinical Practice,* Vol. 15. (Schwartz, W. J., ed.), Karger, Basel, pp. 117–142.

128. Lydic, R. (1987) State-dependent aspects of regulatory physiology. *FASEB J.* **1,** 6–15.

129. Kubin, L., Tojima, H., Davies, R. O., and Pack, A. I. (1992) Serotoninergic excitatory drive to hypoglossal motoneurons in the decerebrate cat. *Neurosci. Lett.* **139,** 243–248.

130. Kubin, L., Reignier, C., Tojima, H., Taguchi, O., Pack, A. I., and Davies, R. O. (1994) Changes in serotonin level in the hypoglossal nucleus region during carbachol-induced atonia. *Brain Res.* **645,** 291–302.

131. Hershenson, M., Brouillette, R. T., Olsen, E., and Hunt, C. E. (1984) The effect of chloral hydrate on genioglossus and diaphragmatic activity. *Pediatr. Res.* **18,** 516–519.

132. Nicoll, R. A. and Madison, D. V. (1982) General anesthetics hyperpolarize neurons in the vertebrate central nervous system. *Science* **217,** 1055–1057.

133. Lydic, R., Fleegal, M. A., Burak, C., and Mortazavi, S. (1998) NMDA channel blockers applied to the medial pontine reticular formation decrease acetylcholine release, inhibit REM sleep, and depress respiratory rate. *Soc. Neurosci. Abstr.* **24,** A823.

134. Shyr, M. H., Tsai, T. H., Yang, C. H., Chen, H. M., Ng, H. F., and Tan, P. P. (1997) Propofol anesthesia increases dopamine and serotonin activities at the somatosensory cortex in rats: a microdialysis study. *Anesth. Analg.* **84,** 1344–1348.

135. Flood, P., Ramirez-Latorre, J., and Role, L. (1997) Alpha 4 beta 2 neuronal nicotinic acetylcholine receptors in the central nervous system are inhibited by isoflurane and propofol but alpha 7–type nicotinic acetylcholine receptors are unaffected. *Anesthesiology* **86,** 859–865.

136. Hales, T. G. and Lambert, J. J. (1991) The actions of propofol on inhibitory amino acid receptors of bovine adrenomedullary chromaffin cells and rodent central neurons. *Br. J. Pharmacol.* **104,** 619–628.

137. Kshatri, A. M., Baghdoyan, H. A., and Lydic, R. (1998) Increased tail flick latency evoked by cholinomimetics, but not morphine, from pontine reticular regions regulating rapid eye movement sleep. *Sleep* **21,** 677–685.

138. Kikuchi, T., Wang, Y., Sato, K., and Okumura, F. (1998) In vivo effects of propofol on acetylcholine release from the frontal cortex, hippocampus and striatum studied by intracerebral microdialysis in freely moving rats. *Br. J. Anaesth.* **80,** 644–648.

139. Smith, J. C., Ellenberger, H. H., Ballanyi, K., Richter, D. W., and Feldman, J. L. (1991) Pre-Botzinger complex: a brain stem region that may generate respiratory rhythm in mammals. *Science* **254,** 726–729.

140. St. John, W. M. (1996) Medullary regions for neurogenesis of gasping: noeud vital or noeuds vitals? *J. Appl. Physiol.* **81,** 1865–1877.

141. Reinoso-Barbero, F., and de Andres, I. (1995) Effects of opioid microinjections in the nucleus of the solitary tract on the sleep-wakefulness cycle in cats. *Anesthesiology* **82,** 144–152.

142. Dampney, R. A. L. (1994) Functional organization of central pathways regulating the cardiovascular system. *Physiol. Rev.* **74,** 323–362.

143. Yang, C.-Y., Luk, H.-N., Chen, S.-Y., Wu, W.-C., and Chai, C.-Y. (1997) Propofol inhibits medullary pressor mechanisms in cats. *Can. J. Anaesth.* **44,** 775–781.

144. Ernsberger, P., Arango, V., and Reis, D. J. (1988) A high density of muscarinic receptors in the rostral ventrolateral medulla of the rat is revealed by correction for autoradiographic efficiency. *Neurosci. Lett.* **85,** 179–186.

145. Snir-Mor, I., Weinstock, M., Davidson, J. T., and Bahar, M. (1983) Physostigmine antagonizes morphine-induced respiratory depression in human subjects. *Anesthesiology* **59,** 6–9.

146. Guo, T. Z., Jiang, J. Y., Buttermann, A. E., and Maze, M. (1996) Dexmedetomidine injection into the locus coeruleus produces antinociception. *Anesthesiology* **84,** 873–881.

147. Rabin, B. C., Guo, T. Z., Gregg, K., and Maze, M. (1996) Role of serotonergic neurotransmission in the hypnotic response to dexmedetomidine, an alpha 2-adrenoceptor agonist. *Eur. J. Pharmacol.* **306,** 51–59.

148. Buttermann, A. E., Reid, K., and Maze, M. (1998) Are cholinergic pathways involved in the anesthetic response to alpha2 agonists? *Toxicol. Lett.* **100–101,** 17–22.

149. Burton, M. D., Johnson, D. C., and Kazemi, H. (1990) Adrenergic and cholinergic interaction in central ventilatory control. *J. Appl. Physiol.* **68,** 2092–2099.

150. Champagnat, J., Denavit-Saubie, M., Henry, J. L., and Leviel, V. (1979) Catecholaminergic depressant effects on bulbar respiratory mechanisms. *Brain Res.* **160,** 57–68.

151. Benhamou, D., Veillette, Y., Narchi, P., and Ecoffey, C. (1991) Ventilatory effects of premedication with clonidine. *Anesth. Analg.* **73,** 799–803.

152. Penon, C., Ecoffey, C., and Cohen, C. E. (1991) Ventilatory response to carbon dioxide after epidural clonidine injection. *Anesth. Analg.* **72,** 761–764.

153. Sauerland, S. K., and Harper, R. M. (1976) The human tongue during sleep: electromyographic activity of the genioglossus muscle. *Exp. Neurol.* **51,** 160–170.

154. Parkis, M. A. and Berger, A. J. (1997) Clonidine reduces hyperpolarization-activated inward current in rat hypoglossal motoneurons. *Brain Res.* **769,** 108–118.

155. O'Halloran, K. D., Herman, J. K., and Bisgard, G. E. (1999) Differential effects of clonidine on upper airway abductor and adductor muscle activity in awake goats. *J. Appl. Physiol.* **87,** 590–597.

156. O'Halloran, K. D., Herman, J. K., and Bisgard, G. E. (1999) Nonvagal tachypnea following alpha-2 adrenoceptor stimulation in awake goats. *Respir. Physiol.* **118,** 15–24.

157. Kohn, L. T., Corrigan, J. M., and Donaldson, M. S. (eds). (1999) *To Err is Human. Building a Safer Health System.* Washington, DC: Institute of Medicine, National Academy Press.

158. Beecher, H. K. and Todd, D. P. (1954) A study of the deaths associated with anesthesia and surgery. *Ann. Surg.* **140,** 2–35.
159. Morell, R. C. and Eichhorn, J. H. (eds). (1997) *Patient Safety in Anesthetic Practice.* Churchill Livingstone, New York, NY.
160. Quine, M. A., Bell, G. D., McCloy, R. F., Charlton, J. E., Devlin, H. B., and Hopkins, A. (1995) Prospective audit of upper gastrointestinal endoscopy in two regions of England: safety, staffing, and sedation methods. *Gut* **36,** 462–467.
161. Joas, T. A. (1998) Sedation and anesthesia in the office setting. *Aesthetic Surg. J.* **18,** 300–301.
162. Allen, M. Albany study finds perils in surgery in doctors' offices. *The New York Times* 1999;March 8, B6.
163. Coté, C. J., Notterman, D. A., Karl, H. W., Weinberg, J. A., and McCloskey, C. (2000) Adverse sedation events in pediatrics: a critical incident analysis of contributing factors. *Pediatrics* **105,** 805–814.
164. Grazer, F. M. and de Jong, R. H. (1999) Fatal outcomes from liposuction: census survey of cosmetic surgeons. *Plas. Reconstr. Surg.* **105,** 436–446.
165. MacKenzie, R. A. (2000) Office-based surgery and anesthesia: A continuing challenge. *Am. Soc. Anes. News* **64,** 2.
166. Voelker, R. (1995) Anesthesia-related risks have plummeted. *J. Am. Med. Assn.* **273,** 445–446.
167. Keifer, J. C., Baghdoyan, H. A., and Lydic, R. (1992) Sleep disruption and increased apneas after pontine microinjection of morphine. *Anesthesiology* **77,** 973–982.
168. Lydic, R. Baghdoyan, H. A., and Zwillich, C. W. (1989) State-dependent hypotonia in posterior cricoarytenoid muscles of the larynx caused by cholinergic reticular mechanisms. *FASEB J.* **3,** 1625–1631.
169. Lydic, R. and Baghdoyan, H. A. (1989) Cholinoceptive pontine reticular mechanisms cause state-dependent changes in respiration. *Neurosci. Lett.* **102,** 211–216.
170. Lydic, R., Baghdoyan, H. A., Wertz, R., and White, D. P. (1991) Cholinergic reticular mechanisms influence state-dependent ventilatory response to hypercapnia. *Am. J. Physiol.* **261,** R738–R746.

2

Practice Guidelines for Pediatric Sedation

David M. Polaner, MD, FAAP

1. INTRODUCTION

The sedation of children for diagnostic and therapeutic procedures has undergone quite an evolution from the days of "DTP (demerol, thorazine, phenergan) cocktail" without monitoring. Although the use of sedation for infants and children is often motivated by a desire to avoid both physical and psychological trauma, these goals must be tempered by the realities of risk and safety. Prior to the 1980s, there was often little or no awareness of the potential consequences of effects and interactions of sedating drugs, outside the specialty of anesthesiology. Practitioners had minimal recognition of the potential hazards of oversedation, including loss of airway, aspiration, and cardiorespiratory compromise. Concerns about recovery and premature discharge were either rarely acknowledged or ignored. Unfortunately, such an attitude may persist today, although there has been increasing recognition that sedation of infants and children can carry the same inherent risks as general anesthesia. In response to the publicity surrounding "sedation disasters," specialized societies dedicated to the care and safety of children have developed guidelines to provide a framework for the safe provision of sedation. The guidelines deal with the use of various sedating agents, as well as the environment in which the sedation is administered, monitoring of patients, patient selection, and the responsibilities of practitioners who administer the agents. There has been an attempt to tighten and restrict the use of terminology and definitions that have been used loosely and inaccurately in the medical literature. Several different sets of guidelines have been promulgated by different specialty groups, which have attempted to address the issues of safety and standards of care. These guidelines are not all the same, however, and it is instructive and important to understand the differences between them and to recognize their potential shortcomings and limitations. This chapter examines the practice guidelines written specifically for pediatric sedation and discusses how they should be

From: *Contemporary Clinical Neuroscience: Sedation and Analgesia for Diagnostic and Therapeutic Procedures*
Edited by: S. Malviya, N. N. Naughton, and K. K. Tremper © Humana Press Inc., Totowa, NJ

used in developing an institutional policy and plan, and how the systems or organizational approach to the implementation of sedation guidelines may decrease risk and increase safety.

2. HISTORY AND BACKGROUND

Until the 1980s, there was little oversight or attempt to organize and scrutinize the practice of sedation. Prompted by a series of disastrous outcomes following sedation during dental procedures, the American Academy of Pediatrics (AAP) requested that its Section on Anesthesiology offer guidance in developing a set of guidelines that were eventually published by the Academy in 1985. This document was authored by representatives from the Section on Anesthesiology, the Committee on Drugs, and the American Academy of Pediatric Dentistry (AAPD), and was entitled "Guidelines for the Elective Use of Conscious Sedation, Deep Sedation, and General Anesthesia." This title was chosen to emphasize that there was a continuum between these three states. It became clear to the Academy and to the authors of the original document that a revision was needed to address other concerns and issues that were not adequately clarified. It was apparent that discharge criteria were a major problem, and that a number of adverse outcomes could be blamed on inadequate recognition of when a child was "street ready" *(1)*. For this reason, the title of the revised document was changed to reflect the importance of applying the guidelines both during and after the administration of the sedating agents *(2)*. There were also a plethora of papers appearing in the medical literature on the subject that stretched the definition of "conscious sedation" beyond credulity *(3,4)*. The use of numerous anesthetic agents at doses that result in varying planes of general anesthesia was commonly described as sedation in an apparent attempt to extend the boundaries of practice *(5,6)*. For this reason, the strict definitions of "conscious" and "deep" sedation were given special emphasis. Many other aspects of the guidelines were revised to reflect the reports of complications that were culled from the literature, adverse drug reports, and popular press, in an attempt to address the systems problems that led to adverse outcomes.

The guidelines were not met with uniform acceptance. Many of the prescribers of sedation believed that the guidelines were overly burdensome and represented an intrusion on practices they believed to be safe based on historical impressions, despite mounting data to the contrary. Clearly, the purchase of monitoring equipment and the use of trained observers imposed additional costs on both individual practitioners and institutions. Ever-increasing financial pressures from diminishing third-party reimbursement added to this problem. The reference in the title of the guidelines to "general anesthesia" unfortunately led to the impression by some physicians that the guidelines did not apply to them because they did not administer general anesthesia (this led to the change in the title of the revised guidelines of 1992). Other specialties and subspecialties published their own sets of guidelines in response to the AAP guidelines *(7–9)*. It is the belief of some physicians that these latter sets of guidelines are attempts to redefine the standards of practice to fit within the traditionally accepted practices of those specialties *(10)*. Whether there are data to support these alternative guidelines, or whether the potential consequences of adopting looser standards are worth the risks in situations where adequate data are not available, will be examined later in this chapter. It should be recognized from the outset that clinical and outcomes-based considerations are clearly not the only factors involved here, and that several specialties have staked out claims to what has traditionally long been the purview of the anesthesiologist. This has created an environment that is laden with political and financial implications, which have tended to cloud the objectivity of much of the "research" that has been published.

3. WHY GUIDELINES?

The need for guidelines has been disputed, in most cases by clinicians who have been prescribing sedating medications for years without recognized or perceived mishaps. In many cases, the development of national guidelines has been viewed as an intrusion and a limitation of medical practice and physician autonomy. There is little outcome-based data on which to base many of the guidelines, and that which exists has significant limitations of power and methodology. So why promote them at all? It is recognized by all that adverse events in sedation are infrequent *(11)*. An individual clinician may see them only rarely, although the precipitating events that have the potential to lead to catastrophic outcomes may occur, albeit unrecognized, far more often *(12)*. This is a particular problem in infants and children, especially in adult or general hospitals, where the volume of pediatric cases may not approach that of a large children's hospital. Furthermore, adverse events may be defined differently by clinicians with various levels of risk acceptance. At a recent hospital sedation committee meeting, the author was stunned to discover that one group of clinicians did not consider respiratory depression severe enough to require the use of naloxone as an adverse event—this was simply considered routine practice. Such perceptions clearly impact on the reporting of complication rates.

Many of the improvements in patient safety, and the reduction of adverse events in medicine over the past 25 years, have come through advances in anesthesia practice. The report of the Institute of Medicine (IOM) not only recognizes this, but suggests that similar methodologies and strategies can be generalized to other areas of medical practice as well *(13)*. Two prime factors in the reduction of risk in anesthesia have been (i) the advances in monitoring technology and the routine application of monitoring to provide early detection of adverse events before they affect physiologic stability and (ii) the aggressive use of risk reduction strategies in patient care. The philosophy in anesthesia practice has been to be exceedingly cautious in addressing various potentially risky situations, whether it is the patient with the risk of a full stomach, the use of halothane in adults, or the routine use of succinylcholine in children. This same philosophical view is embodied in the idea of using guidelines for the practice of sedation in pediatric patients. The overriding approach embodies several axioms:

1. Adverse events occur rarely, but inevitably.
2. Although an individual practitioner may not see a significant number of these events, in the national aggregate they occur frequently enough, or have severe enough preventable sequelae, that a change in practice is deemed desirable.
3. Because these events will invariably occur, a systems approach to prevention and detection is most effective.
4. In order to reduce adverse outcomes, practices must be implemented that will reduce the incidence of these events and provide early detection of the events. This means both avoiding and eliminating practices with excessive risk and using appropriate observation and monitors.

Guidelines are a foundation of the systems approach, which seeks to promote safe practices that result in both risk reduction and early detection of adverse events.

4. PRACTICE GUIDELINES

Numerous sedation guidelines have been promulgated in the United States by various organizations. Only two deal specifically with pediatric patients, and both are from physician specialty organizations. There are other guidelines that impact on pediatric patients, two from physician specialty organizations and one from the Joint Commission on the Accreditation of Health Care Organizations (JCAHO). This section examines the AAP guidelines as a prototype—because it was the first document to specifically address the sedation of children, and thus served as template for others that followed, and also because several of the subsequent documents were published as reactions to the AAP guidelines. This chapter examines the AAP guidelines in detail, and discusses the other guidelines and how they differ. The guidelines not written specifically for pediatric patients are addressed elsewhere in this volume, but issues especially relevant to pediatric practice are discussed here, particularly when they are in conflict with the AAP guidelines.

4.1. American Academy of Pediatrics Guidelines (1992 revision)

The current AAP guidelines, authored by the Committee on Drugs, have attempted to deal with issues that were left ambiguous or were not addressed in the first version. Monitoring—the use of observation and devices for the early detection of adverse events—and the skills and responsibilities of the clinician, are the primary focus of this document. The guidelines emphasize that sedation is a continuum, which ranges from "conscious sedation" to general anesthesia, and that monitoring must be geared to the depth of sedation. The crucial complications of respiratory depression and loss of airway reflexes and stability are explicitly acknowledged as potential events in any infant or child who is sedated. These risks are emphasized, not minimized, so that the practitioner is encouraged to maintain a heightened sense of vigilance at all times. Monitoring standards must not be selected solely on the basis of the anticipated usual effect of the drug administered, but rather based on the actual effect observed. This is an essential point in the AAP guidelines that cannot be overemphasized. The guidelines require that the monitoring reflect the level of consciousness of the child, and that the monitoring be used to detect early events that might progress to significant complications without intervention. The guidelines further recognize the inability of a single person to both perform the procedure and simultaneously closely observe the patient. The importance of an independent observing clinician is emphasized.

The guidelines first clearly define the terms that are used in the document. This is crucial, since ambiguities in terminology, both intentional and unintentional, became a rampant problem in the literature that followed the initial AAP guidelines. The AAP defines three levels of sedation:

- *Conscious sedation*, a state in which consciousness is medically depressed, but a patent airway and protective airway reflexes are maintained independently at all times. The patient exhibits appropriate and purposeful responses to stimuli or verbal command. These responses do not include reflex withdrawal.
- *Deep sedation*, a state in which the patient is not easily aroused and may be unconscious. There may be partial or complete blunting of protective reflexes, and the patient may or not be able to independently maintain a patent airway. Purposeful response to stimuli may not be present.
- *General anesthesia* is defined as "a medically controlled state of unconsciousness accompanied by a loss of protective reflexes, including the inability to maintain a patient airway independently and respond purposefully to physical stimulation or verbal command."

This classification scheme was not promulgated to strictly classify the condition of a sedated patient. The guidelines emphasize that these levels are in reality a continuum, and that a patient may easily pass from one level to the next. The levels are identified in order to define appropriate levels of physiologic monitoring, not to strictly categorize the effects of a particular drug or sedation regimen. This distinction is an important difference from several other sedation guidelines. The AAP guidelines recognize that no particular agent can be expected to produce consistent results in every patient, and that it is the response to an agent, not the use of a specific drug, that determines the patient's level of sedation and thereby dictates the level of monitoring. The definition of general anesthesia may be problematic, as some have inferred from the guidelines that a state of general anesthesia does not exist if a patient has the ability to independently maintain a patent airway, a contention that is obviously not accurate. Such an implication was not the intent of the definition, but it demonstrates that these definitions, even when very carefully crafted, can create ambiguities that the authors did not anticipate. Despite the clarity and precision of the definition of terms, the use of "conscious sedation" remains problematic, because the term has entered the lexicon, where it continues to be frequently misused to describe deeper states of sedation *(14)*. It would probably be best if this oxymoron is retired and replaced with "moderate sedation," the term adopted in the most recent JCAHO standards *(15)*.

The guidelines also clearly define the levels of imperatives in the language of the document: which items are mandated, and which items are suggested, yet may have alternatives that can be employed.

The AAP guidelines are directed at personnel who provide sedation and are not trained in anesthesiology, and thus advise that patients undergoing sedation be American Society of Anestesiologists (ASA) physical status I or II, and that physical status III and IV patients require special consideration. Back-up facilities and services must also be clearly identified; these systems must be in place so that a defined plan of action can be immediately implemented if complications develop. The proper and appropriately sized equipment to provide resuscitation from both respiratory and circulatory complications is required in the sedating location. These items include a system for the delivery of positive pressure ventilation and supplemental oxygen ($FiO_2 > 0.90$), suction apparatus, airway equipment in varied sizes, and drugs necessary for resuscitation. It is emphasized that the equipment and supplies must be immediately available to the sedating clinician, and that they must be regularly checked and maintained. A list of suggested drugs and equipment is appended to the guidelines.

Documentation of both the pre-sedation evaluation and the intra-operative events are mandated by the guidelines. Proper informed consent must be obtained, as the administration of sedating drugs is not without risk, and the parent or guardian must understand the benefits and risks in order to permit the administration of these agents. A history, physical examination (with special attention paid to the airway) and review of the patient's medications is required. The ASA Physical Status score (listed in an appendix) should be assigned. The parent or guardian must be issued instructions regarding the care required following the completion of the sedation, and they must be able to contact medical help at any time should problems arise in the post-sedation period.

Fasting (NPO) status is referenced in the appendix of the document. The risks of sedation, loss of airway reflexes, and aspiration of gastric contents are acknowledged. The standard recommendations for NPO times in elective cases are cited, with 2-h fasting times for clear fluids, and 4-, 6-, and 8-h fasting times for other foods and liquids for ages 0–6 mo, 6– 36 mo, and greater than 3 yr, respectively. These recommendations are well supported by data in the literature *(16–18)*. The problem of a full stomach in emergency cases is discussed. The AAP guidelines recommend (i) delaying the sedation, (ii) the use of pharmacological means to enhance gastric emptying and raise gastric pH, or (iii) consider securing the airway when the case cannot be postponed and the stomach cannot be effectively emptied.

From the time sedation commences until discharge criteria are met, documentation of vital signs and the level of consciousness, drugs administered, and inspired oxygen concentration is required, using a time-based record. The record must also document any significant clinical events that occur during this period. At recovery, the record must document return to baseline vital signs and level of consciousness, and a note stating that the child is deemed ready for discharge from care must be entered in the chart. The criteria for discharge are found in an appendix to the guidelines, and include the return to baseline mental status and cardiovascular stability. The responsible adult must be issued post-sedation instructions. Strict criteria for discharge are particularly important in view of the number of sedation complications that have been reported from premature discharge and subsequent airway obstruction and respiratory arrest *(12)*.

The AAP document next describes specific guidelines for the three levels of sedation previously defined. The continuum of sedation concept is reiterated, and the clinician is reminded to be prepared to escalate the level of monitoring if that occurs. Both conscious and deep sedation require an independent monitor to observe the patient, assess vital signs, administer drugs, and attend to the airway. For conscious sedation, the guidelines list this person under the heading of "support personnel", and for deep sedation this person is listed under "personnel", implying a greater level of vigilance and dedication to that single task. The conscious sedation requirements include the practitioner performing the procedure in question as part of the monitoring and sedation care team; for deep sedation, the practitioner is not mentioned, and all of the sedation tasks fall to the independent sedating clinician. The emphasis on "constant observation" in the deep sedation section and the emphasis on the observation of the airway further reinforce that idea, and the wording of requirements for conscious sedation imply that the monitoring person may be involved in other tasks during the procedure. The increased vigilance demanded by a deeper state of sedation requires that the monitoring clinician be completely devoted to that task, without distraction. Both deep and conscious sedation require that one person be trained in at least pediatric basic life support. Deep sedation also requires that the monitoring person possess skills in pediatric airway management; pediatric advanced life support skills are "strongly encouraged." The level of care required during the procedure is described, and should include continuous monitoring of oxygen saturation and heart rate, and intermittent measurement of respiratory rate and blood pressure. Attention to the airway is again emphasized, and for deep sedation, more intensive monitoring of respiration and airway patency is required, such as the use of capnometry or a precordial stethoscope. In settings where it may not be possible to readily detect transitions in the depth of consciousness—for example, in the magnetic resonance imaging (MRI) scanner—it may be prudent to implement a higher level of monitoring even if minimal or conscious sedation is the goal. Documentation of drug administration and vital signs on a time-based record is mandated. Either vascular access or the ability to immediately obtain it is necessary during deep sedation. Cautions about the potential for toxicity from local anesthetics and the special risks entailed with the use of nitrous oxide, especially the problems of synergy when used in conjunction with other sedating agents, are cited. The monitoring problems in MRI are mentioned, but there are no specific cautions about the particular difficulty in assessing adequacy of respiration and airway patency in that environment. The risks of thermal injury caused by induction currents with electronic monitoring cables in the high-gauss magnetic field are noted.

The AAP guidelines do not directly address the issue of credentialling and the qualifications of the personnel administering sedation and monitoring the patient except to advise regarding the training and certification in pediatric life support (mentioned previously). These difficult issues are left to the individual institution to decide *(19)*.

4.2. American Academy of Pediatric Dentistry Guidelines (1998 revision)

AAPD first published its own set of guidelines for sedation in 1985. These were revised in 1996, and further revised in 1998 to include a section on general anesthesia. The document describes the guidelines as "systematically developed recommendations," which may be "adopted, modified or rejected according to clinical needs and constraints." The AAPD explicitly states that the guidelines are not to be construed as setting standards or requirements. This caveat is similar or identical to other guidelines, but is in some contrast to the disclaimers in the introduction to the AAP guidelines, which state that they "reflect our current understanding of appropriate monitoring needs," and that they may be *exceeded* at any time, based on the judgement of the responsible physician" [emphasis added]. The language used in the AAP guidelines appears to be a greater call for compliance by the clinician, although these, are guidelines and not practice standards, and these semantic differences are highly nuanced. The language in the AAPD document, by eliminating the term "exceeded," may potentially weaken the impact on practice patterns by individual clinicians. The practice settings for pediatrics and for dentistry may be quite different. It is likely that a greater percentage of dental care under sedation is administered in an individual office, unlike the use of sedation in pediatric medical practice, which is more likely to be hospital-based and under the greater oversight mandated by JCAHO standards. There are no data to show if this results in any difference in compliance with the guidelines by dentists.

The guidelines begin with a section of definitions. Like the AAP guidelines, the document is careful to define levels of imperatives contained in the guidelines. They delineate three levels of sedation (conscious, deep, and general anesthesia), but also subdivide the conscious sedation category into three sublevels, thus resulting in five levels. The descriptions of the levels are defined as both behavioral goals and as levels of responsiveness. A table in the appendix to the document details the definition and the personnel and monitoring equipment appropriate for each level. Level 1 is anxiolysis; the patient is totally awake, and only clinical observation is necessary. In Level 2, the patient has a minimally depressed level of consciousness. They eyes may intermittently close, but the patient is still able to respond to verbal commands. This corresponds to the "conscious sedation" stage described in the AAP guidelines. Pulse oximetry is required, and precordial stethoscope is recommended. The use of the precordial stethoscope to assess aeration is a frequent recommendation (required for levels 3–5) in the AAPD guidelines, and allows the dentist to continually monitor airway patency and respiratory rate without continual visual observation. The AAPD guidelines are unique in their emphasis on the means of monitoring of airway patency, a prominence that is certainly born from the potential interference with the airway by dental interventions. Emphasis on this device in situations where direct observation of the patient is obscured would probably be advisable in the AAP guidelines as well, and may be underemphasized in that document. Like the auditory signal from a pulse oximeter, which falls in pitch as the saturation declines, the precordial stethoscope permits the clinician to focus the eyes on one task and the ears on another. The limitation, of course, is that for full concentration to be focused on the monitoring of the sedated patient, all the senses must be engaged in a task related to monitoring. In the case of the dentist, attention is likely to be focused on the dental procedure, since the monitoring is a secondary task. This is unlikely to be a problem for patients sedated to Levels 1 and 2, but with Level 3, as discussed in the next paragraph, or for patients who unintentionally descend to a greater depth of sedation, one may be distracted from adequate vigilance. The goal is that the auditory cues will alert the clinician that something is wrong with the airway, which will then result in refocusing of attention. This type of vigilance is a skill that needs development and experience. Furthermore, the noise of the handpiece and suction device may obscure the breath sounds or heart sounds heard through the precordial stethoscope. Capnometry has been validated as an early warning device for airway patency and respiratory depression in several settings, but requires that attention be given to the waveform trace *(20–22)*.

Level 3, which the AAPD still defines as within the boundaries of conscious sedation, results in "moderately depressed levels of consciousness" that "mimics physiologic sleep." Despite the description of this state as conscious sedation, patients may not respond to verbal stimuli, may respond to moderately painful stimuli with only reflex withdrawal, and may require chin thrust to maintain the airway. It is this part of the AAPD guidelines that most radically differs from the AAP document. The categorization of this state is clearly inaccurate. If the patient is sedated to the point where he or she does not respond to verbal stimuli, the patient is not conscious, and the resulting state cannot honestly be described as conscious sedation. The main problem with this categorization is that although blood pressure and the option of capnometry are added to the monitoring, "conscious sedation" does not require an independent monitoring clinician. Certainly, the use of continuous auscultation via a precordial stethoscope or capnometry is useful, but distractions are a concern when the monitoring clinician is busy concentrating on other complex tasks. The AAP guidelines and JCAHO standards would require an independent monitoring clinician for children who have reached this stage of sedation.

Level 4 sedation is defined as deep sedation, with the patient expected to require constant monitoring and frequent management of the airway. Recommended monitoring devices include the full array of noninvasive physiologic monitors, including precordial stethoscope, capnometry, ECG, noninvasive blood pressure, and oximetry. The presence of emergency equipment, such as a defibrillator, is recommended. Patients in this state of sedation have a "deeply depressed level of consciousness" and are not expected to be responsive to most stimuli, but may respond to pain with reflex withdrawal. An independent monitoring clinician with training in airway management is required.

Level 5 is general anesthesia. According to the guidelines, a dentist who has completed training in oral and maxillofacial surgery is qualified to administer general anesthesia. The duration of training in general anesthesia for these practitioners is usually about 3 mo. The adequacy of such training to qualify an individual to administer general anesthesia is an issue that is beyond the scope of this chapter.

A preoperative evaluation is required for all patients, and standard NPO recommendations are cited. Consent is required, and must be documented. The guidelines permit the administration of minor pre-procedure tranquilizers such as diazepam or hydroxyzine by a responsible adult at home, but not chloral hydrate or narcotics. Because even these drugs may have considerable variation in effect from patient to patient, there is some risk in permitting the use of benzodiazepines in younger children and in many older children with developmental or neurological problems. The use of sedating medications outside of a medical facility was one of the risk factors cited by Coté et al. that increases the risk of adverse sedation events *(12)*. Record keeping is mandated for all levels of sedation, and adequacy of recovery must be documented prior to discharge. The criteria for discharge are similar to the AAP guidelines, and continuous observation and monitoring during recovery by a qualified individual experienced in recovery care is emphasized. A responsible parent or guardian must be given appropriate discharge instructions. Explicit and proactively determined emergency procedures are mandated. This is particularly important for the dental setting, where sedation is commonly administered in a private office, remote from a hospital where additional assistance such as a "code team" is readily available.

One would not think that the differences between the AAP and AAPD guidelines are difficult to reconcile, and that the acceptance by the AAPD of the few additional aspects of the AAP guidelines would be so onerous. There are clearly "turf" issues at play here, but the most glaring difference—that of the definition of AAPD Level 3 as conscious sedation—actually has greater implications, both financial and logistic, than one would notice at first glance. Level 3 sedation has considerable latitude and breadth of definition, and it is not difficult to stretch most deeper levels of sedation to fit within this rubric. It is likely that a large proportion of sedation performed in the dental office may fall under this category. Levels 1 and 2 are often inadequate to deal with the needs of the majority of children who require more intensive dental interventions. Thus, the additional requirement of an independent monitoring clinician actually imposes an obligation on the dentist that has significant financial and personnel implications. We are faced with the decision of risk vs expediency, and must decide how much risk one is willing to accept to prevent or allow early detection of a relatively uncommon event. Since those events have the potential for serious or life-threatening complications, and they are preventable with commonly available technology or procedures, both the AAP and JCAHO have come down on the side of minimizing risk, and the AAPD guidelines appear to offer some degree of compromise in this regard.

4.3. The American College of Emergency Physicians (ACEP)

The American College of Emergency Physicians (ACEP) guidelines were designed to cover sedation of all patients in the emergency room, not just infants and children *(9)*. The ACEP has also published a position paper on the use of sedation and analgesia in pediatrics, but this policy statement is not a set of guidelines, and makes no specific recommendations regarding management, monitoring, or personnel, other than in very broad generalities *(8)*. There are no statements in the ACEP clinical policy that address the unique needs of children or consider them separately from adults. Much of the data referenced in the document are from adult studies, and may not be applicable to infants and children. They have entitled their document a clinical policy," and acknowledge that many of the statements in the policy are at odds with JCAHO criteria. They offer the clinical policy as a challenge, as it were, to the JCAHO and others, to reinterpret which criteria should be considered in sedation standards.

The ACEP clinical policy is clearly an outgrowth of the unique needs of emergency physicians, who are called upon to provide care for unprepared patients in urgent situations. The patients are often frightened or uncooperative, and either require interventions that cannot be postponed, or the logistics and management issues in running the emergency room are considered to take precedence over the ability to postpone an intervention. The emergency room is a rapid turnover environment in which efficiency is crucial to avoid unmanageable back-ups and delays in care for other unstable patients. Several of the cornerstones of the AAP document are at odds with these administrative matters, and thus the ACEP was faced with either having common practices in many emergency rooms be out of compliance with the AAP and JCAHO guidelines, or write new standards of their own that contested those that had been promulgated by others. Again, the questions that arise are in many ways related to this central issue: at what point is one willing to draw the lines that set the boundaries between patient safety and expediency? Does one give priority to protecting a status quo standard of practice over preventing an infrequent but possible adverse event? How much risk is one willing to accept? These are the real questions posed by the ACEP clinical policy, but they are not discussed in this document. Rather, the ACEP document attempts to refocus the discussion in evidence-based terms, and contest the authenticity of those risks.

The ACEP document begins with a statement that charges other guidelines with not being evidence-based, and implies that at least some of the recommendations contained in those other documents are biased. The authors claim that the ACEP clinical policy will be evidence-based, and will only make recommendations that are founded on such data. However, under scrutiny, there is a clear agenda underlying much of this document. The authors clearly wish to shift the emphasis of guidelines from minimizing risk to permitting certain practices because they have not, in the eyes of the ACEP, been definitively proven as hazardous. Unfortunately, many of the statements made in the document in this regard are not well-supported by the cited data, or do not consider relevant data from the non-emergency medicine literature. It appears from the description of methodology that the ACEP views the Emergency Room as fundamentally different from any other venue in medicine, and therefore excludes virtually all data obtained in other settings from consideration in their "evidence-based" policy statement. This enables them to state repeatedly that there are no evidence-based standards for numerous issues. The two areas of greatest deviation from the AAP guidelines are with regard to the unprotected airway in a patient with a full stomach, and in issues of airway management. Other issues that are contested are informed consent, monitoring standards, personnel and drug choice, and administration.

The ACEP does not accept the long-held contention that the full, or potentially full stomach, is a sufficient risk to avoid using deeper levels of sedation without a secured airway. They believe that there are inadequate data to prove that an unfasted patient in the emergency room is at increased risk of aspiration during sedation. This is in large part based on the assertion that "procedural sedation and analgesia in the [emergency department] is not reasonably expected to result in the loss of protective reflexes." This statement is based on studies that do not specifically look at that question, or contain a requisite number of patients from which to draw that conclusion. A Type II statistical error, in which it is assumed that a numerator of zero implies absence of risk, is the problem here *(23)*. They also assume that the clinician is able to predict with a reasonable degree of certainty whether a given sedation technique is likely to result in the loss of airway reflexes, thus minimizing risks of aspiration. The data do not provide adequate evidence to prove that the risk is as negligible as the clinical policy or original papers imply.

Airway issues, such as oxygen desaturation and respiratory depression, are largely dismissed by the ACEP policy, as they do not accept the contention that hypoxia has a significant potential to lead to adverse outcomes during sedation. This has particular implications for pediatric patients, as the majority of cardiac arrests in children outside of the operating room setting begin as respiratory events. The policy again largely ignores the problem of inferring safety from studies of small numbers of patients.

4.4. American Society of Anesthesiologists (ASA)

The ASA published *Practice Guidelines for Sedation and Analgesia by Non-Anesthesiologists* in 1996 *(24)*. They have been referenced by JCAHO *(15)* and adopted by the Governing Board of the American Society for Gastrointestinal Endoscopy. The guidelines use similar language to the AAPD guidelines in the preamble defining their goals and limitations, but insert the term "exceed" with regard to the recommendations. They also clearly reject the term "conscious sedation" in favor of "sedation and analgesia." The ASA guidelines are unique in that a comprehensive review of over 1,300 scientific articles was undertaken by the authors. 269 Articles selected from all disciplines were found to have direct linkage to evidence to support or reject the hypotheses regarding fourteen parameters of sedation care, including pre-procedure evaluation, monitoring, training of personnel, record keeping, drug administration, oxygen administration, airway management, and special considerations. These papers were subject to review and statistical analysis to determine recommendations for clinical practice. In addition, these recommendations were reviewed by non-anesthesiologists who were asked to evaluate the effect on their practices, including time and effort. Even economic impact was considered, although the personnel costs may be considerably underestimated, depending on the particulars of a given institution *(25)*. It must be emphasized that the depth of sedation that is intended by this set of guidelines would have the patient remain communicative at all times. This has some limits in its applicability in pediatrics, where greater depths of sedation are often needed, but further emphasizes the need for diligence in monitoring and care.

There are no pediatric-specific recommendations in the ASA guidelines, other than in general terms the need to consider special patient needs at the extremes of age. The importance of this document, however, is that a painstaking methodology was applied to evaluating the need for a wide range of care parameters that cut across all medical disciplines. This document remains the most scientifically rigorous set of sedation guidelines published to date.

4.5. Joint Commission for Accreditation of Healthcare Organizations (JCAHO)

The JCAHO standards *(15)* differ in both scope and purpose from the guidelines discussed thus far. Like the ASA and ACEP guidelines, they do not specifically address the care of pediatric patients. Their primary distinction is that unlike the guidelines, these are a set of standards that a hospital or institution must adhere to in order to obtain accreditation. The JCAHO also maintains a policy regarding patient safety and the institutional responses to sentinel events. Such events are defined as:

> unexpected occurrence[s] involving death or serious physical or psychological injury, or the risk thereof. Serious injury specifically includes loss of limb or function. The phrase, "or the risk thereof" includes any process variation for which a recurrence would carry a significant chance of a serious adverse outcome *(15)*.

This standard has clear implications for an institutional policy regarding sedation, in that it mandates a review and quality assurance program, and requires continual significant oversight of all sedation practices within an institution. Failure to follow this mandate can result in punitive action by the JCAHO both when accreditation is reviewed, and, were an adverse event to occur, if an investigation is begun. Guidelines such as those promulgated by the ACEP are not alternatives that the JCAHO accepts. The JCAHO references the ASA guidelines as the prototype document that should be used by institutions in setting up their own sedation guidelines.

The JCAHO has defined four levels of sedation. They have chosen to dispose of the term "conscious sedation" and have replaced it with terms that are more descriptive. The first level, called *minimal sedation or anxiolysis*, describes a drug-induced state of altered cognition in which consciousness is not impaired, hemodynamic and ventilatory responses and equilibrium are not affected, and patients maintain verbal responsiveness. *Moderate sedation* replaces the category previously termed conscious sedation. In this state, patients still respond purposefully as described for minimal sedation, although consciousness is more impaired. The airway remains stable without intervention, and hemodynamic status is "usually" unaffected. During *deep sedation/analgesia*, patients "cannot be easily aroused but respond purposefully following repeated or painful stimulation." Although hemodynamic function is usually unaffected, airway patency and adequacy of ventilation may be adversely impacted, resulting in the need for ventilatory intervention. The last level, *anesthesia*, consists of general and major regional anesthesia. The most important characteristic of general anesthesia in this framework is the inability to be aroused even in response to a painful stimulus. The importance of this classification system is that the most important characteristic of "grading" the level of sedation is the response of the patient to stimulus. The idea that a given patient is not anesthetized because certain drugs were or were not used, or because the airway and ventilation remains intact without intervention is rejected. The guidelines also note that reflex withdrawal to stimulus is not considered a purposeful response.

The JCAHO mandates seven specific standards for moderate and deep sedation and anesthesia, spanning the entire continuum of the patient's care.

1. The individual providing the care must be "qualified." The standards for qualification must include the following criteria:
   • training in the administration of drugs to produce a desired sedation level, i.e., titration of sedating drugs to effect, and in carefully monitoring of patients in order to maintain a stable and appropriate level of sedation.
   • appropriate credentialling for the management of patients "at whatever level of sedation or anesthesia is achieved, *either intentionally or unintentionally*" [emphasis added]. This means that a clinician that is administering moderate sedation must be qualified to rescue a patient who unintentionally becomes deeply sedated, including the ability to manage an unstable airway. The clinician who is permitted to administer deep sedation must be qualified to rescue a patient who enters the level of general anesthesia.
   • competency-based education, training, and experience commensurate with the skills described here.
   • There must be adequate staffing of trained personnel in addition to the clinician performing the procedure so that pre-sedation medical evaluation, drug administration, and monitoring during the procedure, and recovery and discharge can be executed.
2. There must be appropriate resuscitation and monitoring equipment available. Monitoring must include continuous measurement of heart rate, pulse oximetry, and respiratory rate and adequacy of ventilation, and blood pressure mea-

surement at regular intervals. Electrocardiogram monitoring is required for patients with cardiovascular disease or in situations where dysrhythmias might occur.

3. All patients must undergo an evaluation before receiving moderate or deep sedation in order to assess the patient's status and formulate the sedation plan. Each patient must have a plan of sedation individualized for his or her underlying medical condition and appropriate for the procedure to be performed.

4. The JCAHO requires that the plans, options, and risks of the sedation plan are discussed with the patient or guardian and that informed consent is obtained.

5. While the sedation is administered, monitoring of the patient's physiologic status appropriate to the patient's condition, the level of sedation, and the complexity of the procedure must be performed.

6. The patient's status must similarly be assessed during the emergence period in an appropriate post-anesthesia or post-sedation recovery area.

7. The patient must be discharged from care by a "qualified licensed independent practitioner, or according to criteria approved by the medical staff."

Compliance with these standards is evaluated during the JCAHO site visits for accreditation. Revisions and updates to the standards occur frequently. These, and clarifications of the intent of the standards, can be found at the JCAHO website (www.jcaho.org).

5. EFFICACY

Has the use of guidelines led to changes in outcome for sedated children? Are there data to suggest that the implementation of risk-reduction strategies, improved monitoring, or observation by trained personnel have decreased the incidence of adverse events? (11) At this time, hard data are still lacking. Because the incidence of those events is relatively small, virtually all of the studies that purport to demonstrate the safety of various sedation recipes or sedation systems lack the statistical power to draw those conclusions. Until a controlled study measuring the incidence of complications and outcome in many tens of thousands of patients can be performed, we are not likely to have population-based information about safety that is meaningful. Furthermore, studies that focus on incidence alone may not provide the information necessary to draw conclusions about the application of guidelines in clinical practice. It may, however, be more useful to focus on a different approach to determining best or safest practice, by using a systems approach to analyze various practices and determine which are best able to minimize risk. The best available data using this approach come from the study by Coté et al., a retrospective analysis of adverse outcomes in children who underwent sedation (12). This study did not intend to measure incidence, prevalence, or the "safety" of any one system, but instead focused on determining if there were specific systems or practices that could be associated with adverse outcomes.

The authors, a group of pediatric anesthesiologists, pediatric intensivists, and emergency pediatrics specialists, analyzed 95 reports of critical incidents during sedation, and sought to define practices that were shared among the adverse events. In addition to identifying problematic practices, the authors sought to identify factors that led to positive outcomes. This is particularly important, since, as discussed earlier, adverse events inevitably occur, and it is a primary goal of guidelines to maximize the likelihood of rescue from a complication. Factors that were recognized as common to adverse outcomes included sedation in a non-hospital setting, inadequate medical evaluation prior to sedation, lack of an independent observer, medication errors, and inadequate recovery procedures. The use of monitoring devices alone, despite their warning of oxygen desaturation, were associated with better outcomes specifically only when the alarms were answered by trained personnel. In respiratory arrests that occurred in non-hospital facilities, the risk of permanent neurological injury or death was three times as likely as in a hospital, suggesting that the availability of trained personnel responding to an emergency had a major impact on outcome. This conclusion was strengthened by the finding that out of hospital respiratory events were much more likely to be followed by cardiac arrests and inadequate resuscitation than in hospital events. This was the case even though the initiating respiratory events occurred equally among hospital and non-hospital patients. These findings appear to validate the systems and practices recommended in the AAP guidelines. They add strength to the idea that such systems have universal application, and that they should be applied across specialties and settings. The institution of such systems is likely to have the greatest impact on safety and outcome if done as an integrated approach with all departments and practitioners so that every patient will benefit.

6. CONCLUSIONS

Sedation guidelines are likely to engender controversy and opposition until all groups of physicians and practitioners acknowledge that there is an advantage to working from the common viewpoint of a systems approach to minimizing risk. This has been designed as a primary goal in the current decade by the Institute of Medicine reports of the past two years *(13,26)*. This approach also requires that one accept that scientific proof of the efficacy of many interventions and procedures will be difficult or impossible to obtain. Risk-reduction strategies offer the best answer to improving safety, and have proven beneficial and effective in industry and other professions such as commercial aviation. In the hospital venue, the JCAHO standards are likely to override other interests in maintaining a stricter view of safe and prudent practice. Continuing refinements of guidelines will tighten the interpretation of language and practice, and systems-based approaches have enormous potential to improve both safety and efficiency. A major factor in implementing safe practice will continue to be the considerable cost associated with independent clinician observers and limited resources in an era of shrinking medical funds and reimbursement. It is clear that the JCAHO mandates will provide the rubric under which most, if not all, hospitals and health care institutions will need to operate. The AAP guidelines, supplemented by those promulgated by the ASA, appear to offer the most effective approach to compliance with accreditation standards, together with the goal of promoting safe systems for the sedation care of infants and children. The ongoing identification of lowest-risk practices and continuing assessment will be ongoing projects for the future.

REFERENCES

1. Malviya, S., Voepel-Lewis, T., Prochaska, G., and Tait, A. R. (2000) Prolonged recovery and delayed side effects of sedation for diagnostic imaging studies in children. *Pediatrics* **105(3)**, E42.
2. Guidelines for monitoring and management of pediatric patients during and after sedation for diagnostic and therapeutic procedures. (1992) *Pediatrics* **89(6)**, 1110–1115.
3. Manuli, M. A. and Davies, L. (1993) Rectal methohexital for sedation of children during imaging procedures. *AJR Am. J. Roentgenol.* **160(3)**, 577–580.
4. Hopkins, K. L., Davis, P. C., Sanders, C. L., and Churchill, L. H. (1999) Sedation for pediatric imaging studies. *Neuroimaging Clin. N. Am.* **9(1)**, 1–10.
5. Lawson, G. R. (2000) Controversy: Sedation of children for magnetic resonance imaging. *Arch. Dis. Child.* **82(2)**, 150–153.
6. Bauman, L. A., Kish, I., Baumann, R. C., and Politis, G. D. (1999) Pediatric sedation with analgesia. *Am. J. Emerg. Med.* **17(1)**, 1–3.
7. Guidelines for the elective use of conscious sedation, deep sedation, and general anesthesia in pediatric patients. (1986) *ASDC J. Dent. Child.* **53(1)**, 21–22.
8. Use of pediatric sedation and analgesia. (1997) American College of Emergency Physicians. *Ann. Emerg. Med.* **29(6)**, 834–835.
9. Clinical policy for procedural sedation and analgesia in the emergency department. (1998) American College of Emergency Physicians. *Ann. Emerg. Med.* **31(5)**, 663–677.
10. Coté, C. J. (1994) Sedation protocols—why so many variations? Pediatrics **94(3)**, 281–283.
11. Coté, C. J. (1995) Monitoring guidelines: do they make a difference? *AJR Am. J. Roentgenol.* **165(4)**, 910–912.
12. Coté, C. J., Notterman, D. A., Karl, H. W., Weinberg, J. A., and McCloskey, C. (2000) Adverse sedation events in pediatrics: a critical incident analysis of contributing factors. *Pediatrics* **105(4 Pt 1)**, 805–814.

13. Committee on Quality of Health Care in America LTK (1999) *To Err Is Human: Building a Safer Health System.* (Corrigan, Janet M., and Donaldson, Molla eds.), National Academy Press, Washington, DC, Institute of Medicine.
14. Maxwell, L. G. and Yaster, M. (1996) The myth of conscious sedation. *Arch. Pediatr. Adolesc. Med.* **150(7),** 665–667.
15. Revisions to Anesthesia Care Standards Comprehensive Accreditation Manual for Hospitals Effective January 1, 2001. Standards and Intents for Sedation and Anesthesia Care. http://www.jcaho.org/standards_frm.html.
16. Splinter, W. M., Schaefer, J. D., and Zunder, I. H. (1990) Clear fluids three hours before surgery do not affect the gastric fluid contents of children. *Can. J. Anaesth.* **37(5),** 498–501.
17. Schreiner, M. S., Triebwasser, A., and Keon, T. P. (1990) Ingestion of liquids compared with preoperative fasting in pediatric outpatients. *Anesthesiology* **72(4),** 593–597.
18. Ingebo, K. R., Rayhorn, N. J., Hecht, R. M., Shelton, M. T., Silber, G. H., and Shub, M. D. (1997) Sedation in children: adequacy of two-hour fasting. *J. Pediatr.* **131(1 Pt 1),** 155–158.
19. Bozadjian, E. M. (1999) Quality improvement, credentialing, and competency. *Int. Anesthesiol. Clin.* **37(4),** 47–57.
20. Croswell, R. J., Dilley, D. C., Lucas, W. J., and Vann, W. F., Jr. (1995) A comparison of conventional versus electronic monitoring of sedated pediatric dental patients. *Pediatr. Dent.* **17(5),** 332–339.
21. Tobias, J. D., Flanagan, J. F., Wheeler, T. J., Garrett, J. S., and Burney, C. (1994) Noninvasive monitoring of end-tidal CO2 via nasal cannulas in spontaneously breathing children during the perioperative period. *Crit. Care Med.* **22(11),** 1805–1808.
22. Hart, L. S., Berns, S. D., Houck, C. S., and Boenning, D. A. (1997) The value of end-tidal CO_2 monitoring when comparing three methods of conscious sedation for children undergoing painful procedures in the emergency department. *Pediatr. Emerg. Care* **13(3),** 189–193.
23. Hanley, J. A. and Lippman-Hand, A. (1983) If nothing goes wrong, is everything all right? Interpreting zero numerators. *JAMA* **249(13),** 1743–1745.
24. Practice guidelines for sedation and analgesia by non-anesthesiologists. (1996) A report by the American Society of Anesthesiologists Task Force on Sedation and Analgesia by Non-Anesthesiologists. *Anesthesiology* **84(2),** 459–471.
25. Conscious sedation raises safe staffing concerns. (1999) *Dimens. Crit. Care Nurs.* **18(1),** 35.
26. Richardson, W. C., Berwick, D. M., Bisgard, J. C., Bristow, L. R., Buck, C. R., Cassel, C. K., et al. (2000) The Institute of Medicine Report on Medical Errors: misunderstanding can do harm. Quality of Health Care in America Committee. *Med. Gen. Med.* E42.

3

Practice Guidelines
for Adult Sedation and Analgesia

Randolph Steadman, MD and Steve Yun, MD

1. INTRODUCTION

The goal of sedation and analgesia is to ensure patient comfort and safety and allay anxiety during diagnostic and therapeutic procedures (1). A corollary of improved patient comfort is improved cooperation, and as a result, the enhanced potential for the timely completion of the procedure under optimal conditions. The rapid growth of new technologies has led to the increased use of novel, less invasive approaches to diagnosis and treatment outside the operating room, and many of these require the use of sedation and analgesia for a successful outcome. Anesthesiologists are logically called upon to provide services; however, the volume of procedures in most institutions exceeds the anesthesiologists' availability because of operating room duties and other commitments (2). This has increasingly led to the provision of sedation services by non-anesthesiologists from a variety of disciplines. The Joint Commission on the Accreditation of Healthcare Organizations (JCAHO) has recognized the need for comparable standards throughout the hospital, suggesting in a sample policy accompanying their standards that sedation policies and procedures "shall be monitored and evaluated by the Department of Anesthesia" (3). This chapter, with a focus on these regulatory standards and other guidelines (4–10) relating to the provision of adult sedation and analgesia, will review the evidence upon which they are based and offer recommendations on the development of hospital policies.

2. LEVELS OF SEDATION: DEFINITIONS

Conscious sedation is a minimally depressed level of consciousness in which the patient retains the ability to maintain a patent airway and to respond appropriately to physical stimulation and verbal command. *Deep sedation* is

From: *Contemporary Clinical Neuroscience: Sedation and Analgesia for Diagnostic and Therapeutic Procedures*
Edited by: S. Malviya, N. N. Naughton, and K. K. Tremper © Humana Press Inc., Totowa, NJ

a medically controlled state of depressed consciousness from which the patient is not easily aroused. It may be accompanied by a partial or complete loss of protective reflexes, and may include the inability to maintain a patent airway independently.

In 1996, the American Society of Anesthesiologists (ASA) published "Practice Guidelines for Sedation and Analgesia by Non-Anesthesiologists," in which the term "sedation and analgesia" was preferred over "conscious sedation," as the former "more accurately defines the therapeutic goal than does the more commonly used but imprecise term 'conscious sedation'" *(4)*. In this document, a cautionary note was issued that "reflex withdrawal from a painful stimulus" amounted to more than sedation and analgesia, but this Task Force stopped short of defining or suggesting guidelines for deeper levels of sedation.

In 1999, the ASA House of Delegates, recognizing that sedation is a continuum, defined terms for the range of sedation beginning with *minimal sedation* ("anxiolysis"), progressing to *moderate sedation/analgesia* ("conscious sedation"), *deep sedation/analgesia,* and finally, *general anesthesia*. These terms are defined by the patients' response to various stimuli *(11)* (Table 1). These states have implications for airway management: *moderately sedated* ("conscious sedation") patients should not require interventions, and more deeply sedated patients may not be able to maintain a patent airway or adequate ventilation without assistance. Cardiovascular function is usually maintained during *deep sedation,* but may be impaired during *general anesthesia*.

3. SCOPE

Sedation policies are used in patients receiving sedation/analgesia to decrease anxiety, discomfort, and/or movement while undergoing procedures, whether the procedures are diagnostic or therapeutic, noninvasive or invasive. The JCAHO specifically includes as examples percutaneous aspirations and biopsies, cardiac and vascular catheterizations, and endoscopies. Examples of noninvasive procedures include radiologic studies such as computerized tomography (CT) and magnetic resonance imaging (MRI).

Situations typically excluded from sedation policies include pre-operative premedication given prior to transport to the operating room, general or regional anesthesia administered outside the operating room by anesthesiologists (these areas are addressed by department of anesthesia policies) *(2)*, postoperative analgesia (including patient-controlled analgesia) and sedation/analgesia administered in the intensive care unit (ICU) to facilitate mechanical ventilation.

Table 1
Continuum of Depth of Sedation
Definition of General Anesthesia and Levels of Sedation/Analgesia*

	Minimal sedation (Anxiolysis)	Moderate sedation/analgesia ("conscious sedation")	Deep sedation/analgesia	General anesthesia
Responsiveness	Normal response to verbal stimulation	Purposeful ** response to verbal or tactile stimulation	Purposeful** response following repeated or painful stimulation	Unarousable even with painful stimulus
Airway required	Unaffected	No intervention required	Intervention may be required	Intervention often
Spontaneous ventilation	Unaffected	Adequate	May be inadequate	Frequently inadequate
Cardiovascular function	Unaffected	Usually maintained	Usually maintained	May be impaired

Continuum of Depth of Sedation ©1999 website (http://www.asahq.org/standards/20.tm) and is reprinted with permission of the American Society of Anesthesiologists.

* Monitored Anesthesia Care does not describe the continuum of depth of sedation; it describes "a specific anesthesia service in which an anesthesiologist has been requested to participate in the care of a patient undergoing a diagnostic or therapeutic procedure."
** Reflex withdrawal from a painful stimulus is NOT considered a purposeful response.

The JCAHO states that "the standards for anesthesia care apply when patients receive, for any purpose, by any route, sedation which may be reasonably expected to result in the loss of protective reflexes" which the *Accreditation Manual for Hospitals* defines as the inability to handle secretions without aspiration or to maintain a patent airway independently. The Commission's Accreditation Manual points out that it is "not often possible to predict how a patient will respond to sedation" *(12)*.

4. PERSONNEL/PRIVILEGING

Studies have not yet determined whether the number and training of staff affects patient outcomes. However, the JCAHO and the ASA Task Force appreciate that an individual who performs a procedure cannot adequately monitor a patient's condition. Both organizations agree that the minimum number of personnel required during procedures in which sedation or analgesia is administered is two—the individual performing the procedure and the individual monitoring the patient. Both providers should be practicing within their scope of practice as defined by law and hospital policy. One of the two providers must be a licensed independent practitioner (physician, podiatrist, dentist, or oral surgeon) with legal authority to administer conscious sedation. The licensed independent practitioner has primary responsibility for patient care, for sedation/analgesia medication orders, and for the supervision and management of the patient's response to sedation. The health care provider monitoring the patient may administer the sedative and/or analgesic medication under written or verbal order from the licensed independent practitioner if their scope of practice permits. During conscious sedation, the provider monitoring the patient may assist the operator as needed, with brief, interruptible tasks. During deep sedation, this is no longer the case, and a third individual is required if the operator needs assistance *(13)*.

4.1. Training

Health care providers involved in the administration of sedation should be trained in clinical pharmacology and in airway management. Specific concerns of the ASA Task Force regarding safe drug use include the potential for drug combinations to potentiate respiratory depression, too-frequent dosing resulting in a cumulative overdose, and a lack of familiarity with sedative and opioid antagonists *(4)*. Airway management training should focus on establishing a patent airway and maintaining oxygenation and ventilation using positive pressure. Additional resources, such as respiratory support equipment and a practitioner skilled in tracheal intubation and advanced life-support, should be readily available. During procedures involving deep

Table 2
Equipment Needs for Sedation/Analgesia

Present at the location

- Pulse oximeter, automated blood pressure cuff, temperature monitor (patients < 5 kg)
- Suction
- Oxygen source and appropriate delivery devices (nasal cannula, face mask, non-rebreathing mask)
- Bag-valve-mask devices with appropriate masks
- Reversal agents as appropriate to the drugs administered

Immediately available

- Defibrillator
- EKG machine
- Intubation equipment
- ACLS drugs and procedural equipment
- Personnel adequately trained to provide ACLS

sedation, the need for airway management training is greater, and a higher level of skill should be required prior to privileging.

5. EMERGENCY EQUIPMENT

Numerous reports support the fact that respiratory depression and apnea can occur as complications of sedation. Iber reported 10 episodes of apnea or cardiopulmonary arrest, primarily involving patients over 60 years of age, during the performance of 10,000 endoscopies *(14)*. Bailey noted that 78% of the 80 deaths reported after the use of midazolam were respiratory in nature; many of these were precipitated by concurrent opioid administration *(15)*. These and other reports of respiratory events suggest that the availability of emergency equipment will reduce the risk of an adverse outcome during sedation. Equipment should be immediately accessible, and in good working order, and should meet the needs of the particular patient population served—e.g., adult or pediatric. Such equipment includes a self-inflating positive-pressure oxygen delivery system with appropriate sized masks, a vacuum source, suction supplies, oxygen source and delivery equipment, tracheal intubation supplies, resuscitation and reversal medications, an electrocardiographic monitor, and a defibrillator (Table 2). The ASA Task Force noted that there is insufficient evidence to support the need for defibrillators, yet strongly supports their availability. Standard physiologic monitoring equipment is discussed in Subheading 7.

6. PATIENT CARE: PRE-PROCEDURAL ASSESSMENT

A recent (per medical staff policy) history and physical examination by a physician and an assessment by the qualified health care provider administering the sedation/analgesia must be available prior to each procedure in which sedation/analgesia is given. This assessment should include the patient's age, any known allergies or drug reactions, current medications, tobacco, alcohol or substance use, current health problems, and review of systems with specific note of any airway or cardiopulmonary problems. Additionally, the patient's last food intake should be assessed for compliance with institutional policies for elective procedures. The physical examination should include vital signs, weight and height, an airway and sedation-directed evaluation, and a risk stratification using the ASA Physical Status classification (Tables 3, 4). The risk assessment allows outcome monitoring (a JCAHO requirement) to be stratified by pre-existing illness. Finally, the patient should be informed of the benefits, risks and alternatives to sedation as part of the planned procedure (Table 5).

7. MONITORING AND CARE DURING THE PROCEDURE

During the procedure, the patient's heart rate and oxygen saturation should be continuously monitored; the level of consciousness, blood pressure, and respiratory rate should be monitored intermittently at a frequency determined by the depth of sedation/analgesia. Because the risk of loss of protective reflexes, the monitoring of intermittently assessed variables should be more frequent during deep sedation than the minimum requirement of every 15 min for conscious sedation *(16)*. The same monitoring and documentation frequency during deep sedation as during general anesthesia—every 5 min during the procedure—is used by some hospitals even for conscious sedation *(2)*. Table 6 contains recommendations for the frequency of monitoring during sedation/analgesia.

7.1. *Level of Consciousness*

Level of consciousness monitoring assures a level of patient responsiveness sufficient to maintain an open upper airway and gag reflex. Patient responsiveness allows an assessment of the effect of previously administered sedative and analgesic agents and assists in determining, along with the drugs' pharmacokinetic profile (time to peak effect), whether further titration of sedation/analgesia is required. In procedures in which the patient's verbal response is precluded, such as endoscopy, an alternate means of signaling responsiveness such as a "thumbs up" sign should be used. Sedation administered for procedures, in which lack of patient motion is desired,

Table 3
Pre-Procedural Assessment

History

A recent (per institutional policy) H&P by a physician

An assessment by the health care provider administering the sedation/analgesia prior to the procedure

Patient age

Allergies or drug reactions

Current medications

Tobacco, alcohol, or substance use

Current health problems

Review of systems with specific note of any airway or cardiopulmonary problems

Last food intake assessed for compliance with institutional policies for elective procedures

Physical

Vital signs

Weight and height

An airway and sedation directed evaluation

Risk stratification using the ASA Physical Status classification

Informed consent

Including benefits, risks, and alternatives to sedation

such as MRI, carries a higher risk, particularly in uncooperative patients. Drugs and dosing schemes used during such procedures should have a wide margin of safety.

7.2. Pulse Oximetry

Oxygen saturation monitoring has been extensively studied under a variety of conditions. Oral surgeons *(17,18)*, plastic surgeons *(19)*, interventional radiologists *(20)*, endoscopists *(21)*, and colonoscopists *(22)* have all noted clinically significant hypoxemia diagnosed by pulse oximetry before "clinically detectable signs of respiratory depression" *(20)* and earlier than with other

Table 4
American Society of Anesthesiologist Physical Class

	Risk stratification
Class I	Normal, healthy patient
Class II	Mild systemic disease
Class III	Severe systemic disease
Class IV	Life-threatening illness
Class V	Moribund patient

Table 5
Sample Consent

(May be incorporated with procedural consent)

For the procedure you are to undergo, sedation and analgesic medications are frequently required. The benefit of sedative and analgesic medication is to allow the safe, comfortable completion of your procedure. The primary risk of these medications is respiratory depression (decreased breathing effort), which can be serious or even fatal if not treated. This risk is minimized by careful administration of these medications and by close monitoring of your blood pressure, heart rate, and breathing. You may be asked to take a deep breath periodically during the procedure and/or administered oxygen. Infrequently, allergic reactions to medications can occur. If you are known to be allergic to any medications or have any concerns about receiving sedation/analgesia, please let us know so that we may address your concerns directly. You may decline the administration of sedatives and analgesics or wish to discuss other alternatives, which include general anesthesia, regional anesthesia, or local anesthesia. If you elect to receive sedation and analgesia, by signing below, you consent to allow us to administer, as appropriate, the medication required for the comfortable completion of your procedure.

Table 6
Recommendations for Frequency of
Monitoring and Documentation During Sedation/Analgesia

	Conscious sedation	Deep sedation
Heart rate	Continuous	Continuous
Oxygen saturation	Continuous	Continuous
Respiratory rate	Minimum of every 15 min	Minimum of every 5 min
Noninvasive blood pressure	Minimum of every 15 min	Minimum of every 5 min
Level of consciousness	Minimum of every 5 min	Minimum of every 5 min

methods of monitoring *(19)*. In a study evaluating nursing interventions for hypoxemia, knowledge of the oxygen saturation influenced the timing of interventions and was believed to improve quality of care when compared to a second group of patients whose oxygen saturation values were revealed only if they fell below 85% *(23)*.

The accuracy and reliability of pulse oximeter values have also been evaluated. At low saturation values (below 80%), the pulse oximeter overestimates the true value as measured by co-oximeter *(24)*. Variations in accuracy between manufacturers occur below saturation values of 70% *(25,26)*. This is probably most clinically relevant in patients with cyanotic heart disease, for whom co-oximetry should be used to verify the pulse oximeter. Situations producing low signal-to-noise ratios, such as patient motion, may produce artifactual pulse oximetry values. Recently introduced signal extraction technology reduces the incidence of erroneous and dropped readings *(27,28)*.

Despite these minor limitations, pulse oximetry is strongly advised in all sedation settings because of its considerable benefit, low cost, and negligible risk. However, pulse oximetry should not be viewed as a substitute for monitoring ventilatory function.

7.3. Respiratory Rate

As drug-induced respiratory depression is the primary cause of morbidity associated with sedation/analgesia, ventilation monitoring by observation or auscultation should be assessed on all patients *(4)*. A decreasing respiratory rate may represent the earliest warning of medication overdose, particularly during oxygen administration, when desaturation may be a late indicator of respiratory depression *(4)*. In situations that require access to the patient, the evaluation of exhaled carbon dioxide can serve as an indicator of upper airway obstruction *(29)* or apnea.

7.4. Heart Rate and Blood Pressure

Autonomic stimulation occurring during procedures may indicate inadequate sedation/analgesia; conversely, sedation/analgesia may blunt appropriate responses to procedural stress or hypovolemia. In a study of 100 patients undergoing endoscopy, 20 developed a tachycardia of over 120 beats per minute (bpm) *(30)*. During colonoscopy, 16% of 223 patients had vasovagal reactions manifested by bradycardia to 60 bpm, hypotension, or diaphoresis *(31)*. The only predictors of such a reaction were a higher mean dose of midazolam (4.6 mg vs 3.9 mg) and a higher rate of diverticulosis in those experiencing vasovagal reactions. About one-third of patients with vasovagal reactions required treatment. Electrocardiographic monitoring is not routinely used in all ages, but is recommended in the elderly or in patients with known or suspected cardiovascular disease. Matot studied 29 patients over the age of 50 undergoing elective fiberoptic bronchoscopy and found that five patients (17%) had myocardial ischemia lasting 20 ± 8 min, associated with a mean increase in heart rate of 30 bpm (to 120 bpm) and a decrease in saturation from 95–90%, in the absence of blood pressure changes *(32)*. He warned against the dangerous combination of hypoxemia and tachycardia, suggesting routine oxygen administration and avoidance of routine atropine usage.

The routine monitoring of heart rate and blood pressure is recommended for all patients undergoing sedation/analgesia.

7.5. Temperature

Although care should be taken to avoid hypo- or hyperthermia, there is no evidence that routine temperature monitoring improves outcome in adults. Temperature should be monitored in small infants or in children who are placed under warming lights.

7.6. Oxygen Administration

Routine oxygen administration has repeatedly been shown to be beneficial during sedation/analgesia when used to avoid or delay the onset of hypoxemia. During endoscopy, oxygen administered at 2 L/min was as effective as 3 L/min and oral administration via a bite guard was as effective as nasal cannula-administered oxygen *(33)*. In patients over the age of 60 undergoing endoscopic retrograde cholangiopancreatography (ERCP), the group randomized to receive nasal oxygen at 2 L/min required fewer interventions for hypoxemia and maintained significantly higher oxygen saturations throughout the procedure than the group that did not receive oxygen *(34)*. The higher oxygen saturations did not protect patients who received oxygen from tachycardia, as both groups had short periods of significant tachycardia.

Bowling found similar results during endoscopy in patients over 60 yr of age: oxygen saturation values improved with supplemental oxygen administration, but the frequency of ventricular and supraventricular ectopic beats was not decreased *(35)*. During colonoscopy in patients sedated with midazolam (2.6 ± 0.2 mg) and meperidine (48 ± 3 mg), those receiving oxygen at 3 L/min were less likely to desaturate to less than 90% than those breathing room air (10 of 28 vs 22 of 28) *(36)*. The authors concluded that supplemental oxygen decreases the risk of, but does not prevent, hypoxemia. The period of risk for hypoxemia does not end with the completion of the procedure. Hardeman showed that 20 of 100 patients breathing room air became hypoxemic in the postanesthesia recovery room (vs 3 of 100 patients receiving supplemental oxygen) after intravenous (iv) sedation for oral surgery *(37)*.

The clinical significance of the frequent finding of hypoxemia during sedation/analgesia is unclear. In fact, decreases in oxygen saturation to less than 90% occurred during sleep in 43% of asymptomatic men (13% had oxygen saturations <75%) *(38)*. There are no studies showing that detection of a decrease of oxygen saturation alone, in the absence of other findings such as unresponsiveness, has an effect on patient outcome *(39)*. However, because of the known risk of cardiopulmonary complications during sedation/analgesia and the fact that such complications represent more than 50% of the reported complications during gastrointestinal (GI) endoscopy *(5)*, monitoring for—and the prevention of—hypoxemia should be routine. Because oxygen administration decreases the incidence and magnitude of hypoxemia, its routine administration should be strongly encouraged, particularly in elderly patients or patients with co-existing disease. However, as its administration delays the recognition of respiratory depression by pulse oximetry, another means of evaluating ventilation—such as assessment of the quality and rate of respirations—should be routinely employed.

7.7. Drugs

Knowledge of onset time, appropriate dosing frequency, the potential for side effects, and the appropriate agents to reverse respiratory depression are essential when administering sedation/analgesia. When inhalational agents such as nitrous oxide are used the maintenance of an adequate oxygen concentration must be assured. (*See* Chapters 6 and 7 in this book for a detailed discussion of the drugs commonly used for sedation/analgesia.) Table 7 provides suggestions regarding drug use during sedation/analgesia.

Hospitals may define dosages of drugs that require the application of the sedation policy. For example, the JCAHO sample policy does not require adherence to sedation guidelines for adults who receive benzodiazepines in doses below a predetermined threshold, such as 5 mg of midazolam in patients under 60 yr of age. However, this sample policy applies to adults who receive any narcotic or combination of drugs and all pediatric (18-yr-old) patients *(40)*.

7.8. Intravenous Access

In adult patients receiving iv medications for sedation/analgesia, vascular access should be maintained throughout the procedure and until the patient is no longer at risk for sedation-related respiratory depression. In patients who have received sedation/analgesia by non-intravenous routes or whose iv line is no longer functional, the decision to establish or reestablish iv

Table 7
Drug Principles for Sedation and Analgesia

1. Avoid making changes to a successful drug regimen.
2. When a drug regimen for adults must be changed, use the safest intravenous drug with the shortest duration of effect appropriate for the procedure.
3. Avoid suggesting drugs that require infusion pumps for safe administration.
4. Benzodiazepines alone rarely cause apnea.
5. Benzodiazepines produce anxiolysis and amnesia, not analgesia.
6. The shortest-acting benzodiazepines have durations of action considerably longer than the shortest-acting opioids.
7. Opioid-induced apnea frequently responds to tactile stimulation.
8. Opioids produce analgesia, not amnesia. They may produce apnea prior to sedation.
9. Benzodiazepines markedly potentiate opioid-induced respiratory depression.
10. Flumazenil antagonizes benzodiazepines; naloxone antagonizes opioids.
11. Ketamine and propofol are intravenous general anesthetics, and their use should be restricted to individuals with the expertise and privileges to use such agents.

access should be considered on a case-by-case basis. In all instances, an individual with the skills to establish iv access should be immediately available *(4)*.

8. DOCUMENTATION

Documentation should include the patient's diagnosis, planned procedure, the sedation/analgesia plan, the pre-, intra- and post-procedural assessment, the care provided, monitoring results, and discharge information.

9. RECOVERY AND DISCHARGE

In the post-procedural period, the removal of stimulation exposes the patient to the unopposed effects of residual sedation. This is illustrated by a report of apnea occurring after reduction of a shoulder dislocation *(41)*. When sedation/analgesia is administered to outpatients, the clinician should assume that they will not have immediate access to medical care or advice after discharge. Therefore, patients should have returned to their pre-procedural level of consciousness and no longer be at risk for respiratory depression, have stable vital signs, be adequately hydrated without active vomiting, have minimal discomfort, and be able to ambulate. If reversal of narcotics or benzodiazepines has been used, the observation period should be sufficient to assure that resedation does not occur. Patients should be given instructions for follow-up care and guidelines for when and how to seek emergency

Table 8
Recommendations for Discharge Criteria

	Inpatient	Outpatient
Stable vital signs	Required	Required
Independently maintains a patent airway	Required	Required
Return to baseline level of consciousness	Not required	Required
Ambulation	Not required	Required
Absence of nausea/vomiting	Preferable	Required
Pain well-controlled	Preferable	Required

care should problems arise. Patients should be discharged accompanied by a responsible adult and instructed not to drive for 24 h. Inpatients should not require assistance to maintain a patent airway and should have stable vital signs before discharge. If vital signs are unstable, admission to an acute care area is indicated. Table 8 contains a summary of suggested discharge criteria.

10. GUIDELINES FOR ANESTHESIA CONSULTATION

Consultation with appropriate specialists should be considered prior to sedation if the patient's condition requires expertise or skills beyond those of the practitioner performing the procedure. Patients with neurological, cardiopulmonary, or other organ system disease believed to represent a significant hazard may be at increased risk during sedation/analgesia. Morbid obesity, sleep apnea, pregnancy, drug or alcohol abuse, and concerns related to airway management, fasting status, or extremes of age also warrant consideration for consultation before the procedure. For patients who are likely to develop complications during sedation/analgesia or those who experience difficulty achieving optimal sedation/analgesia, consultation with an anesthesiologist is recommended.

11. OUTCOMES

11.1. Failed Sedation

Very little documentation exists regarding the frequency of failed sedation/ analgesia. Inadequate sedation/analgesia can result in cancellation of the procedure, a suboptimal evaluation, procedural complications, or the need for general anesthesia. Many factors can influence the probability of a procedure's successful completion, including patient age, ability to cooperate, co-existing disease, tolerance to drugs, and the nature of the procedure.

During cerebral angiography and embolization, the consequences of patient movement (such as during the "hot flush" that occurs during injection of contrast media) include cerebral infarction and hemorrhage. Neurological assessment may provide the first clue to the development of ischemia during interventional neuroradiology *(42)*.

Of 1200 endoscopic retrograde cholangiopancreatographies (ERCP) performed over a 2-yr period, 65 patients required general anesthesia, the major indication being substance abuse *(43)*. The complication rate of ERCP during general anesthesia was believed to be comparable or lower than that of ERCP performed under sedation/analgesia.

11.2. Hypoxemia

The incidence of hypoxemia is determined by the characteristics of the patient, the procedure, the sedatives or analgesics given (dose, frequency, single drug or combination of medications), the oxygen concentration of the inspired gas and stimulation provided by the health care providers. The incidence of hypoxemia ($SaO_2 < 90\%$) during endoscopy has been reported to be 4% of 508 patients (with four episodes of apnea) *(44)*. During ERCP the mean saturation in 132 sedated patients decreased from 95 ± 2% to 88.9 ± 6.4%, and the same author reported saturations falling from 97 ± 1.9% to 93.9 ± 3.3% in non-sedated endoscopy patients *(45)*. During cardiac catheterization 11 (38%) of 29 patients had episodes of hypoxemia ($SaO_2 < 90\%$) *(46)*. The minimum oxygen saturation was directly related to the baseline saturation and inversely related to the duration of the procedure and the ventricular end-diastolic volume. Fifty-four of 100 patients undergoing colonoscopy became hypoxemic *(22)*, and age, body-surface area, drug dose, smoking, and cardiac or pulmonary history did not predict which patients would become hypoxemic. Woods et al. have also investigated variables associated with hypoxemia during sedation; during ERCP, age and weight appeared to be most significantly associated *(47)*. Others have not found the same variables to be good predictors of hypoxemia *(48,49)*.

In trials comparing sedated patients with patients not receiving sedation during upper gastrointestinal endoscopy, hypoxemia was noted to occur in both groups, although less frequently in the group without sedation (16% of sedated vs 11% of non-sedated patients had SaO_2 values < 92%) *(50)*. In 481 non-sedated patients, desaturation to 90% occurred in 6.4% of patients and was associated with basal SaO2 values < 95% (odds ratio 67), respiratory disease (odds ratio 30), more than one endoscopic intubation attempt (odds ratio 39), an emergent procedure (odds ratio 15), and ASA Physical Status III or IV (odds ratio 4) *(51)*. Hypoxemia has also been shown to occur in dental patients who received only topical lidocaine anesthesia *(52)* and in patients undergoing bronchoscopic procedures who received topical lidocaine and intramuscular atropine *(53)*.

11.3. Morbidity and Mortality

Morbidity incidence data have been extensively evaluated during gastrointestinal procedures. The complication rate for upper endoscopy is about 0.1%; for colonoscopy: 0.2%; procedural complications (bleeding, perforation, and infection) and sedation-related complications are included in these rates *(5)*. Cardiopulmonary complications are believed to account for more than 50% of reported complications, with aspiration, oversedation, hypoventilation, vasovagal reactions and airway obstruction accounting for most of these events *(54)*. The complication rate of therapeutic procedures (such as ERCP, polypectomy, or stent placement) and emergency procedures is higher than the complication rate of non-emergent diagnostic procedures *(54,55)*. This higher rate of complications is the result of bleeding, infection, pre-existing disease, the condition being treated, the increased procedural duration, and/or the need for deeper levels of sedation. In reviewing morbidity data, it is apparent that the exact frequency of complications caused by sedation/analgesia (vs the procedure) is unknown.

In the 1974 survey of endoscopists reported by Silvis, 17 deaths occurred in a series of over 240,000 GI procedures (about 1 in 15,000); excluding deaths attributed to perforation *(4)*, bleeding *(1)* and cholangitis/sepsis *(4)*, eight of the deaths remain as *possibly* sedation-related (an incidence of 1 in 30,000) *(54)*. These eight deaths were caused by cardiac arrest (six), myocardial infarction (one), and aspiration (one). Conceivably, any or all of these deaths may have been related to underlying disease, topical anesthesia predisposing to aspiration, or inadequate rather than excessive sedation/analgesia.

McCloy pointed out that "exact data on the morbidity and mortality of endoscopy are surprisingly sparse," but estimated the mortality at 0.5 to 3 per 10,000 (about 1 in 3000 to 1:20,000), and agreed that most are cardiopulmonary *(56)*. Although he concedes that many factors may be related to procedural safety, he emphasized the role of sedation, stating that "successful sedation should achieve anxiolysis and amnesia rather than ptosis and hypnosis." He points out the 24–57-h plasma elimination half-life of diazepam (with an active metabolite with a 5-d half-life), noting that it is commonly used for diagnostic endoscopy lasting 5–10 min. Other issues he raised regarding safety include infrequent use of continuous iv access during the procedure (43% of cases in England) and the use of opioids in conjunction with benzodiazepines (5% of cases in the United Kingdom and 87% of cases in the United States). He noted the overall mortality for general anesthesia in the

Table 9
Continuing Quality Improvement Indicators

If any of the following occur and are caused by the sedatives and/or analgesics administered, and not the pre-existing and underlying disease or its treatment, a review of the chart will be performed and appropriate action taken:

1. Oxygen saturation 90% and a drop of 5% from baseline for greater than 1 min
2. Use of opioid or benzodiazepine reversal agents
3. A decrease in blood pressure or heart rate requiring pharmacologic intervention or rapid fluid administration
4. Failure to respond to physical stimulation
5. Assisted ventilation and/or unanticipated endotracheal intubation
6. Unplanned admission
7. Cardiac or respiratory arrest

United Kingdom at the time of his report (1992) to be 1:185,000; current estimates of mortality for general anesthesia range between 1:250,000 and 1:400,000 *(57)*.

In another retrospective survey of oral and maxillofacial surgeons in Massachusetts, there were no mortalities reported of the 1.5 million office treatments conducted during the 5 yr (1990–1994) covered by the survey *(58)*. An Illinois survey of oral surgeons and dentists holding permits for deep sedation/general anesthesia (86% of respondents, 97% of these did not routinely intubate) or conscious sedation (14% of respondents) revealed one death in a patient with cardiac disease during just over 150,000 anesthetics *(59)*. In a closed-claims analysis of 13 dental cases resulting in death or permanent injury, the majority of patients had pre-existing conditions such as morbid obesity, or cardiac, pulmonary, or neurological disease; and most were at the extremes of age. Hypoxemia resulting from airway obstruction and/or respiratory depression was the most common cause of adverse outcome *(60)*.

In order to improve patient safety and determine the incidence of adverse events, the outcome of all procedures requiring sedation/analgesia should be monitored (*see* Table 9 for suggested outcome variables). By auditing the outcome of each procedure requiring sedation, performance improvement can be evaluated by department, procedure, and provider.

12. FUTURE DIRECTIONS

12.1. Patient-Controlled Sedation

In an uncontrolled pilot study, 16 healthy patients received a mixture of alfentanil and propofol (alfentanil :12 mcg; propofol: 5 mg per dose) via patient-controlled infusion pump during colonoscopy; all tolerated the procedure and found the pump easy to use *(61)*. A trial of patient-controlled sedation comparing two different doses of propofol (20 mg/dose, 0.3 mg/kg/dose) with a propofol-alfentanil mixture (propofol: 0.2 mg/kg/dose; alfentanil: 4 mcg/kg/dose) concluded that propofol alone was inadequate for pain relief, but the propofol-alfentanil combination was acceptable. The authors noted that most patients had recall *(62)*. Ten patients in a dental fear clinic who were given midazolam via patient-controlled sedation received more midazolam, were less anxious, and moved less during treatment than patients given iv boluses or intranasal midazolam *(63)*.

12.2. Capnography

In the Australian Incident Monitoring Study, pulse oximetry and capnography were the most useful monitors for incident detection in patients undergoing general anesthesia *(64)*. Fifty-two percent of 2000 incidents were detected first by a monitor; oximetry (27%) and capnography (24%) detected over one-half of the monitor-detected incidents. In a U.S. closed claims analysis, pulse oximetry and capnography were believed to be most useful in preventing adverse outcomes. However, the efficacy of these two monitors varied between those patients who were given regional anesthesia (a situation more closely resembling sedation/analgesia) compared to those given general anesthesia. Capnography was believed to be useful in only 17% of preventable adverse outcomes during regional anesthesia, but in 60% of preventable adverse outcomes during general anesthesia. Pulse oximetry theoretically would have prevented 80% of preventable regional anesthesia mishaps, but only 32% of preventable general anesthesia events *(65)*.

In an emergency department evaluation of 27 patients, capnography, obtained via nasal cannula, was believed to be useful. It identified post-procedure apnea in one patient, although the nurse observer also detected apnea. The author noted the benefit of the detection of respiratory pattern changes by the waveform of the capnograph, but concluded that further research and experience were required before routine use could be recommended *(66)*.

Cost, lack of portability, and lack of familiarity with the technology has slowed acceptance of capnography during sedation/analgesia in areas outside of the operating room. Whether the benefits of capnography outweigh the risks (misinterpretation, technology-caused distraction) or the disadvantages (cost of equipment, training) is unknown.

12.3. BIS Monitor

For four decades, anesthesiologists have attempted to catalog electroencephalographic changes induced by anesthetic drugs *(67)*. The Bispectral Index (BIS) is a number derived from a processed EEG signal using proprietary technology. Higher numbers (the maximum value of 100 corresponds to an awake state) indicate less sedation than lower ones. Some evidence suggests that BIS scores measure sedation/analgesia *(68)*. Studies conducted in the ICU suggest that BIS may be useful to guide sedation/analgesia in this setting, particularly for patients who are receiving mechanical ventilation and neuromuscular blocking drugs *(69)*. The cost of the sedation/analgesia used in the ICU for this purpose makes the BIS monitor an intriguing option.

12.4. Assessment of the Need for Sedation

In a randomized trial in Finland, two groups receiving either iv midazolam or iv placebo were compared with a third group (control) without iv access during colonoscopy. There was a difference between the sedation and placebo (iv saline) groups in how they rated the difficulty of the exam on a visual analog scale (30 vs 40 mm respectively on a 100-mm scale; 0 = not difficult; 100 = difficult). However, there was no difference between the midazolam and control (no iv cannulation) groups *(70)*. In a study in the United Kingdom, where iv sedation is routinely used, 50 patients received midazolam 5 mg if under 65 years of age (3 mg if older) and another 50 patients were randomized to receive no sedation during upper GI endoscopy. Both received topical oropharyngeal local anesthesia. The group given no sedation had shorter, easier procedures (per the endoscopists' assessment), although the difference was not significant. The group given sedation reported greater comfort, but both groups preferred any future procedure repeated in a similar fashion *(71)*. In the United States, where sedation is routine, 70 of 250 patients (28%) agreed to participate in a randomized trial of routine vs as-needed sedation. Interestingly, 16 of the 250 patients declined to enroll because they preferred no sedation. In the "sedation as needed" group, 94% completed colonoscopy without sedation but had higher pain scores. Three of the sedation-as-needed group rated the experience as less than optimal and all patients in the routine sedation group were very satisfied *(72)*. In another study of 80 patients who elected to have colonoscopy without sedation, 18% believed they would request sedation on repeat exam, 10% were undecided; and 73% would undergo a repeat procedure without sedation although 54% of these patients described their pain as "moderate to severe" *(73)*. The authors concluded that "sedation by choice is more cost-effective, may be safer, and should be offered."

13. CONCLUSIONS

Numerous societies and organizations have issued guidelines regarding sedation and analgesia administered for procedures. The intent of these guidelines is to provide a safe, uniform level of care when procedures are performed. Although conclusive evidence of improved patient safety is still needed, guidelines such as those described provide a deliberate, rational step toward a safer environment during sedation/analgesia. Although following the described guidelines does not guarantee prevention of an adverse outcome, adherence to them makes it less likely. However, the ultimate responsibility for patient protection lies with the practitioner, not with the policy, the assistant, or the monitors.

REFERENCES

1. Lind, L. J., and Mushlin, P. S. (1987) Sedation, analgesia and anesthesia for radiologic procedures. *Cardiovasc. Interventional Radiol.* **10,** 247–253.
2. Holzman, R. S., Cullen, D. J., Eichhorn, J. H., and Philip, J. H. (1994) Guidelines for Sedation by nonanesthesiologists during diagnostic and therapeutic procedures. *J. Clin. Anesth.* **6,** 265–276.
3. Joint Commission on Accreditation of Healthcare Organization (JCAHO) 1999 (Jan.) *Comprehensive Accreditation Manual for Hospitals: The Official Handbook.* Oakbrook Terrace, IL, JCAHO, TX–74.
4. American Society of Anesthesiologists Task Force, Practice (1996) Guidelines for sedation and analgesia by non-anesthesiologists. *Anesthesiology* **84(2),** 459–471.
5. American Society for Gastrointestinal Endoscopy (1995) Sedation and monitoring of patients undergoing gastrointestinal endoscopic procedures. *Gastrointest. Endosc.* **42:6,** 626–629.
6. Iverson, R. E. (1999) Sedation and analgesia in ambulatory settings. American Society of Plastic and Reconstructive Surgeons Task Force on sedation and analgesia in ambulatory settings. *Plast. Reconstr. Surg.* **104:5,** 1559–1564.
7. American College of Emergency Physicians. (1998) Clinical policy for procedural sedation and analgesia in the emergency department. *Ann. Emerg. Med.* **31:5,** 663–677.
8. Innes, G., Murphy, M., Nijssen-Jordan, C., Ducharme, J., and Drummond, A. (1999) Procedural sedation and analgesia in the emergency department. Canadian Consensus Guidelines. *J. Emerg. Med.* **17:1,** 145–156.
9. Association of Operating Room Nurses. (1997) Recommended practices for managing the patient receiving conscious sedation/analgesia. *AORN* **65:1,** 129–134.
10. Turajek, S. K. (1999) Office based anesthesia standards. American Association of Nurse Anesthetists. *AANA J.* **67:2,** 115–120.
11. http://www.asahq.org/Standards/20.htm.
12. Joint Commission on Accreditation of Healthcare Organization (JCAHO) (1999) *Accreditation Manual for Hospitals.* Oakbrook Terrace, IL, JCAHO, TX–15.
13. Joint Commission on Accreditation of Healthcare Organization (JCAHO) (1999) *Accreditation Manual for Hospitals.* Oakbrook Terrace, IL, JCAHO, TX–78.

14. Iber, F. L., Livak, A., and Kruss, D. M. (1992) Apnea and cardiopulmonary arrest during and after endoscopy. *J. Clin. Gastroenterol.* **14:2.** 109–113.

15. Bailey, P. L., Pace, N. L., Ashburn, M. A., Moll, J. W., East, K. A., and Stanley, T. H. (1990) Frequent hypoxemia and apnea after sedation with midazolam and fentanyl. *Anesthesiology* **73:5,** 826–830.

16. Joint Commission on Accreditation of Healthcare Organization (JCAHO) (1999) *Accreditation Manual for Hospitals.* Oakbrook Terrace, IL, JCAHO, TX–74.

17. Sugiyama, A., Kaneko, Y., Ichinohe, T., Koyama, T., Sakurai, S., and Nakakuki, T. (1991) Usefulness of the pulse oximeter as a respiratory monitor during intravenous sedation. *Bull. Tokyo Dent. Coll.* **32:1,** 19–26.

18. Kraut, R. A. (1985) Continuous transcutaneous O_2 and CO_2 monitoring during conscious sedation for oral surgery. *Oral Maxillofac. Surg.* **43:7,** 489–492.

19. Singer, R., and Thomas, P. E. (1988) Pulse oximeter in the ambulatory aesthetic surgical facility. *Plast. Reconstr. Surg.* **82:1,** 111–115.

20. Newland, C. J., Spiers, S. P., and Finlay, D. B. (1991) Technical report: oxygen saturation monitoring during sedation for chemolysis. *Clin. Radiol.* **44:5,** 352–353.

21. Murray, A. W., Morran, C. G., Kenny, G. N., and Anderson, J. R. (1990) Arterial oxygen saturation during upper gastrointestinal endoscopy: the effects of a midazolam/pethidine combination. *Gut* **31:3,** 270–273.

22. McKee, C. C., Ragland, J. J., and Myers, J. O. (1991) An evaluation of multiple clinical variables for hypoxia during colonoscopy. *Surg. Gynecol. Obstet.* **173:1,** 37–40.

23. Hinmann, C. A., Budden, P. M., and Olsen, J. (1992) Intravenous conscious sedation use in endoscopy: does monitoring of oxygen saturation influence timing of nursing interventions? *Gastroenterol. Nurs.* **15:1,** 6–13.

24. Schmitt, H. J., Schuetz, W. H., Proeschel, P. A., and Jaklin, C. (1993) Accuracy of pulse oximetry in children with cyanotic congenital heart disease. *J. Cardiothorac. Vasc. Anesth.* **7:1,** 61–65.

25. Barker, S. J., and Tremper, K. K. (1987) Pulse oximetry: applications and limitations. *Int. Anesthesiol. Clin.* **25,** 155–175.

26. Severinghaus, J. W., and Naifeh, K. H. (1987) Accuracy of response of six pulse oximeters to profound hypoxia. *Anesthesiology* **67:4,** 551–558.

27. Dumas, C., Wahr, J. A., and Tremper, K. K. (1996) Clinical evaluation of a prototype motion artifact resistant pulse oximeter in the recovery room. *Anesth. Analg.* **83:2,** 269–272.

28. Barker, S. J., and Shah, N. K. (1997) The effects of motion on the performance of pulse oximeters in volunteers (revised publication). *Anesthesiology* **86:1,** 101–108.

29. Iwasaki, J., Vann, W. F., Dilley, D. C., and Anderson, J. A. (1989) An investigation of capnography and pulse oximetry as monitors of pediatric patients sedated for dental treatments. *Pediatr. Dent.* **11:2,** 111–117.

30. Hayward, S. R., Sugawa, C., and Wilson, R. F. (1989) Changes in oxygenation and pulse rate during endoscopy. *Am. Surg.* **55:3,** 198–202.

31. Herman, L. L., Kurtz, R. C., McKee, K. J., Sun, M., Thaler, H. T., and Winawer, S. J. (1993) Risk factors associated with vasovagal reactions during colonoscopy. *Gastrointest. Endosc.* **39:3**, 388–391.

32. Matot, I., Kramer, M. R., Glantz, L., Drenger, B., and Cotev, S. (1997) Myocardial ischemia in sedated patients undergoing fiberoptic bronchoscopy. *Chest* **112:6**, 1454–1458.

33. Bell, G. D., Quine, A., Antrobus, J. H., Morden, A., Burridge, S. M., Coady, T. J., and Lee, J. (1992) Upper gastrointestional endoscopy: a prospective randomized study comparing continuous supplemental oxygen via the nasal or oral route. *Gastrointest. Endosc.* **38:3**, 319–325.

34. Haines, D. J., Bibbey, D., and Green, J. R. (1992) Does nasal oxygen reduce the cardiorespiratory problems experienced by elderly patients undergoing endoscopic retrograde cholangiopancreatography? *Gut* **33:7**, 973–975.

35. Bowling, T. E., Hadjiminas, C. L., Polson, R. J., Baron, J. H., and Foale, R. A. (1993) Effects of supplemental oxygen on cardiac rhythm during upper gastrointestinal endoscopy: a randomised controlled double blind trial. *Gut* **34:11**, 1492–1497.

36. Gross, J. B., and Long, W. B. (1990) Nasal oxygen alleviates hypoxemia in colonoscopy patients sedated with midazolam and meperidine. *Gastrointest. Endosc.* **36:1**, 26–29.

37. Hardeman, J. H., Sabol, S. R., and Goldwasser, M. S. (1990) Incidence of hypoxemia in the postanesthetic recovery room in patients having undergone intravenous sedation for outpatient oral surgery. *J. Oral Maxillofac. Surg.* **48:9**, 942–944.

38. Block, A., Boysen, P., Wynne, J., et al. (1979) Sleep apnea hypopnea and oxygen desaturation in normal subjects: a strong male predominance. *N. Engl. J. Med.* **300,** 513–517.

39. American College of Emergency Physicians. (1998) Clinical policy for procedural sedation and analgesia in the emergency department. *Ann. Emerg. Med.* **31:5,** 663–677.

40. Joint Commission on Accreditation of Healthcare Organization (JCAHO) (1999) *Accreditation Manual for Hospitals.* Oakbrook Terrace, IL, JCAHO, TX–73.

41. Wright, S., Chudnofsky, C., Dronen, S., et al. (1993) Comparison of midazolam and diazepam for procedural sedation and analgesia in the emergency department. *Ann. Emerg. Med.* **22,** 201–205.

42. Manninen, P. H., Chan, A. S. H., and Papworth, D. (1997) Conscious sedation for interventional neuroradiology: a comparison of midazolam and propofol infusion. *Can. J. Anaesth.* **44:1,** 26–30.

43. Etzkorn, K. P., Diab, F., Brown, R. D., Dodda, G., Edelstein, B., Bedford, R., and Venu, R. P. (1998) Endoscopic retrograde cholangiopancreatography under general anesthesia: indications and results. *Gastrointest. Endosc.* **47:5,** 363–367.

44. Iber, F. L., Sutberry, M., Gupta, R., and Kruss, D. (1998) Evaluation of complications during and after conscious sedation for endoscopy using pulse oximetry. *Gastrointest. Endosc.* **39:5,** 620–625.

45. Al-Hadeedi, S., and Leaper, D. J. (1991) Falls in hemoglobin saturation during ERCP and upper gastrointestinal endoscopy. *World J. Surg.* **15:1,** 88–94.

46. Dodson, S. R., Hensley FA, J. r., Martin, D. E., Larach, D. R., and Morris, D. L. (1988) Continuous oxygen saturation monitoring during cardiac catheterization in adults. *Chest* **94:1,** 28–31.

47. Woods, S. D., Chung, S. C., Leung, J. W., Chan, A. C., and Li, A. K. (1989) Hypoxia and tachycardia during endoscopic retrograde cholangiopancreatography: detection by pulse oximetry. *Gastrointest. Endosc.* **35:6,** 523–525.

48. O'Connor, K. W., and Jones, S. (1990) Oxygen desaturation is common and clinically underappreciated during elective endoscopic procedures. *Gastrointest. Endosc.* **36:3,** S2–S4.

49. Visco, D. M., Tolpin, E., Straughn, J. C., and Fagraeus, L. (1989) Arterial oxygen saturation in sedated patients undergoing gastrointestinal endoscopy and a review of pulse oximetry. *Del. Med. J.* **61:10,** 533–542.

50. Reed, M. W., O'Leary, D. P., Duncan, J. L., Majeed, A. W., Wright, B., and Reilly, C. S. (1993) Effects of sedation and supplemental oxygen during upper alimentary tract endoscopy. *Scand. J. Gastroenterol.* **28:4,** 319–322.

51. Alcain, G., Guillen, P., Escolar, A., Moreno, M., and Martin, L. (1998) Predictive factors of oxygen desaturation during upper gastrointestinal endoscopy in nonsedated patients. *Gastrointest. Endosc.* **48:2,** 143–147.

52. White, C. S., Dolwick, M. F., Gravenstein, N., and Paulus, D. A. (1989) Incidence of oxygen desaturation during oral surgery outpatient procedures. *J. Oral Maxillofac. Surg.* **47:2,** 147–149.

53. Putinati, S., Ballerin, L., Corbetta, L., Trevisani, L., and Potena, A. (1999) Patient satisfaction with conscious sedation for bronchoscopy. *Chest* **115:5,** 1437–1440.

54. Silvis, S. E., Nebel, O., Rogers, G., et al. (1976) Cardiopulmonary complications are more common than bleeding or perforation during diagnostic procedures. *JAMA* **235,** 928–930.

55. Gilbert, D. A., Silverstein, F. E., Tedesco, F. J., et al. (1981) National ASGE survey on upper gastrointestinal bleeding; complications of endoscopy. *Dig. Dis. Sci.* **26S,** 55–59.

56. McCloy, R. (1992) Asleep on the job: sedation and monitoring during endoscopy. *Scand. J. Gastroenterol.* **27S:192,** 97–101.

57. Doctors Day 1999: Patient Safety. (1999) *ASA Newsletter* **63:2,** 13–14.

58. D'Eramo, E. M. (1999) Mortality and morbidity with outpatient anesthesia: the Massachusetts experience. *J. Oral Maxillofac. Surg.* **57:5,** 531–536.

59. Flick, W. G., Green, J., and Perkins, D. (1998) Illinois dental anesthesia and sedation survey for 1996. *Anesth. Prog.* **45:2,** 51–56.

60. Jastak, J. T., and Peskin, R. M. (1991) Major morbidity or mortality from office anesthetic procedures: a closed-claim analysis of 13 cases. *Anesth. Prog.* **38:2,** 39–44.

61. Roseveare, C., Seavell, C., Patel, P., Criswell, J., and Shephard, H. (1998) Patient-controlled sedation with propofol and alfentanil during colonoscopy; a pilot study. *Endoscopy* **30:5,** 482–483.

62. Heiman, D. R., Tolliver, B. A., Weis, F. R., O'Brien, B. L., and DiPalma, J. A. (1998) Patient-controlled anesthesia for colonoscopy using propofol: results of a pilot study. *South. Med. J.* **91:6,** 560–564.

63. Kaufman, E., Davidson, E., Sheinkman, Z., and Magora, F. (1994) Comparison between intranasal and intravenous midazolam sedation (with or without patient control) in a dental phobia clinic. *J. Oral Maxillofac. Surg.* **52:8,** 840–843.

64. Webb, R. K., Van der Walt, J. H., Runciman, W. R., et al. (1993) Which monitor? An analysis of 2000 incident reports. *Anesthesiol. and Int. Care* **21:5,** 529–542.

65. Tinker, J. H., Dull, D. L., Caplan, R. A., et al. (1989) Role of monitoring devices in prevention of anesthetic mishaps: a closed claims analysis. *Anesthesiology* **71,** 541–546.

66. Wright, S. W. (1992) Conscious sedation in the Emergency Department: the value of capnography and pulse oximetry. *Ann. Emerg. Med.* **21,** 551–555.

67. Shapiro, B. A. (1999) Bispectral index: better information for sedation in the intensive care unit? *Crit. Care Med.* **27:8,** 1663–1664.

68. Glass, P., Gan, T. J., Sebel, P. S., et al. (1995) Comparison of the Bispectral Index (BIS) and measured drug concentrations for monitoring the effects of propofol, midazolam, alfentanil and isoflurane. *Anesthesiology* **83S3A,** A374.

69. Shah, N., Clack, S., Tayong, M., et al. (1996) The Bispectral Index of EEG can predict response in intensive care patients. *Anesthesiology* **85S3A,** A281.

70. Ristikankare, M., Hartikainen, J., Heikkinen, M., and Janatuinen, E. (1999) Is routinely given conscious sedation of benefit during colonoscopy? *Gastrointest. Endosc.* **49:5,** 566–572.

71. Fisher, N. C., Bailey, S., and Gibson, J. A. (1998) A prospective, randomized controlled trial of sedation vs. no sedation in outpatient upper gastrointestinal endoscopy. *Endoscopy* **30:1,** 21–24.

72. Rex, D. K., Imperiale, T. F., and Portish, V. (1999) Patients willing to try colonoscopy without sedation: associated clinical factors and results of a randomized controlled trial. *Gastrointest. Endosc.* **49:5,** 554–559.

73. Hoffman, M. S., Butler, T. W., and Shaver, T. (1998) Colonoscopy without sedation. *J. Clin. Gastroenterol.* **26:4,** 279–282.

4
Procedure and Site-Specific Considerations for Pediatric Sedation

Shobha Malviya, MD

1. INTRODUCTION

The appropriate management of anxiety and pain for diagnostic and therapeutic procedures in children frequently requires the administration of drugs with sedative properties. Sedation for these procedures has been associated with considerable risk for adverse events *(1–3)*. In light of reports of life-threatening adverse events, the American Academy of Pediatrics (AAP) *(4)*, American Society of Anesthesiologists (ASA) *(5)*, and Joint Commission on the Accreditation of Health Care Organizations (JCAHO) *(6)* have mandated guidelines in order to reduce continuing variability in practice, and the risk associated with sedation. These guidelines, as detailed in Chapter 2, emphasize the importance of uniformity of monitoring and care for sedated children, regardless of the nature of the procedure and the setting in which it is performed or the intended depth of sedation. Despite the availability of nationally publicized guidelines, there is great variability in sedation practice.

The general goals of sedation for any procedure are listed in Table 1. With these goals in mind, the needs for sedation for painful procedures are different than for nonpainful procedures. Most cooperative adults are able to undergo noninvasive procedures such as computerized tomography (CT), bone scans, and echocardiography without sedation. Children, on the other hand, frequently require sedation even for such painless procedures to allay their anxiety, to facilitate their cooperation and to enable them to lie still for the procedure. This chapter reviews practical approaches to the sedation of children in diverse settings and addresses specific considerations relevant to the administration of sedatives and analgesics in children for commonly performed diagnostic and therapeutic procedures.

From: *Contemporary Clinical Neuroscience: Sedation and Analgesia for Diagnostic and Therapeutic Procedures*
Edited by: S. Malviya, N. N. Naughton, and K. K. Tremper © Humana Press Inc., Totowa, NJ

Table 1
Goals of Sedation for Diagnostic and Therapeutic Procedures

Analgesia
Anxiolysis
Amnesia
Enhance patient comfort
Facilitate cooperation/immobilization
Promote patient safety

2. RADIOLOGIC PROCEDURES

The use of neuroimaging studies such as CT and magnetic resonance imaging (MRI) has dramatically increased over the last two decades as a diagnostic tool for many pediatric neurological and other disorders. Although these procedures are painless, children frequently require sedation to decrease apprehension and to facilitate immobilization, thereby minimizing the deleterious effect of movement on diagnostic information. Non-pharmacological measures such as reassurance, presence of a parent, and distraction techniques may permit completion of short painless procedures in some children. However, the majority of painless and virtually all painful procedures in children require the use of sedative and/or analgesic agents. Furthermore, most children require deep sedation to assure scans of diagnostic quality, since mild and moderate planes of sedation do not consistently provide the extent of immobilization needed to perform these studies.

2.1. Personnel and Practitioner Issues

Most diagnostic radiologic procedures are associated with little to no risk; however, sedation for these procedures adds considerable risk for adverse events, some of which may pose the threat of permanent sequelae and even death. Despite the recognition of these risks, children who are sedated for radiologic procedures receive varying levels of care at different institutions—and frequently even within the same institution depending on the time of day, staffing levels, and acuity of the patient. The responsibility of providing sedation care may therefore be assigned to the practitioner ordering the test, the radiologist, or to the anesthesiologist. Although the practitioner ordering the test is most familiar with the patient's underlying medical history, this individual is usually not present at the diagnostic site where the test is performed. Therefore, radiologists frequently assume the responsibility for provision of sedation care to children. This may be viewed as a burden by the radiologist who is required to review the medical history of all sedated children, order the sedative medications, and be immediately available for a procedure that would otherwise have been performed by a technician alone. The advantage of this approach, however, is minimization of variability in sedation practice and immediate availability of the physician ordering the sedative drugs in case of an adverse event. At the author's institution, all practitioners ordering procedures with sedation are required to provide a detailed history and physical examination (H&P) prior to the day of the scheduled test. Sedatives are ordered by the radiologist after reviewing the H&P, and administered by a pediatric nurse trained in the use of sedatives, airway management, and monitoring and resuscitation techniques. This approach may be practical and fiscally sound at institutions where a large number of procedures are performed using sedation. However, at smaller centers where sedation is performed less frequently, it may be prudent to relegate the care of sedated children to anesthesiologists or to designated trained personnel who perform these services throughout the institution. Medina et al. have described a novel approach to train and evaluate radiologists' responses to critical incidents in sedated patients *(7)*. This approach utilizes interactive computerized simulators with 13 different clinical scenarios, and incorporates several critical incidents including hypoxemia, aspiration, and cardiac arrest. The user must make appropriate and timely interventions to save the simulated patient.

The risks of sedation are further heightened by unique considerations that are very specific for individual procedures. It is very important for practitioners who are responsible for sedation to be familiar with these considerations to assure the safety of children sedated for such procedures.

2.2. Magnetic Resonance Imaging

MRI is a noninvasive procedure that provides multiplanar, high-contrast images that are sensitive to myelin maturation and blood flow. The MRI also produces excellent contrast between gray and white matter and permits easy differentiation between normal and pathologic tissues of the central nervous system (CNS) *(8)*. It has therefore become the imaging technique of choice, particularly for non-traumatic pediatric neurologic conditions. Despite the noninvasive and painless nature of this procedure, the majority of children between 6 mo and 8 yr of age require deep sedation to facilitate MRI scans. Prior to undertaking sedation in the MRI scanner, the practitioner must be aware of specific considerations, which are listed in Table 2. The pounding noise generated by the scanner and the claustrophobic sensation that may be experienced by patients within the enclosed tunnel of the MRI unit present a frightening environment for most young children and even some older children and adults. In addition, scanning time typically requires 45–60 min for each site to be scanned. Furthermore, the quality of the image

Table 2
Specific Considerations for MRI

Patient considerations	Noisy/claustrophobic environment
	Implanted devices may preclude MRI
	Obesity—space constraints
Safety issues	Poor visibility of patient
	Limited access
	Strong magnetic fields, non-ferromagnetic equipment
	Monitoring limitations
Quality of scans	Complete immobility
	Degradation of image quality because of electronic devices

obtained is very sensitive to patient motion. The management of sedation in the MRI suite is complicated by the fact that the MRI equipment prevents easy access to the patient. Depending on the size of the patient and the area to be scanned, the head of the patient lies several feet within the housing of the electromagnetic coils of the scanner. Thus, poor visibility of and difficult access to the patient are the primary issues that limit the safety of children who are sedated for MRI.

In addition to these limitations, the strong magnetic field and radiofrequency (RF) pulses interfere with the function of monitoring equipment comprised of ferromagnetic parts, and electric and electronic controls. Artifacts produced by electronic devices and monitoring cables may also adversely affect the image quality. These problems have been largely overcome with the development of a variety of MRI-compatible monitoring devices including electrocardiographs, pulse oximeters, capnographs, and noninvasive blood pressure monitors. Additionally, anesthesia machines and airway equipment with non-ferromagnetic materials have been devised for use within the MRI suite.

The strong magnetic field precludes the use of MRI as a diagnostic study in certain patients (Table 3), including those with implanted metallic devices such as cerebral aneurysm clips, metal spiraled reinforced tracheostomy tubes such as the Bivona tubes, cochlear implants, and metallic foreign bodies. The magnetic field may further reset implanted electromechanical devices such as pacemakers and automatic defibrillators, and the presence of such devices constitutes an absolute contraindication for an MRI scan. The first trimester of pregnancy is another contraindication for the use of MRI. On the other hand, the presence of metallic limb prostheses, prosthetic cardiac

Table 3
Contraindications for MRI

Implanted metallic devices*
   Cerebral aneurysm clips
   Cochlear implants
   Metallic foreign bodies
Implanted electromagnetic devices
   Pacemakers
   Automatic defibrillators
Pregnancy

* Metal spiraled reinforced tracheostomy tubes (Bivona) need to be replaced and pulmonary artery catheters need to be removed prior to MRI scan.

valves, metallic sutures, and spine fusion rods are not considered contraindications for MRI. All patients who present for a MRI scan should be meticulously screened for these conditions prior to scheduling the scan. In addition, all medical personnel and family members of the patient who enter the MRI suite should be similarly screened prior to entry into the scanner. Finally, any objects containing ferromagnetic material must be left outside the MRI scanner because these may be pulled into the magnetic field, with a risk of patient injury. Indeed, failure to observe these precautions recently resulted in fatal head trauma to a 6-yr-old boy from a metal oxygen tank being pulled into the magnet *(9)*.

2.2.1. MRI-Compatible Monitoring

The safety of the child who is sedated for an MRI scan depends on careful patient selection, titration of sedative agents with a wide therapeutic margin of safety, and appropriate monitoring by trained personnel. Several MRI-compatible monitors are now available for monitoring, including electrocardiograms (ECG), pulse oximeters, blood pressure monitors, and capnograms that work well with 1.5-Tesla (T) scanners. Most of these monitors are comprised largely of non-ferromagnetic materials, and incorporate a variety of shielding mechanisms and filters to prevent distortion of the monitoring signal and of scanned images. Although some monitors may be affected by the strong magnetic field when placed close to the magnet, they may function adequately if placed beyond the 50-Gauss line (usually 15–20 ft) using long cables. ECG is usually transmitted through fiberoptic cables installed for cardiac gated images. To minimize image distortion, carbon-fiber ECG leads must be used and placed in a single line in close proximity to each other. The electrical currents induced in all conductive materials exposed to the

RF energy of the magnetic field during imaging may cause a rise in temperature of monitoring cables, placing patients at risk for thermal injuries. Pulse oximeter probes and ECG leads must be placed with caution because full-thickness burns have been reported if the cable adjoining the probe is placed within the bore of the magnet *(10)*. Pulse oximeter sensors must be placed as far from the imaging site as possible, and thermal insulation should be placed between any essential wires or cables and the patient's skin. Finally, the wires and cables should be periodically inspected for potential fraying, which can occur with repeated use. MRI-compatible monitoring is addressed in greater detail in Chapter 8.

2.2.2. Sedation Techniques

Since complete immobility is necessary to obtain a diagnostic study, some large centers have specific sedation protocols in place that take into consideration the child's age, previous sedation experience, underlying medical history, and anticipated duration of the procedure *(11–14)*. These protocols have been used with a high degree of success. Chloral hydrate (75–100 mg/kg orally) is commonly used to sedate children for MRI scans, and has been found to be adequate in 93–95% of cases *(1,15–17)*. However, its use has been associated with delayed recovery and prolonged side effects such as motor imbalance, agitation, and nausea and vomiting *(18,19)*. Furthermore, the incidence of failed sedation for MRI scans with chloral hydrate has been found to be inversely proportional to age, with a higher incidence of sedation failures after 3 yr of age *(1,17)*. Therefore, several centers use pentobarbital (2–6 mg/kg intravenously) in older children to facilitate sedation for MRI *(12,20–22)*. The advantage of pentobarbital is that it produces a rapid and more predictable onset of sedation, thereby facilitating patient throughput and efficient use of the MRI scanner. However, its use has also been associated with severe oxygen desaturation, paradoxical excitement, sedation failure, and delayed recovery *(12,23,24)*.

The failure rate with chloral hydrate and pentobarbital and their unpredictable duration of action have led to an interest in the use of short-acting agents such as propofol to facilitate MRI *(20)*. In most centers, the use of this agent is restricted to anesthesiologists because of its narrow therapeutic margin and high likelihood to cause apnea.

2.2.3. Cardiopulmonary Resuscitation in the MRI Scanner

The strong magnetic field and limited access to the patient precludes adequate cardiopulmonary resuscitation in the MRI scanner. In the event of a life-threatening adverse event such as cardiac or respiratory arrest, the patient must be immediately taken out of the scanning room to an adjoining proce-

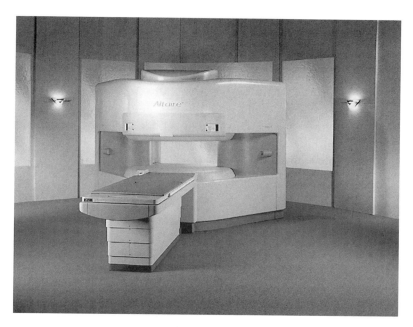

Fig. 1. The open, low-field MRI scanner is open on three sides, affords greater access to and visibility of the patient, and minimizes anxiety related to claustrophobia. Reproduced with permission from Hitachi Medical Systems America, Inc., Twinsburg, Ohio.

dure room. This will permit the use of resuscitation equipment such as defibrillators, which do not work near the magnet. Furthermore, it affords members of the "cardiac arrest team" access to the patient without the need for screening prior to entering the scanning room. It is faster to remove the patient from the MRI scanning room than to turn off the magnetic field, since it takes several minutes to completely eliminate the magnetic field. Additionally, when the magnetic field is turned back on, it takes several hours to re-establish the magnetic field strength, resulting in prolonged downtime of the scanner.

2.2.4. Recent Advances in MRI Technology

Recent technological advances such as open MRI scanners (Fig. 1) and ultrafast MRI may limit the need for sedation in some children undergoing MRI scans. Indeed, Rupprecht et al. found that only 74 of 274 (27%) children with a median age of 9 yr required sedation for an open low-field MRI system compared to 47% of a sample of children undergoing closed MRI *(25)*. However, unless further advances eliminate the problems arising from movement, the need for sedation to facilitate these procedures will continue for at least some children. Open MRI scanners circumvent the problems of claustrophobia and anxiety and allow easier access to the patient. Additionally, the open scanner has extended the use of MRI to the morbidly obese patient who would have to forgo a MRI study because of the space constraints in the closed high-field systems. Further advances with the open MRI systems are likely to include the possibility of performing surgical procedures under continuous MRI guidance.

The development of a MRI-compatible audiovisual system has further reduced the need for sedation, particularly in older children. This system is compatible with magnets up to a strength of 4 Tesla, and is comprised of goggles and a headphone unit that permits patients to view a videotape of their choice on a small binocular headset *(26)*. Harned et al. reported an 18% reduction in the need for sedation for MRI following installation of this system, with a significant potential for cost savings *(26)*.

2.3. Computerized Tomography

Since the original introduction of CT in 1973, it has become an important technique for the evaluation of several pediatric diseases. As for MRI, an immobile patient is important for optimal imaging with CT scanning. Conventional CT techniques are associated with long image acquisition times, with most scans typically lasting 30–45 min, depending on the number of areas to be scanned. The CT scanner, however, does not present as frightening an environment as the MRI scanner, since the scanning table is less confining and the procedure is less noisy. Yet some children may require sedation to ensure the immobility needed to obtain a diagnostic scan. The use of helical CT technology that became available in the mid 1990s has significantly reduced the scanning time, and thereby the need for sedation *(27,28)*. Indeed, Kaste et al. reported a 49% decrease in the frequency of sedation with the use of helical CT compared to conventional CT *(27)*. More recent availability of multisection helical CT scanners have further improved scanning efficiency with a three- to fivefold decrease in scanning time and a similar decrease in frequency of sedation *(29)*.

Unlike MRI, the risk of radiation exposure during CT scanning precludes the continuous presence of health care workers or family members in the room. Intermittent remote observation of the sedated child during periods of radiation exposure requires a high degree of vigilance and positioning of the monitoring devices so that they can be viewed from the control room. Also, children who are undergoing abdominal and pelvic CT scans frequently require oral contrast solutions that may increase the risk of pulmonary aspiration in a sedated patient. Some contrast solutions, such as 1% Hypaque, are clear. Barium sulphate, however, is an opaque, white liquid, which should not be considered a clear fluid. Data regarding the gastric emptying times of oral contrast materials are insufficient. The risk of aspiration of oral contrast material is greater in patients who require emergent CT scans following trauma, and in one study was found to be 2% *(30)*. Optimizing the quality of the scan while minimizing the risk of aspiration requires a careful assessment for each patient by balancing the potential for vomiting and aspiration with the timing of the procedure and target depth of sedation. In some cases, it may be prudent to administer contrast materials via a nasogastric tube placed following induction of general anesthesia and endotracheal intubation. In such cases, the administration of metoclopramide may hasten the passage of the contrast material through the gastrointestinal tract and allow adequate quality of the scans.

2.3.1. Sedation Techniques

Chloral hydrate (50–100 mg/kg PO) remains the most commonly used agent for sedation of children for CT scans, with reported success rates of 93–98% *(1,31,32)*. Since CH has been found to be unpredictable in its onset and duration of action, pentobarbital (3–8 mg/kg iv) has been used in an effort to improve success. It has been associated, however, with similar failure rates and prolonged duration of action as chloral hydrate *(33)*. Methohexital, a shorter-acting barbiturate (25 mg/kg to a maximum of 500 mg rectally) has been used with 95% success and a recovery time of 79 ± 31 min from drug administration to discharge *(34)*. However, significant hypoxemia occurred in 6% of children, with oxygen saturations as low as 70% in 2% of cases. All children who experienced hypoxemia required airway manipulation, including bag-and-mask ventilation in 3% of cases. This study illustrates the risks of using agents with a narrower margin of safety by personnel without anesthesia training. Midazolam has also been administered intravenously (0.2 mg/kg) or orally (0.5 mg/kg), but its use has been associated with very high failure rates, with 19–50% of children requiring supplementation with other sedatives *(35,36)*. Therefore, until a sedative agent with a quick and reliable onset of action, a short duration of action, and with minimal potential to produce respiratory depression becomes available, chloral hydrate and pentobarbital remain good choices for sedation for nonpainful procedures such as CT scanning.

2.4. Interventional Radiologic Procedures

Invasive radiologic procedures that require sedation include angiography, embolization, arteriography, myelography, percutaneous insertion of drains, nephrostomy tubes and gastrostomy tubes, and CT-guided procedures such as biopsies or abscess drainage. These procedures involve varying degrees of pain and discomfort for the patient. The anxiety associated with these procedures, particularly in children, further heightens the perception of pain and decreases their ability to cooperate. The goals of sedation for these procedures, therefore, include anxiolysis, analgesia, and amnesia, especially for children who require repeated procedures. Adequate anxiolysis and analgesia facilitate the patient's cooperation and ability to remain immobile, and greatly enhance their comfort during these procedures. Administration of sedation in the interventional radiology suite frequently poses a challenge for a number of reasons. The radiologic equipment greatly restricts access to the patient. The procedures are often performed in varied positions—including prone and lateral—to maximize imaging while allowing access to the site of the procedure. Positioning and restricted space may allow minimal to no access to the patient's airway. Furthermore, potential radiation exposure may place the sedation care provider at a distance, further limiting direct physical or verbal contact with the patient. This limits the ability of the monitoring individual to judge the depth of sedation and detect changes in level of consciousness, or to monitor the adequacy of ventilation. Additionally, patients who present for these procedures have comorbid conditions such as intracranial pathology and hepatic and/or renal failure, which may place the patient at increased risk for sedation-related adverse events. For these reasons, the responsibility of sedation for these procedures is relegated to anesthesiologists in most centers. The decision to use sedation or general anesthesia is influenced by the availability of trained personnel to monitor the patient, the experience of the interventional radiologist in managing pediatric sedation, the child's medical history, and the anticipated duration and complexity of the procedure.

2.4.1. Sedation Techniques

Sedation for interventional radiologic procedures requires the administration of anxiolytics, systemic analgesics, and local anesthetic infiltration in combination. A variety of drug combinations have been used with success. Midazolam, a short-acting benzodiazepine, may be administered via the oral, intranasal, and iv routes for its anxiolytic and amnestic effects. It is supplemented with incremental doses of fentanyl to provide analgesia and to improve the tolerance of local anesthetic infiltration. Kaye et al. have touted the safety and efficacy of pentobarbital, fentanyl, and midazolam used in combination. They report an incidence of <5% for minor complications such as paradoxical reaction, skin rash, mild respiratory depression, and bronchospasm, and <0.01% incidence of major complications such as cardiac arrest, respiratory arrest, and aspiration *(37)*. Ketamine has been used as a sole sedative because it provides both amnesia and analgesia, maintains airway tone and patency, and is less likely to cause respiratory depression than other sedatives *(38)*. Cotsen et al. have reported a 91% success rate with the use of ketamine for short interventional radiologic procedures in children *(38)*. However, its use was associated with a 5% incidence of transient oxygen desaturation that responded to airway manipulation and supplemental oxygen, and one case of apnea (0.05%) that responded to bag-mask ventilation. These data highlight the risk of serious adverse events with the use of ketamine. Indeed, previous investigators have reported a high incidence of laryngospasm with its use *(39,40)*. In most centers, therefore, the use of ketamine is restricted to personnel with airway management and endotracheal intubation skills because of its potential to rapidly produce a state of general anesthesia or laryngospasm.

3. CARDIOLOGY PROCEDURES

3.1. Cardiac Catheterization

The prevalence of congenital heart disease (CHD) is approximately 1 in every 100 live births. Three infants of every 1000 live births require cardiac catheterization as a diagnostic or therapeutic measure *(41)*. Cardiac catheterization and angiography were introduced as diagnostic tools for CHD in 1947 *(42)*, and interventional catheterizations were first used as therapeutic maneuvers in 1966 *(43)*. Diagnostic cardiac catheterizations are now being performed less frequently because of improved trans-thoracic and trans-esophageal echocardiography (TEE) techniques. However, interventional techniques are being used more often, and the patients who present for these procedures often have complex heart defects. Indications for cardiac catheterization procedures are listed in Table 4.

3.1.1. Specific Considerations

Cardiac catheterization procedures are usually prolonged, and require a cooperative and sometimes motionless child. Table 5 presents specific issues that must be considered when sedating a child for cardiac catheterization. The cardiac catheterization suite and its equipment present a frightening environment to children. Other considerations include limited access to the child and the airway, and the potential for sudden devastating complications such as life-threatening arrhythmias, rupture of a blood vessel, or perforation of a cardiac chamber. Balloon dilatation of valves or blood vessels causes sudden disruption of forward flow for several seconds during balloon expansion that may not be tolerated in children with poor cardiac function.

Changes in oxygen saturation and carbon dioxide tension in children with congenital heart defects may significantly alter pulmonary artery (PA) pres-

Table 4
Indications for Cardiac Catheterization

Diagnostic	
Hemodynamic evaluation	Measurement of chamber pressures
	Pulmonary hypertension and reversibility
	Quantification of shunts
	Calculation of PVR and SVR
Anatomic characterization	Presence of septal defects
	Valve stenosis/regurgitation
Therapeutic	
Occlusion of defects	ASD, PDA, VSD
Coil embolization of vessels	Systemic to pulmonary artery collaterals
Balloon valvuloplasty	Aortic, pulmonary, or mitral valves
Balloon angioplasty	Peripheral pulmonary artery stenosis,
	coarctation of aorta
Stent placement	Pulmonary arteries, conduits, baffle
Treatment of arrhythmias	Radiofrequency ablation

PVR = Pulmonary vascular resistance; SVR = Systemic vascular resistance; ASD = Atrial septal defect; PDA = Patent ductus arteriosus; VSD = Ventricular septal defect.

sure, pulmonary vascular resistance (PVR), and the magnitude and direction of intracardiac shunts. Therefore, for diagnostic catheterizations, most cardiologists prefer to use sedation with the child spontaneously breathing room air so that the hemodynamic data obtained are representative of baseline/awake values. Conversely, most sedation regimens produce clinically significant hypoxemia and hypercarbia with resultant increases in PA pressure and PVR. Indeed, Friesen et al. have demonstrated significant increases in end-tidal carbon dioxide tension and decreases in SpO_2 in children who are deeply sedated for cardiac catheterization *(44)*. Furthermore, these changes were observed more frequently in children with pulmonary hypertension. Sedation for these procedures, therefore, requires careful titration of sedatives and analgesics to promote the comfort of the child while maintaining a patent airway and adequate spontaneous ventilation, thereby avoiding hypoxemia and hypercarbia.

3.1.2. Sedation Techniques

A variety of sedation regimens have been successfully used, but with a varied incidence of adverse events. DPT or "lytic cocktail" is a combination of demerol (meperidine 25 mg/mL), phenergan (promethazine 6.5 mg/mL), and thorazine (chlorpromazine 6.5 mg/mL) that was once extensively used for cardiac catheterization. When administered in doses of 0.02–0.2 mL/kg, this

Table 5
Cardiac Catheterization: Specific Considerations

Comorbidity, high-risk patients
Frightening environment
Limited access to patient
Balance between PVR and SVR
Effects of O_2 and hyperventilation on PVR
Effects of sedative/anesthetic agents on conduction system
Interruption of forward flow with balloon expansion
Potential devastating complications—arrhythmias, vessel rupture

PVR = Pulmonary vascular resistance; SVR = Systemic vascular resistance.

combination reliably produces deep sedation. However, its effects are very prolonged (mean duration ± S.D. of 19 ± 15 h), and frequently outlast the procedure. In addition, its use has been associated with a number of serious side effects including respiratory depression, hypotension, seizures, and death *(24,45–48)*. Therefore, the use of DPT is strongly discouraged, and this regimen has largely been replaced with others that include opioids, benzodiazepines, ketamine, and pentobarbital, usually in combinations of two or more drugs.

Ketamine, in intermittent bolus doses of 0.2–0.5 mg/kg or infusion of 1 mg/kg/h, is a popular choice because it provides intense analgesia and does not cause respiratory depression. Furthermore, it produces minimal hemodynamic effects and is well-tolerated in most children with congenital heart defects. However, it must be used with caution in children with long-standing heart failure because ketamine acts as a direct myocardial depressant in children with depleted catecholamine stores. Additionally, ketamine causes an increase in salivary secretions and depresses airway reflexes, placing patients at risk for laryngospasm *(39)*. This risk may be decreased by concomitant administration of an antisialogogue such as glycopyrrolate. Another undesirable side effect of ketamine is the occurrence of hallucinations and dreaming that may persist for 24 h after its administration. Benzodiazepines given in conjunction with ketamine decrease the incidence of these effects. Although ketamine remains a good choice for children undergoing cardiac catheterization, it must be administered only by individuals skilled in bag-mask ventilation and endotracheal intubation skills and with a high degree of vigilance because of its potential to produce a state of general anesthesia with loss of airway reflexes and the potential for laryngospasm.

A recent expert consensus statement from the North American Society of Pacing and Electrophysiology (NASPE) agrees on the safety, efficiency, and efficacy of sedation for a wide range of electrophysiologic procedures in a wide age range of patients including children *(49)*. However, the NASPE recommends that sedation or general anesthesia for these procedures should be administered by anesthesia providers for children less than 13 yr of age because of their potential for a rapid transition from light sedation to obtundation. Furthermore, most children are unable to lie still for the number of hours needed to complete these procedures unless they are deeply sedated or anesthetized.

The effects of sedative, analgesic, or anesthetic agents on the conduction system including normal atrioventricular and accessory pathways must be considered prior to selection of a sedation regimen for these procedures. Volatile anesthetics have been shown to prolong the refractoriness of the normal as well as the accessory pathways *(50)*. Similarly, droperidol has been found to increase the refractory period of the accessory pathways *(51)*. On the other hand, opioids including fentanyl, sufentanil, and alfentanil, and benzodiazepines including midazolam and lorazepam have been found to have no clinically significant effects on the refractory period of the accessory pathways in patients with Wolff-Parkinson-White Syndrome *(50–52)*.

3.2. Echocardiography

Echocardiography is a fundamental part of the evaluation of a child with suspected or known heart disease, and is used to characterize cardiac anatomy, assess cardiac chamber sizes and dynamics, identify valvular disease, and evaluate cardiac function. Epicardial echocardiography is noninvasive, yet young children frequently require sedation to facilitate cooperation for these procedures. Chloral hydrate is commonly used to provide sedation for epicardial echocardiography. Napoli et al. evaluated the use of chloral hydrate for echocardiography in 405 children with congenital heart defects *(53)*. They reported a 98% success rate, with no clinically significant hemodynamic effects. Six percent of their sample experienced hypoxemia that responded to repositioning of the head or supplemental oxygen. Furthermore, they found that children with trisomy 21 were more likely to become hypoxemic compared with other children. Intranasal midazolam has also been used with some success in children undergoing echocardiography *(54)*.

TEE provides an unobstructed view of the heart because of the proximity of the probe to the cardiac structures, and permits superior visualization of the left atrium and the mitral and aortic valves compared to the epicardial approach. The availability of neonatal TEE probes now permits this procedure to be performed in small infants who weigh 2.4 kg or more. TEE is an invasive procedure, and requires deep sedation or general anesthesia for all children. In most cases, general anesthesia with endotracheal intubation is

Table 6
Dental Procedures: Specific Considerations

Inadequate support services in non-hospital venues
Trauma to surrounding tissue/eye from sudden movement during procedure
Risk of aspiration of blood, secretions, debris in oropharynx
Feeling of suffocation from placement of rubber dam
Increased anxiety, fear caused by noise of handpiece

preferred because of the risks of aspiration and bronchial compression by the probe with resultant hypoxemia.

4. DENTISTRY AND ORAL SURGERY

The prevalence of dental caries has decreased since the 1960s, yet it remains the most common chronic childhood disease. Preschool-aged children and children from low-income groups account for 25–50% of dental caries in children *(55)*. These children frequently present for restorations and extractions of carious teeth, and depending on the age and maturity of the child and the complexity and extent of the planned procedure, many of these children require sedation for successful completion of these procedures. Other dental procedures that require sedation include removal of impacted teeth and minor prosthetic surgery.

4.1. Specific Considerations

Sedation of children for dental procedures poses a tremendous challenge for a number of reasons (Table 6). First, most of these procedures are performed in a non-hospital venue without readily available back-up services in case of an adverse event. Indeed, a recent critical incident analysis of sedation-related disasters including permanent neurologic injury and death found that a disproportionate number of such events occurred in children undergoing dental procedures and that the non-hospital venue was an independent predictor of a poor outcome following sedation *(2)*. Although the Joint Commission on the Accreditation of Health care Organizations (JCAHO) regulates hospital-based sedation, state dental boards regulate sedation in dental offices. Secondly, there is wide variability in the training, skill levels, and extent of specialization among dentists, and in compliance with national sedation guidelines from the American Academy of Pediatrics (AAP) and the American Academy of Pediatric Dentistry (AAPD). The majority of adverse events reported in children who undergo dental procedures occurred as a result of inadequate skill levels, lack of appropriate equipment, insufficient monitoring, or a failure to adequately resuscitate the child once an adverse event had occurred *(2,3,56)*. However, the AAPD contends that they are unaware of any deaths from sedation in dental offices when the AAPD guidelines have been strictly observed.

The dental literature is replete with reports of studies that evaluate the usefulness of pulse oximetry and/or nasal cannula capnography for sedated children *(57–59)*. Verwest et al. reported a 20% incidence of major oxygen desaturation ($\geq$5% decrease from baseline values) in children undergoing dental restorative procedures *(59)*. Additionally, they reported significant interrelationships between hypoxemic episodes and young age (<7 yr), tonsillar hypertrophy, and high lidocaine doses ($\geq$1.5 mg/kg). Other investigators have also demonstrated an inverse relationship between tonsillar size and the ability to spontaneously recover from an obstructed airway in children who are sedated for dental procedures *(60)*. Iwasaki et al. and Croswell et al. found that nasal cannula capnography provided an earlier indicator of respiratory compromise than pulse oximetry *(57,58)*. Croswell et al. reported 85 abnormal capnographic readings in 39 children who are sedated with chloral hydrate, hydroxyzine, and meperidine for dental procedures *(58)*. Although 75 of these incidents were false-positives, 10 cases of obstructive apnea were identified by absence of exhaled CO_2. All 10 incidents were identified and treated by repositioning the head prior to any decrease in oxygen saturation. It is likely that early detection of respiratory compromise and appropriate intervention averted potential episodes of hypoxemia in these patients. Additionally, only three of these incidents were identified by clinical signs such as loss of breath sounds via the precordial stethoscope. These data support the routine use of capnography in conjunction with pulse oximetry in children who are sedated for dental procedures.

Specific procedure-related considerations include the need for cooperation, particularly during local anesthetic injection. Sudden unexpected movement or struggling during injection may result in injury to surrounding structures such as the eye or lip, or even breakage of the needle in the tissue. Therefore, many dentists prefer to use physical restraint in addition to pharmacologic sedation. It is important to minimize psychological trauma in all children, but especially in those who require repeated treatment, since success with subsequent procedures largely depends on previous sedation and dental experiences. The presence of blood, secretions, sponges, pledgets, and other debris in the oropharynx places patients at risk for aspiration and laryngospasm. Therefore, a rubber dam is frequently placed to protect the airway. Some children may experience a feeling of suffocation from placement of the rubber dam, and others fear the sound and sensations generated by the handpiece.

4.2. Sedation Techniques

In the United States, dentists are required to have a permit to administer sedatives intravenously. Most dentists use oral sedative agents alone or in combination with nitrous oxide administered by a nose mask because of the ease of administration and safety profile. Chloral hydrate (50–70 mg/kg) alone or in combination with hydroxyzine, and/or nitrous oxide remains the agent of choice for sedation for dental procedures *(61,62)*. Hydroxyzine (1–2 mg/kg) is frequently added for its antiemetic properties and to potentiate the sedative effects of chloral hydrate. Previous investigators have reported that the addition of hydroxyzine (2 mg/kg) to chloral hydrate (70 mg/kg) significantly reduced crying and movement compared with chloral hydrate alone *(63)*. However, both groups of children experienced a high incidence of hypoxemia (oxygen saturation <90%) that required repositioning of the neck with a trend toward more frequent episodes in children who received chloral hydrate and hydroxyzine. These data highlight the need for continuous pulse oximetry and careful observation by trained individuals to promote the safety of sedated children, particularly those who have received a combination of sedatives.

Since chloral hydrate and hydroxyzine do not have analgesic properties, oral meperidine (1.1–2.2 mg/kg) has been added to the sedative regimen in an effort to minimize the response to noxious stimuli such as local anesthetic injection, placement of the mouth prop, or cavity preparation *(64)*. Using a crossover design, Hasty et al. compared the efficacy and side effects of chloral hydrate (50 mg/kg) and hydroxyzine (25 mg) with and without meperidine (1.5 mg/kg) in children undergoing restorative procedures *(64)*. They reported that the addition of meperidine significantly improved tolerance of and cooperation with the invasive/painful parts of the procedures, with no increase in respiratory depression. However, these investigators did note a trend toward more prolonged drowsiness and disorientation following the procedure with the use of meperidine. They recommended routine supplementation of oxygen, the ready availability of naloxone and airway equipment, and stringent recovery protocols when opioids are added to a sedative regimen.

Nitrous oxide has been extensively used to facilitate dental procedures as a sole agent and as an adjunct to orally or intravenously administered sedatives *(61,65,66)*. Its main attributes are its ease of administration, wide margin of safety, analgesic and anxiolytic effects, and rapid reversibility. Needleman et al. have reported a 74% success rate for dental procedures performed with chloral hydrate and hydroxyzine supplemented with 55% nitrous oxide *(61)*. The incidence of complications included vomiting in

8.1% of cases and oxygen desaturation to <95% in 21% of cases. Other investigators have reported that the addition of 30% or 50% nitrous oxide via face mask to oral chloral hydrate usually produces a state of deep sedation with a significantly higher incidence of hypoventilation compared with the use of chloral hydrate alone *(67)*. It is prudent to extrapolate the results of this study to the dental setting, however, since dentists administer nitrous oxide through a nasal mask that permits the entrainment of room air with dilution of nitrous oxide concentrations. It is advisable to monitor children who receive nitrous oxide in combination with other sedatives with pulse oximetry and to monitor the concentration of nitrous oxide using an oxygen analyzer in accordance with AAP guidelines. Interestingly, a recent large survey of the membership of the AAPD found that 15% of respondents used no monitors and 25% never used pulse oximetry when administering sedative combinations containing nitrous oxide *(66)*. Of greater concern is that 30% of the respondents indicated that they had encountered a compromised airway as a result of deep sedation in children who had received these sedative combinations.

Another caveat with the use of nitrous oxide for sedation is the concern regarding atmospheric contamination and exposure of personnel. In fact, this is the primary reason that nitrous oxide is used very infrequently or not at all for sedation by non-anesthesiologists in other settings such as labor and delivery. In the previously described survey, the majority of respondents *(96%)* used scavenging or some other means of removing exhaled gases. However, 69% of respondents had never tested the ambient levels of nitrous oxide in their offices. Taken together, the results of these studies indicate that nitrous oxide is a valuable adjunct to the sedation armamentarium for dentistry. However, it is imperative for dental practitioners who use this agent to comply with AAP and AAPD guidelines to ensure the safety of both the patients and personnel *(4,68)*.

5. PROCEDURES IN THE EMERGENCY DEPARTMENT

A wide variety of painful procedures are performed in the emergency department (ED). These include laceration repair, abscess drainage, reduction of fractures and dislocations, lumbar puncture, foreign body removal, and endotracheal intubation. Most of these procedures are brief but intensely painful, and the majority of children who undergo these procedures require sedation and analgesia. Previous emergency medicine literature has alluded to the undertreatment of acute pain in the ED due to a number of reasons, including failure to prioritize pain management over other aspects of care and concerns about interfering with the diagnostic assessment of conditions

Table 7
Emergency Department Procedures: Specific Considerations

Full stomach consideration
Chaotic environment
Need for rapid throughput/expediency
Emergent/urgent procedures
Incomplete medical history
Hemodynamic/respiratory instability
Intensely painful procedures

such as abdominal pain and closed head injury *(69,70)*. However, significant progress has been made in the management of acute and procedural pain with the availability of newer and potent, yet short-acting sedatives and analgesics. Sedation and analgesia for procedures in the ED presents a unique set of problems (Table 7).

Most emergency departments present a chaotic and noisy environment, where efficiency is imperative to assure prompt care for patients with conditions of varying acuity. The majority of the procedures performed in the ED cannot be postponed, and all of them are unplanned. Some of the patients such as trauma victims may have been transported by ambulance to the ED and may not be accompanied by parents or caregivers, making it difficult to obtain an adequate medical history. Additionally, some of these patients may present the added risks of hemodynamic or respiratory instability.

The majority of patients who undergo procedures in the ED have not fasted, thereby placing them at risk for aspiration if a sufficiently deep level of sedation with loss of airway reflexes is achieved. This risk is increased in the presence of comorbid conditions such as obesity, gastro-esophageal reflux, tracheoesophageal fistula, ileus, trauma, and pain. The incidence of aspiration in emergency patients who have not fasted is unknown. However, case reports of aspiration in children sedated with ketamine for emergency procedures *(71,72)* underscore the importance of careful consideration of the following issues: risks vs benefits of sedation in children with full stomach considerations, the timing and urgency of the procedure, and the target depth of sedation. In some cases, the use of local anesthetic infiltration in conjunction with nonpharmacologic measures such as distraction may be the safest alternative. Some children may require the addition of mild sedation with preservation of airway reflexes to allow completion of the procedure. Furthermore, the use of pharmacologic prophylaxis including antacids, prokinetic agents (metoclopramide) and H_2-receptor blockers should be strongly considered in patients with conditions that increase the risk of aspiration.

Finally, for some children general anesthesia with endotracheal intubation for airway protection may be the only safe alternative for completion of the procedure.

5.1. Sedation Techniques

Since most of the procedures are painful, it is rarely appropriate to use a sedative agent alone without the concomitant administration of analgesics or infiltration of local anesthetic. The use of nonpharmacologic techniques such as verbal reassurance, parental presence, distraction, guided imagery, or hypnosis may permit some children to tolerate the injection of local anesthetic with subsequent completion of the procedure with minimal to no sedation. The success of this approach largely depends on the age, maturity, and past medical experiences of the child, the duration and nature of the procedure, and the experience and skills of the caregivers to calm an anxious child.

The need for expediency and rapid patient throughput and the short duration of the procedures makes it important to use sedatives and analgesics that have a quick onset and short duration of action. A variety of agents administered via the oral, transmucosal, iv, and inhaled routes have been used to facilitate procedures in the ED. The choice of sedatives used and the frequency of sedation in children vary with the nature of the treatment facility. Previous investigators have demonstrated that sedation is used more frequently, and with a preference for shorter-acting and more potent agents such as fentanyl and ketamine when children are treated in a pediatric hospital ED compared to an ED in a general community hospital *(73)*. Yet regardless of the setting, midazolam administered alone or in combination with an analgesic remains the most common agent used for sedation in the ED *(73)*.

For painful procedures such as fracture reduction, the therapeutic index between adequate sedation and pain relief and the potential for adverse events is very narrow. A large retrospective study evaluated the use of fentanyl (mean dose 1.5 micrograms/kg) and midazolam (mean 0.17 mg/kg) in 338 children undergoing fracture reduction *(74)*. Ninety-one percent of the fractures were successfully reduced. However, 11% of children experienced adverse respiratory events including hypoxemia, airway obstruction, and hypoventilation. Several of these children required intervention, including supplemental oxygen, airway repositioning, verbal breathing reminders, and naloxone. Of greatest concern is that 8% of children were unresponsive to pain and voice because they had progressed beyond a state of deep sedation. The mean time to discharge following the last dose of sedative was 92 min.

Since most of the procedures performed in the ED are rapid in duration, and since emergency physicians are skilled in airway management and cardiopulmonary resuscitation, there has been increasing interest in the use of iv anesthetics including propofol, etomidate, methohexital and ketamine to provide sedation and analgesia in the ED *(75–81)*. Each of the cited studies found a high degree of success with completion of the procedure with shorter induction times, and reported good patient acceptance of the sedative regimen. However, all these studies report a significant incidence of excessive sedation, with some patients exhibiting only reflex withdrawal to pain—a state of sedation in which preservation of airway reflexes is highly unlikely. Furthermore, these studies found a small yet significant incidence of adverse events including hypoxemia, hypoventilation, apnea, severe vomiting, and laryngospasm. Although no patient in any of these studies experienced any permanent sequelae or morbidity, the experience with the use of these potent agents in the emergency department setting is simply not sufficient to justify their routine use, particularly in patients with full stomach considerations.

It remains difficult to balance the goals of providing patient comfort and efficiency, and above all maintaining the safety of children who undergo procedures in the ED. Further evaluation of sedation practices in the ED, with close collaboration between emergency physicians, anesthesiologists, and perhaps hospital administration, is urgently required to assure the safety of sedated children.

6. SUMMARY AND FUTURE DIRECTIONS

Significant progress has been made with regard to sedation practices in both adults and children over the past two decades. These developments have largely encompassed the recognition of risks related to sedation and development of guidelines that emphasize consistency of sedation practices. Recent advances that have reduced the requirement for sedation in selected cases include the availability of open MRI scanners, ultrafast CT scans, and the use of the cyanoacrylate polymer adhesive Dermabond® for laceration repair in lieu of suturing. Existing comparative studies evaluating different sedation regimens lack the power to compare the incidence of adverse events or to capture the occurrence of major complications that are fortunately rare. Large, prospective, multicenter trials are needed for the evaluation of different sedation techniques to delineate their safety profile and identify those regimens that are most suited for individual procedures in terms of safety and efficacy.

With further advances in imaging and other medical technology, children will continue to require sedation with increasing frequency and in more diverse settings. Each of these settings is likely to pose individual and specific considerations and challenges. For each of these procedures, it is necessary to carefully balance the objectives of optimizing patient comfort and allaying anxiety while minimizing potential risks to the patient. The prudent practitioner realizes that regardless of the nature of the procedure, the setting in which it is performed or the need for efficiency, the highest standards of monitoring and vigilance, and the selection of sedative agents with a wide therapeutic margin will enhance the safety of the sedated child.

REFERENCES

1. Malviya, S., Voepel-Lewis, T., and Tait, A. R. (1997) Adverse events and risk factors associated with the sedation of children by nonanesthesiologists [published erratum appears in Anesth Analg 1998 Feb;86(2):227]. *Anesth. Analg.* **85(6),** 1207–13.
2. Coté, C. J., Notterman, D. A., Karl, H. W., Weinberg, J. A., McCloskey, and C. (2000) Adverse sedation events in pediatrics: a critical incident analysis of contributing factors. *Pediatrics* **105(4 Pt 1),** 805–814.
3. Jastak, J. T. and Peskin, R. M. (1991) Major morbidity or mortality from office anesthetic procedures: a closed-claim analysis of 13 cases. *Anesth. Prog.* **38(2),** 39–44.
4. American Academy of *Pediatrics* Committee on Drugs: guidelines for monitoring and management of pediatric patients during and after sedation for diagnostic and therapeutic procedures. (1992) *Pediatrics* **89(6 Pt 1),** 1110–1115.
5. Practice guidelines for sedation and analgesia by non-anesthesiologists. (1996) A report by the American Society of Anesthesiologists Task Force on Sedation and Analgesia by Non-Anesthesiologists. *Anesthesiology* **84(2),** 459–471.
6. Joint Commission on Accreditation of Healthcare Organizations. (2001) Comprehensive Accreditation Manual for Hospitals: The Official Handbook, in JCAHO, Oakbrook Terrace, IL, http://www.jcaho.org/standards_frm.html.
7. Medina, L. S., Racadio, J. M., and Schwid, H. A. (2000) Computers in radiology. The sedation, analgesia, and contrast media computerized simulator: a new approach to train and evaluate radiologists' responses to critical incidents. *Pediatr. Radiol.* **30,** 299–305.
8. Rao, C. C. and Krishna, G. (1994) Anaesthetic considerations for magnetic resonance imaging. *Ann. Acad. Med. Singapore* **23(4),** 531–535.
9. Hospital Lists Safety Lapses in MRI Death. Newsday, Inc. 2001 August 22; Sect. A45.
10. Bashein, G. and Syrory, G. (1991) Burns associated with pulse oximetry during magnetic resonance imaging. *Anesthesiology* **75(2),** 382–383.
11. Sury, M. R., Hatch, D. J., Deeley, T., Dicks-Mireaux, C., and Chong, W. K. (1999) Development of a nurse-led sedation service for paediatric magnetic resonance imaging. *Lancet* **353(9165),** 1667–1671.
12. Bluemke, D. A. and Breiter, S. N. (2000) Sedation procedures in MR imaging: safety, effectiveness, and nursing effect on examinations. *Radiology* **216(3),** 645–652.

13. Keengwe, I. N., Hegde, S., Dearlove, O., Wilson, B., Yates, R. W., and Sharples, A. (1999) Structured sedation programme for magnetic resonance imaging examination in children. *Anaesthesia* **54(11)**, 1069–1072.
14. Egelhoff, J. C., Ball, W. S., Jr., Koch, B. L., and Parks, T. D. (1997) Safety and efficacy of sedation in children using a structured sedation program. *AJR Am. J. Roentgenol.* **168(5)**, 1259–1262.
15. Malviya, S., Voepel-Lewis, T., Eldevik, O. P., Rockwell, D. T., Wong, J. H., Tait, A. R. (2000) Sedation and general anaesthesia in children undergoing MRI and CT: adverse events and outcomes. *Br. J. Anaesth.* **84(6)**, 743–748.
16. Marti-Bonmati, L., Ronchera-Oms, C. L., Casillas, C., Poyatos, C., Torrijo, C., and Jimenez, N. V. (1995) Randomised double-blind clinical trial of intermediate- versus high-dose chloral hydrate for neuroimaging of children. *Neuroradiology* **37(8)**, 687–691.
17. Ronchera-Oms, C. L., Casillas, C., Marti-Bonmati, L., Poyatos, C., Tomas, J., Sobejano, A., et al. (1994) Oral chloral hydrate provides effective and safe sedation in paediatric magnetic resonance imaging. *J. Clin. Pharm. Ther.* **19(4)**, 239–243.
18. Malviya, S., Voepel-Lewis, T., Prochaska, G., and Tait, A. R. (2000) Prolonged recovery and delayed side effects of sedation for diagnostic imaging studies in children. *Pediatrics* **105(3)**, E42.
19. Kao, S. C., Adamson, S. D., Tatman, L. H., and Berbaum, K. S. (1999) A survey of post-discharge side effects of conscious sedation using chloral hydrate in pediatric CT and MR imaging. *Pediatr. Radiol.* **29(4)**, 287–290.
20. Bloomfield, E. L., Masaryk, T. J., Caplin, A., Obuchowski, N. A., Schubert, A., Hayden, J., et al. (1993) Intravenous sedation for MR imaging of the brain and spine in children: pentobarbital versus propofol. *Radiology* **186(1)**, 93–97.
21. Hollman, G. A., Elderbrook, M. K., and VanDenLangenberg, B. (1995) Results of a pediatric sedation program on head MRI scan success rates and procedure duration times. *Clin. Pediatr. (Phila.)* **34(6)**, 300–305.
22. Beebe, D. S., Tran, P., Bragg, M., Stillman, A., Truwitt, C., and Belani, K. G. (2000) Trained nurses can provide safe and effective sedation for MRI in pediatric patients. *Can. J. Anaesth.* **47(3)**, 205–210.
23. Strain, J. D., Campbell, J. B., Harvey, L. A., and Foley, L. C. (1988) IV Nembutal: safe sedation for children undergoing CT. *AJR Am. J. Roentgenol.* **151(5)**, 975–979.
24. Coté, C. J., Karl, H. W., Notterman, D. A., Weinberg, J. A., and McCloskey, C. (2000) Adverse sedation events in pediatrics: analysis of medications used for sedation. *Pediatrics* **106(4)**, 633–644.
25. Rupprecht, T., Kuth, R., Bowing, B., Gerling, S., Wagner, M., and Rascher, W. (2000) Sedation and monitoring of paediatric patients undergoing open low-field MRI. *Acta Paediatr.* **89(9)**, 1077–1081.
26. Harned, R. K., 2nd, and Strain, J. D. (2001) MRI-compatible audio/visual system: impact on pediatric sedation. *Pediatr. Radiol.* **31(4)**, 247–250.
27. Kaste, S. C., Young, C. W., Holmes, T. P., and Baker, D. K. (1997) Effect of helical CT on the frequency of sedation in pediatric patients. *AJR Am. J. Roentgenol.* **168(4)**, 1001–1003.

28. White, K. S. (1995) Reduced need for sedation in patients undergoing helical CT of the chest and abdomen. *Pediatr. Radiol.* **25(5)**, 344–346.

29. Pappas, J. N., Donnelly, L. F., and Frush, D. P. (2000) Reduced frequency of sedation of young children with multisection helical CT. *Radiology* **215(3)**, 897–899.

30. Lim-Dunham, J. E., Narra, J., Benya, E. C., and Donaldson, J. S. (1997) Aspiration after administration of oral contrast material in children undergoing abdominal CT for trauma. *AJR Am. J. Roentgenol.* **169(4)**, 1015–1018.

31. Greenberg, S. B., Faerber, E. N., and Aspinall, C. L. (1991) High dose chloral hydrate sedation for children undergoing CT. *J. Comput. Assist. Tomogr.* **15(3)**, 467–469.

32. Hubbard, A. M., Markowitz, R. I., Kimmel, B., Kroger, M., and Bartko, M. B. (1992) Sedation for pediatric patients undergoing CT and MRI. *J. Comput. Assist. Tomogr.* **16(1)**, 3–6.

33. Pereira, J. K., Burrows, P. E., Richards, H. M., Chuang, S. H., and Babyn, P. S. (1993) Comparison of sedation regimens for pediatric outpatient CT. *Pediatr. Radiol.* **23(5)**, 341–344.

34. Pomeranz, E. S., Chudnofsky, C. R., Deegan, T. J., Lozon, M. M., Mitchiner, J. C., and Weber, J. E. (2000) Rectal methohexital sedation for computed tomography imaging of stable pediatric emergency department patients. *Pediatrics* **105(5)**, 1110–1114.

35. Moro-Sutherland, D. M., Algren, J. T., Louis, P. T., Kozinetz, C. A., and Shook, J. E. (2000) Comparison of intravenous midazolam with pentobarbital for sedation for head computed tomography imaging. *Acad. Emerg. Med.* **7(12)**, 1370–1375.

36. D'Agostino, J., and Terndrup, T. E. (2000) Chloral hydrate versus midazolam for sedation of children for neuroimaging: a randomized clinical trial. *Pediatr. Emerg. Care* **16(1)**, 1–4.

37. Kaye, R. D., Sane, S. S., and Towbin, R. B. (2000) Pediatric intervention: an update—part I. *J. Vasc. Interv. Radiol.* **11(6)**, 683–697.

38. Cotsen, M. R., Donaldson, J. S., Uejima, T., and Morello, F. P. (1997) Efficacy of ketamine hydrochloride sedation in children for interventional radiologic procedures. *AJR Am. J. Roentgenol.* **169(4)**, 1019–1022.

39. Malviya, S., Burrows, F. A., Johnston, A. E., and Benson, L. N. (1989) Anaesthetic experience with paediatric interventional cardiology. *Can. J. Anaesth.* **36(3 Pt 1)**, 320–324.

40. Coppel, D. L. and Dundee, J. W. (1972) Ketamine anesthesia for cardiac catheterisation. *Anaesthesia* **27**, 25–31.

41. Fyler, D. C., et al. (1980) Report of the New England Regional Infant Cardiac Program. *Pediatrics* **65(2 pt 2)**, 375–461.

42. Bing, R. J., Vandam, L. D., and Gray, F. D., Jr. (1947) Physiological studies in congenital heart disease I. Procedures. *Bulletin of Johns Hopkins Hospital* **80**, 107–120.

43. Rashkind, W. J. and Miller, W. W. (1966) Creation of an atrial septal defect without thoracotomy. A palliative approach to complete transposition of the great arteries. *JAMA* **196(11)**, 991–992.

44. Friesen, R. H. and Alswang, M. (1996) Changes in carbon dioxide tension and oxygen saturation during deep sedation for paediatric cardiac catheterization. *Paediatr. Anaesth.* **6(1)**, 15–20.
45. Cook, B. A., Bass, J. W., Nomizu, S., and Alexander, M. E. (1992) Sedation of children for technical procedures: current standard of practice. *Clin. Pediatr. (Phila.)* **31(3)**, 137–142.
46. Nahata, M. C., Clotz, M. A., and Krogg, E. A. (1985) Adverse effects of meperidine, promethazine and chlorpromazine for sedation in pediatric patients. *Clin. Pediatr.* **24**, 558–560.
47. Reier, C. E. and Johnstone, R. E. (1970) Respiratory depression: Narcotic versus narcotic-transquilizer combinations. *Anesth. Analg.* **49**, 119–124.
48. Snodgrass, W. R. and Dodge, W. F. (1989) Cocktail: Time for rational and safe alternatives. *Pediatr. Clin. North Am.* **36**, 1285–1291.
49. Bubien, R. S., Fisher, J. D., Gentzel, J. A., Murphy, E. K., Irwin, M. E., Shea, J. B., et al. (1998) NASPE expert consensus document: use of i.v. (conscious) sedation/analgesia by nonanesthesia personnel in patients undergoing arrhythmia specific diagnostic, therapeutic, and surgical procedures. *Pacing Clin. Electrophysiol.* **21(2)**, 375–385.
50. Sharpe, M. D., Dobkowski, W. B., Murkin, J. M., Klein, G., Guiraudon, G., and Yee, R. (1994) The electrophysiologic effects of volatile anesthetics and sufentanil on the normal atrioventricular conduction system and accessory pathways in Wolff-Parkinson-White syndrome. *Anesthesiology* **80(1)**, 63–70.
51. Gomez-Arnau, J., Marquez-Montes, J., and Avello, F. (1983) Fentanyl and droperidol effects on the refractoriness of the accessory pathway in the Wolff-Parkinson-White syndrome. *Anesthesiology* **58**, 307–13.
52. Sharpe, M. D., Dobkowski, W. B., Murkin, J. M., Klein, G., Guiraudon, G., and Yee, R. (1992) Alfentanil-midazolam anaesthesia has no electrophysiological effects upon the normal conduction system or accessory pathways in patients with Wolff-Parkinson-White Syndrome. *Can. J. Anaesth.* **39**, 816–21.
53. Napoli, K. L., Ingall, C. G., and Martin, G. R. (1996) Safety and efficacy of chloral hydrate sedation in children undergoing echocardiography. *J. Pediatr.* **129(2)**, 287–291.
54. Latson, L. A., Cheatham, J. P., Gumbiner, C. H., Kugler, J. D., Danford, D. A., Hofschire, P. J., et al. (1991) Midazolam nose drops for outpatient echocardiography sedation in infants. *Am. Heart J.* **121(1 pt 1)**, 209–210.
55. Wilson, S. (2000) Pharmacologic behavior management for pediatric dental treatment. *Pediatr. Clin. N. Am.* **47(5)**, 1159–1175.
56. Krippaehne, J. A. and Montgomery, M. T. (1992) Morbidity and mortality from pharmacosedation and general anesthesia in the dental office. *J. Oral Maxillofac. Surg.* **50(7)**, 691–699.
57. Iwasaki, J., Vann, W. F., Jr., Dilley, D. C., and Anderson, J. A. (1989) An investigation of capnography and pulse oximetry as monitors of pediatric patients sedated for dental treatment. *Pediatr. Dent.* **11(2)**, 111–117.
58. Croswell, R. J., Dilley, D. C., Lucas, W. J., Vann, and W. F., Jr. (1995) A comparison of conventional versus electronic monitoring of sedated pediatric dental patients. *Pediatr. Dent.* **17(5)**, 332–339.

59. Verwest, T. M., Primosch, R. E., and Courts, F. J. (1993) Variables influencing hemoglobin oxygen desaturation in children during routine restorative dentistry. *Pediatr. Dent.* **15(1)**, 25–29.
60. Fishbaugh, D. F., Wilson, S., Preisch, J. W., and Weaver, J. M., 2nd. (1997) Relationship of tonsil size on an airway blockage maneuver in children during sedation. *Pediatr. Dent.* **19(4)**, 277–281.
61. Needleman, H. L., Joshi, A., and Griffith, D. G. (1995) Conscious sedation of pediatric dental patients using chloral hydrate, hydroxyzine, and nitrous oxide—a retrospective study of 382 sedations. *Pediatr. Dent.* **17(7)**, 424–431.
62. Houpt, M. (1993) Project USAP the use of sedative agents in pediatric dentistry: 1991 update. *Pediatr. Dent.* **15(1)**, 36–40.
63. Avalos-Arenas, V., Moyao-Garcia, D., Nava-Ocampo, A. A., Zayas-Carranza, R. E., and Fragoso-Rios, R. (1998) Is chloral hydrate/hydroxyzine a good option for paediatric dental outpatient sedation? *Curr. Med. Res. Opin.* **14(4)**, 219–226.
64. Hasty, M. F., Vann, W. F., Jr., Dilley, D. C., and Anderson, J. A. (1991) Conscious sedation of pediatric dental patients: an investigation of chloral hydrate, hydroxyzine pamoate, and meperidine vs. chloral hydrate and hydroxyzine pamoate. *Pediatr. Dent.* **13(1)**, 10–19.
65. Veerkamp, J. S., van Amerongen, W. E., Hoogstraten, J., and Groen, H. J. (1991) Dental treatment of fearful children, using nitrous oxide. Part I: Treatment times. *ASDC J. Dent. Child.* **58(6)**, 453–457.
66. Wilson, S. (1996) A survey of the American Academy of Pediatric Dentistry membership: nitrous oxide and sedation. *Pediatr. Dent.* **18(4)**, 287–293.
67. Litman, R. S., Kottra, J. A., Verga, K. A., Berkowitz, R. J., and Ward, D. S. (1998) Chloral hydrate sedation: the additive sedative and respiratory depressant effects of nitrous oxide. *Anesth. Analg.* **86(4)**, 724–728.
68. Guidelines for the elective use of conscious sedation, deep sedation and general anesthesia in pediatric dental patients. (1998) *Pediatr. Dent.* **21**, 68–73.
69. Wilson, J. E. and Pendleton, J. M. (1989) Oligoanalgesia in the Emergency Department. *Am. J. Emerg. Med.* **7(6)**, 620–623.
70. Selbst, S. M. and Clark, M. (1990) Analgesic use in the emergency department. *Ann. Emerg. Med.* **19(9)**, 1010–1013.
71. Penrose, B. H. (1972) Aspiration pneumonitis following ketamine induction for general anesthesia. *Anesth. Analg.* **51(1)**, 41–43.
72. Sears, B. E. (1971) Complications of ketamine. Anesthesiology **35(2)**, 231.
73. Krauss, B. and Zurakowski, D. (1998) Sedation patterns in pediatric and general community hospital emergency departments. *Pediatr. Emerg. Care* **14(2)**, 99–103.
74. Graff, K. J., Kennedy, R. M., and Jaffe, D. M. (1996) Conscious sedation for pediatric orthopaedic emergencies. *Pediatr. Emerg. Care* **12(1)**, 31–35.
75. Cheng, E. Y., Nimphius, N., and Kampine, J. P. (1992) Anesthetic Drugs and Emergency Departments. *Anesth. Analg.* **74**, 272–275.
76. Havel, C. J., Strait, R. T., and Hennes, H. (1999) A Clinical Trial of Propofol vs Midazolam for Procedural Sedation in a Pediatric Emergency Department. *Academic Emergency Medicine* **6(10)**, 989–997.

77. Dickinson, R., Singer, A. J., and Carrion, W. (2001) Etomidate for pediatric sedation prior to fracture reduction. *Academic Emergency Medicine* **8(1)**, 74–77.
78. Lerman, B., Yoshida, D., and Levitt, M. A. (1996) A prospective evaluation of the safety and efficacy of methohexital in the emergency department. *Am. J. Emerg. Med.* **14(4)**, 351–354.
79. Green, S. M., Nakamura, R., and Johnson, N. E. (1990) Ketamine Sedation for Pediatric Procedures: Part 1, Prospective Series. *Ann. Emerg. Med.* **19**, 1024–1032.
80. Green, S. M. and Johnson, N. E. (1990) Ketamine Sedation for Pediatric Procedures: Part **2**, Review and Implications. *Ann. Emerg. Med.* **19**, 1033–1046.
81. Green, S. M., Hummel, C. B., Wittlake, W. A., Rothrock, S. G., Hopkins, G. A., and Garrett, W. (1999) What Is Optimal Dose of Intramuscular Ketamine for Pediatric Sedation? *Academic Emergency Medicine* **6(1)**, 21–26.

5

Adult Sedation by Site and Procedure

Norah N. Naughton, MD

1. INTRODUCTION

Procedures and diagnostic studies previously reserved for an operating room or intensive care unit (ICU) setting are now performed in outpatient ambulatory care centers, emergency departments, radiology, cardiology, and gastroenterology suites, and dental offices. Procedures of greater complexity and length are performed on patients with increasingly complex co-existing diseases. Elderly patients comprise a greater proportion of the population. This is coupled with the economic pressures to expedite care and maximize utilization of the diagnostic center. Although the practice of sedation analgesia has moved from the operating room to non-anesthesiologists, Joint Commission on the Accreditation of Health Care Organizations (JCAHO) standards of care for the assessment and treatment of patients is identical to that expected of anesthesiologists *(1)*. Essentially, practitioners must consider themselves anesthesiologists and maintain standards associated with their practice similar to those upheld in the operating room.

Certain principles apply to the practice, regardless of the location. The same standard of care must exist in all settings in the same institution *(1)*. Consistently applied and well-understood definitions of moderate and deep sedation and anesthesia must be accepted throughout all settings. Accurate clinical assessment of sedation level by the practitioner is crucial to maintaining the expected standards of care. Anesthesia may be considered deep sedation if the definitions are unclear. This may have an impact on patient safety, and can lead to practitioners practicing anesthesia when they are not credentialed. Countless clinical studies in the literature have addressed the efficacy and safety of a particular sedation "cocktail." These studies should be reviewed critically prior to adoption to clinical practice. Desaturation, airway management, cardiac arrest, and death are frequently evaluated to determine safety of a particular technique. However, the few available studies addressing the incidence of critical events suggest that the overall rate is

From: *Contemporary Clinical Neuroscience: Sedation and Analgesia for Diagnostic and Therapeutic Procedures*
Edited by: S. Malviya, N. N. Naughton, and K. K. Tremper © Humana Press Inc., Totowa, NJ

low. Critical event incident rates have been reported between 0.54 and 1.6% *(2,3)*, and the incident rate associated with death is estimated at 0.03% *(2)*. As a result, few clinical studies are large enough in scale to make accurate statements regarding the safety and efficacy of a particular sedation regime. The introduction of midazolam for sedation in 1986 serves as a cautionary tale. Over a 4-yr period a total of 86 deaths were reported to the Food and Drug Administration (FDA), and all but three occurred outside of the operating room *(4)*. The majority of deaths were associated with the concurrent administration of an opioid. A subsequent volunteer study found that administration of midazolam alone did not cause hypoxemia or apnea; however, co-administration of fentanyl resulted in hypoxemia in 92% of volunteers and apnea in 50% *(4)*. Recognizing the high risk of hypoxemia and apnea in patients receiving the combination of midazolam and opioid took 4 years.

A similar debate on the safety and efficacy of propofol for sedation by non-anesthesiologists continues. The answer is unlikely to be determined in a single study, and caution must be exercised before widespread adoption of its use. In addition to the low incident rate, clinical controlled trials are associated with investigators who are extensively trained in the use of the drug and skills associated with safe patient monitoring and support. This situation may or may not apply to the clinician who contemplates the use of the drug.

Fasting (NPO) guidelines for elective cases should be strictly maintained. The benefits of the procedure should be balanced with the risk of aspiration in urgent cases when the patient has a full stomach. Additional risks for aspiration include co-existing diabetes, trauma, opioid use, extremes of age, and obesity. The competency of the individuals involved in sedation practice must be maintained at the standards expected, regardless of the frequency of cases performed. Provisions for patient care should be a priority for low-volume sites, where maintenance of skills is difficult. Patients who are considered at risk and high risk to develop sedation analgesia-related complications are listed in Table 1. The presence of one or more of these risks warrants consideration of an anesthesiology consultation prior to initiation of the procedure.

2. RADIOLOGY

2.1. Interventional

Procedures associated with interventional radiology practice are listed in Table 2. A 1997 survey of interventional radiologists in academic and private practice revealed that the top three procedures performed were diagnostic angiography, abdominal or chest biopsy, and abscess or fluid drainage *(5)*.

Table 1
Factors Associated with Increased Risk
of Complications Associated with Sedation Analgesia

At-risk

High ASA classification
History of difficult intubation
Mallampati classification of III
Craniofacial abnormalities
Respiratory insufficiency
Sedation analgesia not expected to be successful

High risk

Morbid obesity
Extremes of age
Severe underlying cardiac, pulmonary, renal, hepatic, or central nervous system
  disease
Sleep apnea
Pregnancy

(Presence of one or more may suggest the need for anesthesiology consultation.)

Table 2
Procedures Associated with the Need for Sedation Analgesia

Categories of Interventional Procedures

Category	Procedure
Vascular diagnostic	Peripheral angiography, pulmonary angiography
Therapeutic	Angioplasty, atherectomy, placement of inferior vena cava filter, chemoembolization, transjugular intrahepatic portosystemic shunt (TIPS), vascular stent, venous access placement, and thrombolysis
Visceral diagnostic	Abdominal, retroperitoneal, or chest biopsy; diagnostic thoracentesis, or paracentesis
Therapeutic	Biliary drainage, percutaneous nephrostomy or nephrolithotomy, cholecystostomy, percutaneous abscess drainage, gastrostomy or jejunostomy, placement of biliary or ureteral stent, tube manipulation or change, and drainage of empyema

From ref. *(5)*: Mueller, P. R., Wittenberg, K. H., Kaufman, J. A., and Lee, M. J. (1997) Patterns of anesthesia and nursing care for interventional radiology procedures: A national survey of physician practices and preferences. *Radiology* **202,** 339–343.

In general, investigators found that most diagnostic vascular and visceral procedures required less sedation, usually no greater than moderate. Therapeutic procedures usually required moderate to deep sedation. Examples included TIPS, biliary dilatation and drainage, nephrolithotomy, and stricture dilation. The group of patients that required general anesthesia were those who underwent catheter manipulation through solid organs, such as, transjugular intrahepatic portosystemic shunt (TIPS) and nephrolithotomy. Patients selected for neuroradiological procedures with altered mental status, increased intracranial pressure, and those who are uncooperative, may require general anesthesia *(7)*.

Patients may be positioned supine, lateral, or prone. The patient may be at a distance from the individual responsible for monitoring, making the level of consciousness and airway patency difficult to evaluate. Careful titration of sedation medication is important in these situations.

A prospective survey of patients showed that those who had previously experienced a similar procedure were less anxious, had a greater understanding of the procedure, and anticipated less pain *(6)*. All patients, whether undergoing a vascular or nonvascular procedure, overestimated their anticipated pain. In particular, patients scheduled for diagnostic visceral procedures significantly overestimated their pain. This may have occurred because a high percentage of those patients had no previous experience. In addition, pain and patient satisfaction were not necessarily correlative.

2.2. Noninterventional

Magnetic resonance imaging (MRI) examinations comprise the majority of noninterventional radiographic procedures that require sedation in the adult population. This is primarily because of a history of claustrophobia (3–7%) or anxiety over the unnatural space, movement restrictions, and the loud "drumming" noise of the scanner. Three to 10 percent of examinations cannot be completed because of such stresses *(8)*. This may have a considerable impact on the cost related to utilization of the scanner.

Complying with standards of care as well as the need for personnel and resources necessary for intravenous (iv) sedation require time and money, and may slow the patient flow of scheduled cases. Anticipating who may require sedation before the procedure starts may reduce the number of failed examinations. Factors associated with the need for sedation include gender, women utilizing sedation more than men, patients having a brain MRI, and patients who had undergone prior MRI procedures *(8)*. Several investigators have found that the use of intranasal midazolam significantly reduces the percentage of patients with claustrophobia that required iv sedation *(9,10)*.

Bluemke et al. reviewed a sedation analgesia database of 6,093 scheduled cases between 1991 and 1998 to assess safety, effectiveness, and the effect of the skill level of nurses on the examinations *(11)*. Of this group, 78.1% required sedation, primarily because the majority of patients were in the pediatric age group. However, 20% of patients were adults. They observed a complication rate of 0.42%, and no deaths occurred. The most common complication was oxygen desaturation, and 93.5% of examinations were completed. Specialized nurses took less time to adequately sedate the patient compared to general radiology and inpatient nurses. Inpatient nurses from hospital wards had the longest sedation time and the greatest variability. From these results, one can conclude that sedation for MRI is safe, and effective, and utilization of specialized nurses in a busy center can decrease the cost associated with down time of a scanner.

Challenges are posed by the magnetic field generated by the scanner, and are reviewed in detail in Chapter 8. Patients with cardiac pacemakers, certain heart valves, vascular clips, large metallic prosthetic implants, cochlear implants, ferromagnetic stapedial replacement prostheses, and pregnant women in the first trimester are not candidates for MRI examinations. Loose ferromagnetic objects such as scissors, clipboards, oxygen cylinders, keys, and stethoscopes can become uncontrolled accelerating objects within the magnetic field. Conventional anesthesia machines cannot be used near the magnet, and special monitoring equipment is required to measure blood pressure, oxygen saturation, electrocardiogram (ECG), body temperature, and end-tidal CO_2 *(12)*. Nonetheless, these vital signs must be documented during intended moderate or deep sedation.

3. PULMONARY

3.1. Bronchoscopy

Bronchoscopy is performed for a variety of diagnostic and therapeutic procedures. A postal survey in 1989 of bronchoscopic practice in North America indicated that 74% of physicians either sometimes or routinely administer sedation for fiberoptic bronchoscopy *(13)*. Both anxiety and pain can contribute to the patient's experience. Sixty-two percent of patients are anxious, and fear pain and difficulty in breathing during the procedure *(14)*. Pain is caused by passage of the bronchoscope through the nose and glottis. However, some investigators consider sedation unnecessary to obtain a satisfactory examination and a comfortable patient. Most practitioners directly apply local anesthetics to the nasopharyngeal airway, glottis, and bronchotracheal tree. Good patient satisfaction has been reported using only local anesthesia *(15)*. Bronchoscopy generally lasts between 30 and 40 min, and is performed on an outpatient basis. The argument has been made that sedation for this short procedure may prolong the hospital stay and increase cost. In addition, sedation may be associated with oxygen desaturation. Desaturation episodes occur often during bronchoscopy, regardless of whether sedation is used or not *(16,17)*. The hypoxemia has been attributed to the presence of the fiberoptic bronchoscope itself *(16)* or to the respiratory depressant effects of the sedative medication *(18)*. Sedation may be associated with up to half of the major life- threatening complications associated with bronchoscopy.

Despite these findings, pre-procedure sedation is commonly used. Improved patient tolerance, satisfaction, and acceptance of repeat examinations has been associated with the use of sedation. These benefits are believed to outweigh the risks *(19)*. Interestingly, physicians rated the patients' tolerance much higher than the patients' rating, suggesting that physicians do not fully appreciate patients' responses to the procedure. Agents commonly used by bronchoscopists to facilitate the examination include local anesthesia—usually lidocaine, anti-cholingerics to reduce secretions, codeine as an antitussive, benzodiazepines for anxiolysis and amnesia, and opioids for analgesia. Co-administration of clonidine facilitates sedation, blunts the hemodynamic responses to bronchoscopy, and reduces requirements of other sedative agents. A comprehensive review of these agents and their use in bronchoscopy is beyond the scope of this section; however, a recent review was published by Matot and Kramer *(20)*.

Sedation can be accomplished in a variety of ways using a variety of agents. However, the usual hemodynamic response to bronchoscopy—an increase in heart rate and blood pressure together with episodes of oxygen desaturation—should be anticipated. The incidence and severity of respiratory depression is probably correlated to the medication dose, an effect greater with the combination of benzodiazepines and opioids than either agent used alone *(4)*.

4. GASTROENTEROLOGY

A variety of diagnostic and therapeutic procedures are performed by gastroenterologists, and in some cases, surgeons. Commonly performed procedures include esophagogastroduodenoscopy (EGD), esophageal dilatation, endoscopic retrograde cholangiopancreatography (ERCP), colonoscopy, and flexible sigmoidoscopy *(21)*. Operative endoscopy (esophageal dilatation and stenting, percutaneous endoscopic gastrostomy) which may be painful and unpleasant, and long procedures, specifically ERCP, are usually performed with sedation analgesia. Controversy exists as to whether sedation analgesia is necessary for flexible sigmoidoscopy and colonoscopy. In the

United Kingdom and the United States, the majority of colonoscopies are performed with sedation analgesia, usually a combination of benzodiazepines and opioid. In France, 80% are completed under general anesthesia, and in Germany and Finland, sedation analgesia is rarely if ever used *(22)*. Rex et al, conducted a study in the United States to find factors associated with patients willing to try colonoscopy without sedation *(23)*. Male sex, increasing age, and lack of abdominal pain were associated with undergoing colonoscopy without sedation. Twenty-seven percent of patients approached agreed to be randomized to receive routine sedation with meperidine and midazolam or as-needed sedation only, and 7% requested no sedation.

In the sedation as-needed only group, 94% of examinations were completed. Colonoscopists and patients both rated their pain higher than the routine sedation group. Mean time to discharge was 10.1 min vs 54.6 min respectively, and medical charges were $104 more in the sedation group. Despite having more pain, all patients in this group said they would return to the same endoscopist. The authors contend that 34% of patients were either willing or requested colonoscopy without sedation, and suggested offering sedationless colonoscopy to select patients. Advantages cited for sedationless endoscopy include shorter recovery time, quicker return to work, and decreased use of monitoring, pharmacy, and staff costs, believed to account for 30–50% of overall procedure cost *(24)*. In addition, serious cardiorespiratory complications associated with sedation, estimated to occur at a rate of 5.4/1,000 cases, could potentially be avoided.

Mortality associated with endoscopic procedures is estimated between 0.5 and 3/10,000 procedures and morbidity at 6–54/10,000 *(4)*. Many investigators believe that the benefits of sedation outweigh these risks because patient tolerance and willingness to undergo repeat examinations is improved with sedation *(25)*. In addition, only a minority of patients in the United States are willing to undergo endoscopy without sedation *(26)*.

Cardiopulmonary complications are believed to account for more than 50% of deaths related to endoscopy, although the pathogenic mechanisms are unknown *(27)*. A combination of tachycardia and hypoxia may explain the complications *(22)*. Of patients undergoing colonoscopy under sedation analgesia, 35% exhibited tachycardia (rate > 100), and 45% exhibited arterial oxygen desaturation in a study from Denmark *(28)*. In a study comparing midazolam to propofol sedation for ERCP, 5% of patients experienced temporary desaturations to <85% *(29)*, and almost one-third of patients undergoing endoscopic ultrasonography (EUS) examinations under minimal sedation experienced desaturation to < 90% *(30)*. A direct association between desaturation and myocardial ischemia has not been shown, and supplemental oxygen has not reliably reduced the incidence of these complications. However, the routine use of supplemental oxygen should be seriously considered in all patients, particularly the elderly and those with co-existing cardiopulmonary disease.

A combination of benzodiazepine and opioid is the most common regimen utilized for endoscopic sedation. A variety of agents, administrative routes, and combinations have been suggested to provide successful sedation. The most commonly used agents include midazolam, valium, fentanyl, and meperidine (22).

It is advisable to keep the dose of agent as low as possible for the desired effect; however, this is particularly true for endoscopists who face the patient with cirrhosis. Assy et al. demonstrated the majority of patients with well-compensated cirrhosis had subclinical hepatic encephalopathy that was worsened for a minimum of 2 h with even modest doses of midazolam (mean dose 2 mg) (31).

Propofol, a short-acting anesthetic agent, has been proposed for use in sedation by non-anesthesiologists. Considerable controversy exists concerning its use in this setting. Proponents cite its rapid onset, improved tolerance to the examination, and quicker recovery times as reasons for its use. However, its narrow therapeutic range must be acknowledged. Wehrmann et al. (29) reported on the use of propofol for routine ERCP. Although the advantages cited here were noted, one patient had an episode of apnea lasting 8 min and required management by mask ventilation. It has been stated that the "psychology of the endoscopist needs to be more akin to that of an airline pilot or anaesthetist" to avoid complications associated with sedation (32). This is certainly the case if hypnotic agents such as propofol, with narrow therapeutic ranges, are to be used. It is unlikely that skills similar to those of an anesthesiologist would be universal, or easily maintained by endoscopists to support the routine use of propofol and be associated with an acceptable complication rate. Two recent editorials on the subject of propofol use consider this an anesthetic agent to be used only by anesthesiologists (33,34).

The intended use of opioid and benzodiazepine antagonists should be discouraged. A 1989 American Society for Gastrointestinal Endoscopy (ASGE) survey of endoscopic sedation and monitoring practices showed that 30% of endoscopists regularly use naloxone as part of their sedation analgesia plan (39). The administration of sedation agents should be titrated to the minimum amount to achieve the desired effect. Naloxone administration can be associated with the acute onset of hypertension, myocardial ischemia, and pulmonary edema. Several investigators have advocated the routine use of the benzodiazepine antagonist flumazenil following sedation with midazolam. Postsedation observation times were significantly shortened with flumazenil, an effect that could reduce costs and increase patient throughput in a busy diagnostic center *(22)*. However, when patients were almost fully awake by the end of the procedure, there was no difference in recovery times between patients who did and did not receive the antagonist *(27)*. Therefore, its use is unnecessary when appropriate doses of midazolam or valium are administered. A randomized double-blind crossover study was performed in human volunteers to assess the effects of flumazenil on alertness and psychomotor function. Although alertness had returned to baseline within 60 min of flumazenil administration, gait stability had not *(40)*. The authors recommended that discharge time should not be based on subjective assessment of alertness in patients whose iv midazolam is reversed with flumazenil. Taken together, the results of these studies do not support the routine use of reversal agents as a part of the sedation plan. The use of these agents should be reserved for those patients who inadvertently reach a level of sedation that is deeper than intended and experience cardiorespiratory instability. Furthermore, the use of a reversal agent must not be considered a substitute for standard resuscitative measures that may be indicated. Finally, once a reversal agent is used, the patient must be monitored until the anticipated effects of the sedative agent have worn off, because the half life of most reversal agents is shorter than that of the sedative agents.

Although elderly patients are managed by a variety of specialists, 30% of all patients undergoing upper gastrointestinal endoscopy in the United Kingdom are over 70 yr of age *(35)*. Bell and associates found that the dose of midazolam needed to adequately sedate for upper gastrointestinal endoscopy decreased markedly with age in both sexes *(36)*. The mean dose of midazolam required in patients over 70 was approximately 2.0–5.0 mg, with only 7.2% requiring more than 5.0 mg. Clearly, the potential for accidental overdose is greater in patients over 70 yr of age. The ASGE recently reviewed modifications in endoscopic practice for the elderly *(37)*.

A clinical situation unique to gastroenterology is emergency upper GI endoscopy for gastrointestinal (GI) bleeding. Significant hepatic impairment, hypovolemia, anemia, labile hemodynamics, and the greater risk of vomiting and aspirating blood exist *(21)*. A recently published survey of prominent gastroenterologists examined the practice of intubation, aspiration prevention, and use of sedation analgesia in the patient with an acute GI bleed *(38)*. All of the respondents used sedation analgesia under this circumstance at doses necessary to achieve the required sedation level. Measures used to prevent aspiration in this setting were not mentioned.

As previously mentioned, the cirrhotic patient is at increased risk of complications secondary to sedation analgesia. There is a reduced ability of the liver to metabolize, detoxify, and excrete many of the agents commonly used. Drug elimination half-lives are usually increased. Therefore, drug dosages should be decreased compared to the healthy patient, with longer intervals between redosing. Midazolam in cirrhotics has been shown to have prolonged clearance and sedation up to 6 h following administration. Opioid actions are secondary to the effects on the central nervous system (CNS), and should be used with caution in patients with hepatic encephalopathy. The respiratory depressant effects may be exaggerated in patients with hepatopulmonary syndrome, hepatic hydrothorax, tense ascites, or hepatic encephalopathy. It is recommended to decrease the dose of agents by one-half of that given to a standard healthy patient, and to administer the medication in small increments.

5. DENTISTRY AND ORAL SURGERY

Procedures performed under sedation analgesia include removal of partially impacted teeth, carious teeth restoration, and minor prosthetic surgery. Patients with severe learning disabilities and challenging behavior are frequently managed under general anesthesia. However, a recent review of the literature suggests that sedation analgesia, initially administered via the oral or nasal route to allow for iv cannulation followed by iv maintenance, can result in a high percentage of procedure completion (41). Intravenous techniques combined with local anesthesia represent the most common approach, yetsupplemental inhalation sedation with nitrous oxide is also used. Delivery of concentrations of nitrous oxide less than 50% provide analgesia with minimal respiratory depression. Caution must be exercised when titrating additional iv sedation, as deep sedation may occur.

Two studies have characterized the morbidity and mortality associated with sedation and general anesthesia in the office setting (42,43). A closed-claim analysis of anesthetic related deaths and permanent injuries reviewed 13 cases between 1974 and 1989 (42). A disproportionate number of patients were over the age of 35. The majority were classified as ASA 2 or 3 with multiple co-existing comorbidities including obesity, cardiac disorder (mitral valve disease, uncontrolled cardiac symptoms, hypertensive cardiac disease with cardiomegaly), heavy smoking, epilepsy, and chronic obstructive pulmonary disease (COPD). Use of multiple sedative agents was common. No patients were monitored by a physician anesthesiologist. Intra-operative monitoring revealed a common lack of vigilance. Four patients had no moni-

Table 3
Common Cardiology Procedures that Require Sedation Analgesia

Cardioversions
Permanent pacemaker insertion
Electrophysiology testing
Radiofrequency catheter ablation
Automatic implantable cardioverter-defibrillator (AICD) placement
Cardiac catheterization
Percutaneous transluminal coronary angioplasty
Transesophageal echocardiography

toring, and in three instances, blood pressure and ECG monitoring was available, but only used when an emergency was identified. The main cause of morbid events was hypoxia secondary to airway obstruction or respiratory depression. All patients died except one, who suffered severe brain damage. Ten of 13 cases were considered avoidable, either by improved patient selection or intraprocedure monitoring.

One year later, Krippaehne and Montgomery published their review of morbidity and mortality associated with 43 cases obtained from nine state dental boards *(43)*. The majority of morbidity and mortality occurred in young (mean age 18) healthy (75% ASA 1) patients who received multiple sedative agents with limited monitoring and resuscitative efforts. In these cases, deficiencies in patient management surrounding underused monitoring and resuscitation efforts, rather than poor patient selection, may have led to the undesirable outcomes.

Airway obstruction is a genuine hazard in oral surgery and sedation. Various dental devices occupy the airway, and manipulation of the tongue can lead to swelling. Blood, secretions, and foreign bodies can be aspirated, leading to oxygen desaturation.

6. CARDIOLOGY

Numerous cardiac procedures are performed under sedation analgesia (Table 3) and vary in the sedation depth required for a successful examination. Local anesthesia is commonly used to reduce the pain associated with insertion of cannulas and instruments.

It is common for patients to have serious co-existing medical conditions in addition to their cardiac disease. A cardiac pre-procedural medical review should include assessment of the ECG, left ventricular function, history of angina, peripheral vascular disease, respiratory status, renal/hepatic function, fluid status, and chronic medications. Medications required for control of dysrhythmias, angina, and hypertension should be continued until the time of the procedure.

Diagnostic electrophysiologic studies, pacemaker implantation, cardiac catheterization, and transesophageal echocardiography (TEE) usually require levels of sedation defined as anxiolysis or moderate (sedation analgesia). Deep sedation is rarely, if ever, required *(44)*. This statement is based on how deep sedation is defined. The North American Society of Pacing and Electrophysiology (NASPE) Expert Consensus Document on the use of sedation analgesia by nonanesthesia personnel defines a single category for light (anxiolysis), three subcategories of moderate sedation, and single categories for deep sedation, and general anesthesia *(44)* (Table 4). Advanced sleep is defined as absent response to verbal stimuli, limited response to physical stimuli, present to limited maintenance of a patent airway, and limited respiratory function for a total SED score of 3–4. Deep sedation is defined as absent response to physical stimuli, in addition to absent response to verbal stimuli, and absent to limited patent airway and respiratory function, for a total SED score of 0–2. The Society further states that deep sedation requires the presence of an anesthesiologist or nurse anesthetist. However, the consensus by the JCAHO and American Society of Anesthesiologists (ASA) defines deep sedation to include a response to a vigorous physical stimulus, which by strict interpretation of the NASPE document would be equivalent to advance sleep. The Society recommends cardioversion, radiofrequency (RF) catheter ablation, and automatic implantable cardioverter-defibrillator (AICD) placement be performed under advanced sleep. But is this really deep sedation, and according to the consensus statement, would it require the presence of an anesthesiologist? These examples underscore the importance of universally accepted sedation definitions and rating scales. This would eliminate confusing interpretations of subtle definitions and should result in appropriate monitoring for any given sedation level.

Published experience with the safety and cost-effectiveness of anesthesia delivered by non-anesthesiologists must be interpreted with caution prior to adoption of the practice. Tobin et al. reported on 1,473 consecutive elective cardioversions performed between 1993 and 1995 *(45)*. Methohexital was administered as needed to achieve an asleep and sluggish or unresponsive patient (Ramsey score 5 or 6). The authors concluded that the practice is safe and results in considerable cost savings. However, the sedation analgesia team consisted of one cardiology fellow, one attending cardiac electrophysiologist, and two registered nurses. Physicians had on-the-job training in airway management and formal training in iv sedation analgesia tech-

Table 4
Definition of Sedation Levels by the North American Society of Pacing and Electrophysiology Spectrum/Continuum of Sedation (SED); Scores: 2 = present; 1 = limited; 0 = absent

Level	Consciousness	Responds Purposefully To				Total SED Score
		Verbal stim.	Physical stim.	Airway	Respiration	
		2	2	2	2	8
Light sedation	Near normal	2	2	2	2	8
IV sedation						
A) Sleepy		1–2	2	2	2	7–8
B) Sleep		0–1	1	2	*1–2	4–6
C) Advanced sleep		0	1	†1–2	1	3–4
Deep sedation	Very depressed	0	0	0–1	0–1	0–2
Gen. anesthesia	Unarousable	0	0	0–(–1)	0–(–1)	0–(1–2)

*May need Nasal O_2 to maintain O_2 saturation >90%; should be routine, especially for SED scores <7. Capnography is also proving useful and may become routine.

†May need limited and transient support.

This SED table represents a variation of the Aldrete scoring system (26–28) developed for postanesthetic recovery assessment, and adapted for iv/conscious sedation.

Reproduced with permission from ref. (44): Bubien, R. S., Fisher, J. D., Gentzel, J. A., Murphy, E. K., Irwin, M. E., Shea, J. B., et al. (1998) NASPE expert consensus document: Use of IV (Conscious) sedation/analgesia by nonanesthesia personnel in patients undergoing arrhythmia specific diagnostic, therapeutic, and surgical procedures. *PACE* **21**, 375–385.

niques. Registered nurses completed a formal competency-based education program that was formally reassessed on an annual basis. Practical skills were acquired by on-the-job supervised training. It is possible that many cardiac sedation teams do not have a similar rigorous training program to acquire this level of educational and clinical skills. The complication rate was 0.7% (10/1,473). There were no deaths; however, 30% of patients with complications required endotracheal intubation by an anesthesiologist. The authors emphasized that the availability of emergency anesthesia back-up should be a prerequisite for the administration of general anesthesia by non-anesthesiologists. It is debatable whether this practice is safe, despite the cost savings. What is the acceptable, possibly life-threatening complication rate from sedation for an elective procedure? In my opinion, it should be as close to zero as possible. This is most likely to be achieved when general anesthesia is administered by anesthesiologists. It is currently recognized that deep sedation is required for patient comfort and satisfactory completion of the examination for many cardiac procedures. Currently, most institutions have created credentialing requirements for the practice of moderate and deep sedation by non-anesthesiologists. Staff should agree upon and meet these deep sedation requirements if patients are intentionally rendered responsive only to a deep physical stimulus. Patients who are intentionally rendered under general anesthesia should be managed by an anesthesiologist.

Historically, radiofrequency (RF) catheter ablation and AICD placement were primarily completed with the patient under general anesthesia managed by an anesthesiologist. Reports of successful RF ablation and AICD implantation with patients under moderate to deep sedation managed by non-anesthesiologists have changed this practice (46). Indications for RF catheter ablation are listed in Table 5. This procedure may take an indefinite period of time. Physical sensations experienced by patients range from moderate to severe pain. Back pain may result from lengthy immobilization. RF energy application has been experienced as mild chest discomfort to severe pain (47). Anticipation of the need for general anesthesia in some patients should be part of the preassessment. A review of the electrophysiologic effects of commonly used sedative and analgesic agents has been reviewed; however, the clinical importance appears to be negligible (47). Recent developments in transvenous placement of AICD devices along with placement of the pulse generator in the pectoral region have resulted in successful placement under local anesthesia and moderate sedation. However, patients experience discomfort during defibrillation threshold testing, when multiple discharges are delivered. During these periods, deep sedation and possibly general anesthesia are necessary for patient comfort (48).

Table 5
Indications for RF Ablation

Paroxysmal supraventricular tachycardia
AV nodal reentrant tachycardia
Accessory pathway tachycardia
Atrial tachycardia
Atrial flutter
Atrial fibrillation*
Ventricular tachycardia
Bundle branch reentrant tachycardia
Monomorphic idiopathic tachycardia
Monomorphic tachycardia from CAD

CAD, coronary artery disease.
*May require AV nodal ablation for control.
Reproduced with permission from ref. *(47)*: Rodeman, B. J. (1997) Conscious sedation during electrophysiology testing and radiofrequency catheter ablation. *Critical Care Nursing Clinics of North America* **9(3)**, 313–324.

7. AMBULATORY CENTERS

Cost containment, efficiency in patient management, and a desire for increased control have contributed to the success of ambulatory surgicenters and office-based practice. However, patient assessment and care standards expected by the JCAHO are identical to those expected of a traditional operating room setting and anesthesiologists, surgeons, and nurses. Appropriately credentialed staff and required emergency resuscitation equipment and plan for back-up help is expected. Adequate intraprocedure monitoring and an acceptable recovery area with appropriate discharge criteria are required.

Patient selection is one of the components of a successful operation. Several societies that represent specialists who engage in practice in these settings suggest that only physical status ASA 1 or 2 patients should be managed in the office setting *(50–52)*. Heart rate and mean arterial pressure increased by 3.9% and 4.7%, respectively, in patients undergoing a procedure under local anesthesia. Patients with a history of pre-existing hypertension or cardiovascular disease exhibited increases of 12.0% and 21.4%, and 25.0% and 75.0%, respectively *(50)*. The psychological perspective of the patient should also be considered. Patients should be motivated to have a procedure performed while they are sleepy but responsive, and should understand that the overall experience is different from that expected under major anesthesia.

Intended deep sedation is discouraged and recommended by some to be administered only by an anesthesiologist or nurse anesthetist under the direction of an anesthesiologist *(51)*. The objective is to maintain adequate sedation with minimal risk. A review of 100,000 anesthetic cases showed that those performed under conscious sedation had the highest mortality rate (209/10,000) compared to those performed under general (36/10,000 inhalational with narcotic) or major regional anesthesia (146/10,000 spinal and 112/10,000 epidural) *(53)*. The Federated Ambulatory Surgery Association (FASA) surveyed over 87,000 cases completed among 40 freestanding surgicenters, and found that those performed under local anesthesia with sedation had the highest complication rate compared to those managed with local only, general, or major regional anesthesia *(50)*. Overall, the majority of adverse outcomes associated with sedation analgesia are cardiorespiratory, and this is also true for the ambulatory setting. Another review of 700 incidences of moderate sedation revealed a 28% incidence of significant transient hypoxemia (SaO_2 <90%) *(50)*.

Sedation analgesia can be safely performed in the ambulatory setting. However, careful patient selection, skilled personnel, appropriate monitoring during and after the procedure, and acceptable discharge criteria are required to optimize the outcome and patient satisfaction.

REFERENCES

1. Joint Commission on Accreditation of Healthcare Organizations. (2000) *Comprehensive Accreditation Manual for Hospitals*. The Official Handbook. Oakbrook Terrace, IL.
2. Arrowsmith, J. B., Gerstman, B. B., Fleischer, D. E., and Benjamin, S. B. (1991) Results from the American Society for Gastrointestinal Endoscopy/U. S. Food and Drug Administration collaborative study on complication rates and drug use during gastrointestinal endoscopy. *Gastrointest. Endosc.* **37(4)**, 421–427.
3. Poe, S. S., Nolan, M. T., Dang, D., Schauble, J., Oechsle, D. G., Kress, L., et al. (2001) Ensuring safety of patients receiving sedation for procedures: evaluation of Clinical Practice Guidelines. *Joint Commission Journal on Quality Improvement* **27(1)**, 28–41.
4. Bailey, P. L., Pace, N. L., Ashburn, M. A., Moll, J. W. B., East, K. A., and Stanley, T. H. (1990) Frequent hypoxemia and apnea after sedation with midazolam and fentanyl. *Anesthesiology* **73**, 826–830.
5. Mueller, P. R., Wittenberg, K. H., Kaufman, J. A., and Lee, M. J. (1997) Patterns of anesthesia and nursing care for interventional radiology procedures: a national survey of physician practices and preferences. *Radiology* **202**, 339–343.
6. Mueller, P. R., Biswal, S., Halpern, E. F., Kaufman, J. A., and Lee, M. J. (2000) Interventional radiologic procedures: Patient anxiety, perception of pain, understanding of procedure, and satisfaction with medication—A prospective study. *Patient Perception of Interventional Radiologic Procedures* **215(3)**, 684–688.

7. Hiew, C.Y. Hart, G. K., Thomson, K. R., and Hennessy, O. F. (1995) Analgesia and sedation in interventional radiological procedures. *Australas. Radiol.* **39,** 128–134.
8. Murphy, K. J. and Brunberg, J. A. (1997) Adult claustrophobia, anxiety and sedation in MRI. *Magn. Reson. Imaging* **15(1),** 51–54.
9. Hollenhorst, J., Münte, S., Friedrich, L., Heine, J., Leuwer, M., Becker, H., et al. (2001) Using intranasal midazolam spray to prevent claustrophobia induced by MR Imaging. *American Journal of Radiology* **176,** 865–868.
10. Moss, M. L., Buongiorno, P. A., and Clancy, V. A. (1993) Intranasal midazolam for claustrophobia in MRI. *J. Comput. Assisted Tomogr.* **17(6),** 991–992.
11. Bluemke, D. A. and Breiter, S. N. (2000) Sedation procedures in MR Imaging: Safety, effectiveness, and nursing effect on examinations. *Radiology* **216(3),** 645–652.
12. Rao, C. C. and Krishna, G. (1994) Anaesthetic considerations for magnetic resonance imaging. *Annals Academy of Medicine Singapore* **23,** 531–535.
13. Prakash, U. B. S., Offord, K. P., and Stubbs, S. E. (1991) Bronchoscopy in North America: The ACCP survey. *Chest* **100,** 1668–1675.
14. Poi, P. J. H., Chuah, S. Y., Srinivas, P., and Liam, C. K. (1998) Common fears of patients undergoing bronchoscopy. *Eur. Respir. J.* **11(5),** 1147–1149.
15. Allen, M. B. (1995) Sedation in fibreoptic bronchoscopy. *BMJ* **310,** 872–873.
16. Dubrawsky, C., Awe, R. J., and Jenkins, D. E. (1975) The effect of bronchofiberscopic examination on oxygen status. *Chest* **67,** 137–140.
17. Milman, N., Faurschou, P., Grode, G., and Jorgensen, A. (1994) Pulse oximetry during fiberoptic bronchoscopy in local anesthesia: Frequency of hypoxemia and effect of oxygen supplementation. *Respiration* **61,** 342–347.
18. Shelley, M. P., Wilson, P., and Norman, J. (1989) Sedation for fiberoptic bronchoscopy. *Thorax* **44,** 769–775.
19. Putinati, S., Ballerin, L., Corbetta, L., Trevisani, L., and Potena, A. (1999) Patient satisfaction with conscious sedation for bronchoscopy. *Chest* **115(5),** 1437–1440.
20. Matot, I. and Kramer, M. R. (2000) Sedation in outpatient bronchoscopy. *Respir. Med.* **94,** 1145–1153.
21. Landrum, L. (1997) Conscious sedation in the endoscopy setting. *Critical Care Nursing Clinics of North America* **9(3),** 355–360.
22. Bell, G. D. (2000) Premedication, preparation, and surveillance. *Endoscopy* **32(2),** 92–100.
23. Rex, D. K., Imperiale, T. F., and Portish, V. (1999) Patients willing to try colonoscopy without sedation: associated clinical factors and results of a randomized controlled trial. *Gastrointest. Endosc.* **49(5),** 554–559.
24. Mulcahy, H. E., Hennessy, E., Connor, P., Rhodes, B., Patchett, S. E., Farthing, M. J. G., et al. (2001) Changing patterns of sedation use for routine outpatient diagnostic gastroscopy between 1989 and 1998. *Aliment. Pharmacol. Ther.* **15,** 217–220.
25. Zuccaro, G. (2000) Sedation and sedationless endoscopy. *Gastrointest. Endosc.* **10(1),** 1–20.

26. Early, D. S., Saifuddin, T., Johnson, J. C., King, P. D., and Marshall, J. B. (1999) Patient attitudes toward undergoing colonoscopy without sedation. *Am. J. Gastroenterol.* **94,** 1892–1895.

27. Lazzaroni, M. and Bianchi-Porro, G. (1999) Premedication, preparation, and surveillance. *Endoscopy* **31(1),** 2–8.

28. Holm, C., Christensen, M., Rasmussen, V., Schulze, S., and Rosenberg, J. (1998) Hypoxemia and myocardial ischaemia during colonoscopy. *Scand. J. Gastroenterol.* **33,** 769–772.

29. Wehrmann, T., Kokabpick, S., Lembcke, B., Caspary, W. F., and Seifert, H. (1999) Efficacy and safety of intravenous propofol sedation during routine ERCP: A prospective, controlled study. *Gastrointest. Endosc.* **49(6),** 677–683.

30. Allgayer, H., Pohl, C., and Kruis, W. (1999) Arterial oxygen desaturation during endoscopic ultrasonography: a safety evaluation in outpatients. *Endoscopy* **31,** 447–451.

31. Assy, N., Rosser, B. G., Grahame, G. R., and Minuk, G. Y. (1999) Risk of sedation for upper GI endoscopy exacerbating subclinical hepatic encephalopathy in patients with cirrhosis. *Gastrointest. Endosc.* **49(6),** 690–694.

32. McCloy, R. (1992) Asleep on the job: Sedation and monitoring during endoscopy. *Scand. J. Gastroenterol.* **27 (Suppl 192),** 97–101.

33. Graber, R. G. (1999) Propofol in the endoscopy suite: an anesthesiologist's perspective. Editorial in *Gastrointest. Endosc.* **49(6),** 803–806.

34. Bell G. D. and Charlton, J. E. (2000) Colonoscopy—Is sedation necessary and is there any role for intravenous propofol? *Endoscopy* **32(3),** 264–267.

35. Quine, M. A., Bell, G. D., McCloy, R. F., Charlton, J. E., Devlin, H. B., and Hopkins, A. (1995) Prospective audit of upper gastrointestinal endoscopy in two regions of England: safety, staffing, and sedation methods. *Gut* **36,** 462–467.

36. Bell, G. D., Spickett, G. P., Reeve, P. A., Morden, A., and Logan, R. F. A. (1987) Intravenous midazolam for upper gastrointestinal endoscopy: a study of 800 consecutive cases relating dose to age and sex of patient. *Brit. J. Clin. Pharmacol.* **23,** 241–243.

37. Standards of Practice Committee of American Society for Gastrointestinal Endoscopy. (2000) Modifications in endoscopic practice for the elderly. *Gastrointest. Endosc.* **52(6),** 849–851.

38. Waye, J. D. (2000) Intubation and sedation in patients who have emergency upper GI endoscopy for GI bleeding. *Gastrointest. Endosc.* **51(6),** 768–771.

39. Keeffe, E. B. and O'Connor, K. W. (1990) 1989 A/S/G/E survey of endoscopy sedation and monitoring practices. *Gastrointest. Endosc.* **36(3),** S13–S18.

40. Coulthard, P., Sano, K., Thomson, P. J., and Macfarlane, T. V. (2000) The effects of midazolam and flumazenil on psychomotor function and alertness in human volunteers. *Br. Dent. J.* **188(6),** 325–328.

41. Manley MCG, Skelly, A. M., and Hamilton, A. G. (2000) Dental treatment for people with challenging behaviour: general anaesthesia or sedation? *Br. Dent. J.* **188(7),** 358–360.

42. Jastak, J. T. and Peskin, R. M. (1991) Major morbidity or mortality from office anesthetic procedures: a closed-claim analysis of 13 cases. *Anesth. Prog.* **38,** 39–44.

43. Krippaehne, J. A. and Montgomery, M. T. (1992) Morbidity and mortality from pharmacosedation and general anesthesia in the dental office. *J. Oral Maxillofac. Surg.* **50,** 691–698.
44. Bubien, R. S., Fisher, J. D., Gentzel, J. A., Murphy, E. K., Irwin, M. E., Shea, J. B., et al. (1998) NASPE expert consensus document: Use of IV (Conscious) sedation/analgesia by nonanesthesia personnel in patients undergoing arrhythmia specific diagnostic, therapeutic, and surgical procedures. *PACE* **21,** 375–385.
45. Tobin, M. G., Pinski, S. L., Tchou, P. J., Ching, E. A., and Trohman, R. G. (1997) Cost effectiveness of administration of intravenous anesthetics for direct-current cardioversion by nonanesthesiologists. *Am. J. Cariol.* **79,** 686–688.
46. Tung, R. T. and Bajaj, A. K. (1995) Safety of implantation of a cardioverter-defibrillator without general anesthesia in an electrophysiology laboratory. *The American Journal of Cardiology* **75(14),** 908–912.
47. Rodeman, B. J. (1997) Conscious sedation during electrophysiology testing and radiofrequency catheter ablation. *Critical Care Nursing Clinics of North America* **9:3,** 313–324.
48. Craney, J. M. and Gorman, L. N. (1997) Conscious sedation and implantable devices. *Critical Care Nursing Clinics of North America* **9:3,** 325–334.
49. McGuire, B. M. (2001) Safety of endoscopy in patients with end-stage liver disease. *Gastrointest. Endosc. Clinics of North America* **11(1),** 111–130.
50. Eige, S., Pritts, E. A., Palter, S. F., and Olive, D. L. (1999) Anesthesia for office endoscopy. *Obstet. Gynecol. Clin. N. Am.* **26(1),** 99–108.
51. Iverson, R. E. (1999) Sedation and analgesia in ambulatory settings. *Clinical Guidelines in Plast. Reconstr. Surg.* 1559–1564.
52. Christian, M., Yeung, L., Williams, R., Lapinski, P., and Moy, R. (2000) Conscious sedation in dermatologic surgery. *Dermatology Surgery* **26(10),** 923–928.
53. Cohen, M. M., Doncan, P. G., and Tate, R. B. (1988) Does anesthesia contribute to operative mortality? *JAMA* **260,** 2859.

6

Pharmacology of Sedative Agents

Joseph D. Tobias, MD

1. INTRODUCTION

Over the years, various pharmacologic agents have been developed to provide sedation, anxiolysis, and amnesia. These agents have been used both as therapeutic agents (barbiturates to control intracranial pressure, propofol to treat refractory status epilepticus) and to provide sedation, anxiolysis, and amnesia in various clinical scenarios. In the setting of diagnostic and therapeutic procedures, these agents usually are used to induce amnesia and to provide a motionless patient, which may be required to facilitate a procedure or achieve an accurate radiologic examination. When used during invasive and/or diagnostic procedures, although these agents provide amnesia, anxiolysis, and sedation, most—except for ketamine—possess limited intrinsic analgesic properties and therefore are often combined with an opioid if analgesia is required (*see* Chapter 7). Although the majority of patients experience few and mild cardiorespiratory effects, these agents can be potent respiratory depressants and may have adverse effects on cardiovascular function. Therefore, these agents should be administered only by those who are well-acquainted with their use and pharmacologic properties and only in a controlled, monitored setting (*see* Chapter 8). This chapter reviews the more commonly used sedative agents, including propofol, ketamine, the barbiturates, the benzodiazepines, nitrous oxide, and chloral hydrate.

2. SPECIFIC AGENTS

2.1. Propofol

Propofol is an intravenous (iv) anesthetic agent of the alkyl phenol group. Because of its insolubility in water, it is commercially available in an egg lecithin emulsion as a 1% (10 mg/mL) solution. Its chemical structure is distinct from that of the barbiturates and other commonly used anesthetic induction agents *(1)*. Like the barbiturates, its mechanism of action involves

From: *Contemporary Clinical Neuroscience: Sedation and Analgesia for Diagnostic and Therapeutic Procedures*
Edited by: S. Malviya, N. N. Naughton, and K. K. Tremper © Humana Press Inc., Totowa, NJ

an interaction with the gamma-aminobutyric acid (GABA) receptor system; increasing the duration of time that the GABA molecule occupies the receptor. This results in increased chloride conductance across the cell membrane. Propofol is a sedative/amnestic agent and possesses no analgesic properties. Therefore, it should be combined with an opioid when analgesia is required.

The anesthetic induction dose of propofol in healthy adults ranges from 1.5 to 3 mg/kg with recommended maintenance infusion rates of 50 to 200 mcg/kg/min, depending on the depth of sedation that is required. Following iv administration, propofol is rapidly cleared from the central compartment and undergoes hepatic metabolism to inactive water-soluble metabolites, which are then renally cleared. Propofol's clearance rate exceeds that of hepatic blood flow, suggesting an extrahepatic route of elimination. Propofol's rapid clearance and metabolism account for its beneficial property of rapid awakening when the infusion is discontinued. There is no evidence to suggest altered clearance in patients with hepatic or renal dysfunction.

Following its introduction into anesthesia practice, propofol's pharmacodynamic profile—including a rapid onset, rapid recovery time, and lack of active metabolites—eventually led to its evaluation as an agent for intensive care unit (ICU) sedation (2,3), as well as for procedures outside of the operating room. When compared with midazolam for sedation in adult ICU patients, propofol resulted in shorter recovery times, improved titration efficiency, reduced post-hypnotic obtundation, and more rapid weaning from mechanical ventilation (4). Lebovic et al. demonstrated the beneficial properties of propofol for sedation during cardiac catheterization in children (5). Children received an initial dose of fentanyl (1 mcg/kg) followed by incremental bolus doses of propofol (0.5 mg/kg) until the appropriate level of sedation was achieved. Once an adequate level of sedation was achieved, a propofol infusion was started with the hourly rate equivalent to 3 times the induction dose. When compared with a group who received ketamine, the authors noted significantly less time to full recovery with propofol (24 ± 19 min vs 139 ± 87 min, $p < 0.001$).

In addition to its favorable properties with regard to sedation and recovery times, propofol has beneficial effects on central nervous system (CNS) dynamics including a decreased cerebral metabolic rate for oxygen ($CMRO_2$), cerebral vasoconstriction, and lowering of intracranial pressure (ICP) (6). The latter effect is much the same as that seen with the barbiturates and etomidate. These CNS effects suggest that propofol may be an effective and beneficial agent for sedation in patients with altered intracranial compliance, provided that ventilation is monitored and controlled when necessary to prevent increases in P_aCO_2 related to the respiratory depressant properties of propofol.

The preliminary laboratory and clinical experience with propofol have demonstrated its possible therapeutic role in regulating CNS dynamics and controlling ICP. Nimkoff et al. evaluated the effects of propofol, methohexital, and ketamine on cerebral perfusion pressure (CPP) and ICP in a feline model of cytotoxic and vasogenic cerebral edema *(7)*. Vasogenic cerebral edema was induced by inflation of an intracranial balloon. Cytotoxic cerebral edema was induced by an acute reduction in blood osmolarity using hemofiltration. Propofol lowered ICP and maintained CPP in vasogenic cerebral edema, but had no effect in cytotoxic cerebral edema. The authors theorized that the loss of autoregulatory function with diffuse cytotoxic edema uncoupled $CMRO_2$ from cerebral blood flow (CBF) and thereby eliminated propofol's efficacy.

Watts et al. evaluated the effects of propofol and hyperventilation on ICP and somatosensory evoked potentials (SEPs) in a rabbit model of intracranial hypertension *(8)*. Following inflation of an intracranial balloon to increase the ICP to 26 ± 2 mmHg and produce a $\geq 50\%$ reduction in SEPs, the animals were randomized to: group 1 (propofol followed by hyperventilation) or group 2 (hyperventilation followed by propofol). The ICP decrease was significantly greater in group 1 (final ICP: 12 ± 2 mmHg vs 16 ± 5 mmHg, $p = 0.008$). When comparing propofol with hyperventilation, propofol resulted in a greater ICP decrease: 16 ± 2 mmHg with propofol vs 21 ± 5 mmHg with hyperventilation, $p = 0.007$). When propofol was administered first, there was a significant increase in the amplitude of the SEPs. The mean arterial pressure (MAP) was maintained at baseline levels by the infusion of phenylephrine. More phenylephrine ($p < 0.02$) was required to maintain the MAP with propofol than with hyperventilation.

Despite these encouraging animal studies, the review of the literature concerning propofol in humans provides somewhat contrasting results. Although several studies demonstrate a decrease in ICP, propofol's cardiovascular effects with a lowering of the MAP can result in a decrease in the CPP. Without the maintenance of MAP, a decrease occurs in CPP that may lead to reflex cerebral vasodilation to maintain CBF, which may result in an increase in ICP and negate the decrease in ICP induced by propofol.

Herregods et al. evaluated the effects of a propofol bolus (2 mg/kg administered over 90 s) on ICP and MAP in six adults with an ICP greater than 25 mmHg following traumatic brain injury *(9)*. The mean ICP decreased from 25 ± 3 to 11 ± 4 mmHg ($p < 0.05$). However, there was a decrease in the MAP and consequently a decrease in the CPP from 92 ± 8 mmHg to a low of 50 ± 7 mmHg. The CPP was less than 50 mmHg in four of six patients. No vasoconstrictor agent was administered to maintain the MAP.

Similar results were obtained by Pinaud et al. during their evaluation of the effects of propofol on CBF, ICP, CPP, and cerebral arteriovenous oxygen content difference in 10 adults with traumatic brain injury *(10)*. Although propofol decreased ICP (11.3 ± 2.6 to 9.2 ± 2.5 mmHg, $p < 0.001$), there was also a decrease in MAP, which resulted in an overall decrease in CPP from 82 ± 14 to 59 ± 7 mmHg, $p < 0.01$. Other investigators in patients with traumatic brain injury *(11)* or during cerebral aneurysm surgery *(12)* have noted similar effects of propofol on ICP and MAP with an overall lowering of CPP caused by the greater decrease in MAP than ICP.

Farling et al. reported their experience with propofol for sedation in 10 adult patients with closed head injuries *(13)*. Propofol was administered as a continuous infusion of 2–4 mg/kg/h for 24 h. Additional therapy for increased ICP included mannitol and hyperventilation. The mean rate of propofol infusion was 2.88 mg/kg/h. There was a statistically significant decrease in the mean ICP of 2.1 mmHg from baseline achieved at 2 h following the start of the propofol infusion. No decrease in MAP was noted. The CPP increased during the 24-h study period, and the difference was statistically significant at the 24-h point (CPP increase of 9.8 mmHg, $p = 0.028$). The authors concluded that propofol was a suitable agent for sedation in head-injury patients who required mechanical ventilation.

Spitzfadden et al. reported their experience with the use of propofol to provide sedation and control ICP in two adolescents *(14)*. Dopamine was used to maintain MAP and CPP. Propofol resulted in adequate sedation and control of ICP. When compared with barbiturates, the usual time-honored therapy for pharmacologic control of ICP, the authors suggested that a significant advantage of propofol was a much more rapid awakening. The latter effect may be most evident following prolonged (>48 h) administration of barbiturates.

Further study will be required to fully evaluate the role of propofol in controlling ICP. With control of MAP, the initial clinical and laboratory evidence suggests that propofol can be used to decrease $CMRO_2$, CBF, and ICP. Additional benefits of propofol in patients with altered intracranial compliance include maintenance of CBF autoregulation in response to changes in MAP and P_aCO_2 as well as preliminary evidence that suggests a possible protective effect of propofol during periods of cerebral hypoperfusion and ischemia *(15,16)*. These latter effects are similar to those reported with the use of barbiturates *(17)*. It is postulated that the neuroprotective effects may result from alterations in $CMRO_2$ or propofol's antioxidant properties related to its phenol ring structure.

Following its increased use both in and outside of the operating room, certain adverse effects have been reported with propofol (Table 1). Propo-

Table 1
Adverse Effects Reported with Propofol

Hypotension
    Negative inotropic effects
    Vasodilation
    Bradycardia, asystole
Neurologic sequelae
    Opisthotonic posturing
    Seizure-like activity
    Myoclonus
Respiratory depression, apnea
Anaphylactoid reactions
Metabolic acidosis and cardiac failure (with prolonged
    administration in the pediatric population)
Pain on injection
Bacterial contamination of solution
Hyperlipidemia
Hypercarbia

fol's cardiovascular effects are similar to those of the barbiturates, including an overall lowering of the MAP related to both peripheral vasodilation and negative inotropic properties *(18)*. Propofol also alters the baroreflex responses, thereby resulting in a smaller increase in heart rate for a given decrease in blood pressure. These cardiovascular effects are especially pronounced following bolus administration. Although generally well-tolerated by patients with adequate cardiovascular function, these effects may result in detrimental physiologic effects in patients with compromised cardiovascular function. Tritapepe et al. have demonstrated that the administration of calcium chloride (10 mg/kg) prevented the deleterious cardiovascular effects of propofol during anesthetic induction in patients undergoing coronary artery bypass grafting *(19)*.

In addition to the negative inotropic properties, central vagal tone may be augmented, leading to bradycardia *(20)* or asystole when combined with other medications known to alter cardiac chronotropic function (fentanyl, succinylcholine) *(21)*. Although the relative bradycardia is generally considered a beneficial effect in patients at risk for myocardial ischemia, it may be detrimental in patients with fixed stroke volumes whose cardiac output is heart-rate-dependent.

Unusual neurologic manifestations including opisthotonic posturing, myoclonic movements (especially in children), and seizure-like activity have been reported with propofol administration *(22–25)*. Although some of the initial reports suggested actual seizure activity, these concerns have most likely been overemphasized, since no electroencephalographic evidence of seizure activity has been documented during the abnormal movements seen with propofol administration. Additionally, propofol is considered a valuable agent in the treatment of patients with refractory status epilepticus that is unresponsive to conventional therapy *(26)*.

Although many studies have examined the cardiovascular effects of propofol, the respiratory-depressant effects of propofol should not be overlooked. Although propofol has become a popular agent for deep sedation in the spontaneously breathing patient, reports demonstrate a relatively high incidence of respiratory effects including hypoventilation, upper airway obstruction, and apnea *(27)*. As with any sedative agent, some degree of hypoventilation is likely to occur in all patients breathing spontaneously. These effects may be detrimental related to the alterations in P_aCO_2 and its obvious deleterious effects on CBF, ICP, and CPP. Despite these potential deleterious effects on respiratory function, recent laboratory and clinical studies suggest that propofol may be advantageous when instrumenting the airway of patients with reactive airway disease. In an animal model, Chih-Chung et al. demonstrated that propofol attenuates carbachol-induced airway constriction *(28)*. The mechanism involves a decrease in intracellular inositol phosphate accumulation, thereby limiting intracellular calcium availability. The latter results from a decrease in calcium release from intracellular stores as well as a decrease in transmembrane movement.

In children, a significant issue with the prolonged use of propofol—such as ongoing sedation in the pediatric ICU setting—are reports of unexplained metabolic acidosis, brady-dysrhythmias, and fatal cardiac failure *(29,30)*. The initial report of Parke et al. published in 1992 included five children with respiratory infections and respiratory failure who received prolonged propofol infusions, although in higher than usual doses (up to 13.6 mg/kg/h). Other anecdotal reports subsequently appeared, followed by a review by Bray examining the reports from the medical literature of 18 children with suspected propofol infusion syndrome *(31)*. Risk factors for the syndrome identified by Bray included propofol administration for more than 48 h or doses greater than 4 mg/kg/h. However, several children received doses greater than 4 mg/kg/h for longer than 48 h, suggesting that factors other than dose and duration are necessary for development of the syndrome. Other associated factors included age; 13 of the 18 patients were 4 yr of age or younger, and only 1 of 18 was more than 10 yr of age. Since the review of Bray et al, the syndrome has been reported in a 17-yr-old patient *(32)*. As suggested by the initial report of Parke et al., there may be an association of an respiratory tract infection in the etiology of the syndrome, as 82% of the reported cases have been in children with such infections. In addition to the cardiovascular manifestations, other features have included metabolic acidosis, lipemic serum, hepatomegaly, and muscle involvement with rhabdomyolysis *(32)*. Suggestions for treatment include discontinuation of the propofol followed by symptomatic treatment of the cardiovascular dysfunction. In patients with rhabdomyolysis and renal failure, hemodialysis has been used. Although hemodialysis has been effective in the management of these patients, it is yet to be determined whether its only effect is in the management of the renal dysfunction, or whether it may also have a therapeutic effect through the removal of a suspected toxic metabolite. Until further data are available, caution is suggested with the administration of propofol by continuous infusion in the pediatric ICU patient less than 10–12 yr in doses exceeding 4 mg/kg/h or for longer than 48 h. However, because of the previously described beneficial properties, propofol may have a role in providing short-term sedation in younger patients and for more prolonged use in older patients.

Additional problems with propofol relate to its delivery in a lipid emulsion. The latter is the same lipid preparation as that used in parenteral hyperalimentation. There have been rare reports of anaphylactoid reactions *(33)*. These may be more likely in patients with a history of egg allergy. Pain occurs with propofol administration through a peripheral infusion site. Variable success in decreasing the incidence of pain has been reported with various maneuvers, including the preadministration of lidocaine, pretreatment with thiopental, mixing the lidocaine and propofol in a single solution, diluting the concentration of the propofol, or cooling it prior to bolus administration *(34,35)*. Another alternative is the administration of a small dose of ketamine (0.5 mg/kg) prior to the administration of propofol *(36)*. Since propofol has limited analgesic properties, ketamine and propofol can be administered together to take advantage of the analgesia provided by ketamine and the rapid recovery with propofol. This combination can be used for brief invasive procedures or for ICU sedation. For these purposes, ketamine can be added to the propofol solution to produce a mixture containing 3–5 mg/mL ketamine and 10 mg/mL propofol. For brief procedures, incremental doses of 0.1 mL/kg can be administered, resulting in the delivery of 0.3–0.5 mg/kg of ketamine and 1 mg/kg of propofol.

Unlike many other medications, the initial formulation of propofol did not contain preservatives. Laboratory investigation has demonstrated that the lipid emulsion is a suitable culture medium for bacteria *(37)*. Systemic bacteremia and postoperative wound infections have been linked to extrinsically contaminated propofol *(38)*. A modification of the initial preparation by

AstraZeneca Pharmaceuticals, manufacturer of propofol, included the addition of ethylenediaminetetraacetic acid (EDTA) as a preservative, which may limit the risk of bacterial contamination and growth. Recently, another preparation of propofol, manufactured by Baxter Pharmaceuticals, has been released for clinical use. This latter preparation contains sodium metabisulfite as a preservative. There remains some controversy over the possible association of sodium metabisulfite with allergic reactions, especially in patients with asthma and other atopic conditions. Despite the recent changes, meticulous aseptic technique is required when using propofol. Opened but unused vials should be disposed of promptly and not saved for later use. When used by continuous infusion for ICU sedation, the vial and tubing should be changed every 12 h.

Additional problems related to the high lipid content of the solution have included hypertriglyceridemia *(39)*. A case report suggests the anecdotal association of high-dose propofol infusion with an increasing $PaCO_2$ during prolonged mechanical ventilation in the ICU setting *(40)*. The latter report describes a patient that required up to 200 mcg/kg/min of propofol to maintain an adequate level of sedation. This resulted in a total caloric intake of 4500 calories/d (53% from the lipid in the propofol diluent). The $PaCO_2$ increased from 67 mmHg to a maximum value of 78 mmHg, despite increasing the minute ventilation from 11 to 13 L/min. The lipid content of propofol should be taken into consideration when calculating the patient's daily caloric intake. A propofol infusion of 2 mg/kg/h provides roughly 0.5 gm/kg/d of fat. Possible solutions to these problems include the potential production of a 2% solution to limit the total lipid administration.

2.2. Ketamine

Ketamine is a sedative/analgesic agent that is structurally related to phencyclidine. It was introduced into clinical practice in the 1960s *(41)*. A unique feature of ketamine, which makes it particularly attractive for sedation during procedures, is the provision of both amnesia and analgesia. Its molecular structure contains a chiral center at the C_2 carbon of the cyclohexanone ring, resulting in both a (+) and (–) enantiomer. Ketamine's anesthetic/analgesic properties result from its interactions with the limbic/thalamic systems, resulting in what has been termed dissociative anesthesia. Additional postulated sites/mechanisms of action include the NMDA receptor as well as subgroups of opioid receptors.

Commercially available ketamine is a racemic mixture of these two optical (+,–) isomers. It is available in three different concentrations, including 1% (10 mg/mL), 5% (50 mg/mL), and 10% (100 mg/mL). Preliminary data suggests that the (+) isomer may possess some clinical advantages, including a more potent anesthetic/analgesic effect with a more limited duration of action allowing for a more rapid awakening and a more rapid return to normal cognitive function *(42)*.

Metabolism occurs primarily by hepatic N-methylation to various metabolites, including norketamine, which is further metabolized via hydroxylation pathways with subsequent urinary excretion. Norketamine retains roughly one-third of the analgesic and sedative properties of the parent compound. Bioavailability is 100% following iv/intramuscular administration. However, the bioavailability is markedly decreased with oral or rectal administration because of limited absorption and a high degree of first-pass metabolism. Higher concentrations of norketamine are noted following oral/rectal administration because of the greater degree of first-pass hepatic metabolism and may account for a significant part of the anesthetic effect following oral/rectal administration. As ketamine is primarily dependent on hepatic metabolism, doses should be reduced in patients with hepatic dysfunction.

The beneficial properties of ketamine include preservation of cardiovascular function and limited effects on respiratory mechanics. These properties make it an effective agent for the provision of amnesia and analgesia during painful, invasive procedures while allowing the maintenance of spontaneous respiratory function *(43)*.

In the majority of clinical scenarios, ketamine results in a dose-related increase in heart rate and blood pressure, which are mediated through the sympathetic nervous system response with the release of endogenous catecholamines *(44,45)*. In most clinical circumstances, ketamine results in increased heart rate and blood pressure, which can increase myocardial oxygen consumption. These effects can alter the balance between myocardial oxygen demand and delivery, inducing ischemia in patients with ischemic heart disease. The hypertension and tachycardia that occur with ketamine administration can be decreased by the administration of ketamine with a benzodiazepine, a barbiturate, propofol, or synthetic opioids (fentanyl or sufentanil). Ketamine's indirect sympathomimetic effects generally overshadow its direct negative inotropic properties. However, hypotension may occur in patients with diminished myocardial contractility *(46,47)*. In these patients, it is postulated that ketamine's direct negative inotropic properties predominate because the endogenous catecholamine stores have been depleted.

Although somewhat controversial, ketamine may adversely effect pulmonary vascular resistance (PVR), and should be used with caution in adults with diminished right ventricular function or altered PVR. This issue remains controversial, as varying results have been reported in the literature, especially when considering both adult and pediatric patients. The initial studies were performed during spontaneous ventilation, and the alterations in PVR may have been related to increases in $PaCO_2$ and not the direct effects of ketamine on the pulmonary vasculature. Following ketamine administration to infants with congenital heart disease during spontaneous ventilation, Morray et al. noted statistically significant increases in pulmonary artery pressure (from a mean of 20.6 mmHg to 22.8 mmHg) and increases in PVR *(48)*. In contrast, Hickey et al. found no change in PVR in intubated infants with minimal ventilatory support (4 breaths/min and an F_iO_2 of 0.4) *(49)*. The latter study included 14 patients—7 with normal and 7 with elevated baseline PVR. Pending further investigations, ketamine should be used cautiously in patients with pulmonary hypertension, especially during spontaneous ventilation. However, the available literature in children with cyanotic and noncyanotic congenital heart disease continues to show beneficial effects of ketamine on overall cardiovascular performance and oxygen saturation *(50)*.

One significant advantage of ketamine over many other sedative/analgesic agents is its lack of significant effects on respiratory function. Functional residual capacity, minute ventilation, and tidal volume remain unchanged following ketamine administration *(51)*, while other investigators have demonstrated improved pulmonary compliance, decreased resistance, and prevention of bronchospasm *(52)*. These effects on respiratory mechanics have been partially attributed to effects from the release of endogenous catecholamines *(53)*. Although minute ventilation is generally maintained, elevations of P_aCO_2 and a rightward shift of the CO_2 response curve have been reported *(54)*, and there remains controversy concerning ketamine's effects on protective airway reflexes. Although clinical use and experimental studies suggest that airway reflexes are maintained, aspiration and laryngospasm have been reported following ketamine in spontaneously breathing patients without a protected airway *(55)*. In higher doses or in severely compromised patients, ketamine can cause apnea, proving again that all sedative/analgesic agents, especially when administered to critically ill patients, should be administered only in a controlled environment with appropriate monitoring. An additional effect that may influence airway patency is increased oral secretions. The concomitant administration of an anti-sialogogue such as atropine or glycopyrrolate is recommended. Ketamine increases salivary and bronchial gland secretion through stimulation of central cholinergic receptors. Ketamine increases CBF/ICP, and should be avoided in patients with altered intracranial compliance *(56,57)*. The effects on ICP are the result of direct cerebral vasodilatation, mediated through central cholinergic receptors. They are not secondary to alterations in the $CMRO_2$ or changes in $PaCO_2$ *(58,59)*.

Perhaps the most well-known adverse effect related to ketamine is the occurrence of emergence phenomena or hallucinations. Emergence phenomena are dose-related, occurring more commonly in adolescents and adult patients. Their incidence can be decreased by the pre- or concomitant administration of a barbiturate, propofol, or benzodiazepine *(60)*. It is postulated that emergence phenomena result from the alteration of auditory and visual relays in the inferior colliculus and the medical geniculate nucleus, leading to the misinterpretation of visual and auditory stimuli *(60)*. The administration of a benzodiazepine (lorazepam or midazolam) 5 min prior to the administration of ketamine is generally effective in preventing emergence phenomena, and may allow for the use of ketamine even in older patients. The combined use of propofol and ketamine has been previously discussed.

Another option with ketamine is to use non-intravenous routes of delivery. Intramuscular (im) administration in doses of 3–4 mg/kg can be used in uncooperative patients who lack venous access. Although the bioavailability of im administration is 100%, the onset of action will be delayed, requiring 10–15 min to achieve a peak effect. Alternatively, in the pediatric population, both intranasal and rectal administration of ketamine have been reported for premedication for the operating room *(61)*, and oral administration has been reported for sedation/analgesia during bone marrow aspiration and for the suturing of lacerations in the emergency room setting *(62,63)*. When the non-parenteral routes are used, larger doses of 6–10 mg/kg are required, since the bioavailability is only 10–20%.

Although it is most often administered in intermittent bolus doses, there are limited reported clinical experiences with the use of ketamine for sedation of the ICU patient. Tobias et al. reported their anecdotal experience with the use of ketamine infusions for sedation in five pediatric ICU patients *(64)*. Four of the patients had experienced adverse cardiorespiratory effects following the administration of benzodiazepines and/or opioids. Hartvig et al. used a ketamine infusion to provide sedation and analgesia following cardiac surgery in 10 infants and children ranging in age from 1 wk to 30 mo *(65)*. A continuous infusion of ketamine in a dose of 1 mg/kg/h was administered to five of the patients, and the other five received 2 mg/kg/h. Both groups received intermittent, as-needed doses of midazolam. The mean plasma clearance of ketamine was 0.94 ± 0.22 L/kg/h with an elimination half-life of 3.1 ± 1.6 h. Norketamine demonstrated an elimination half-life of 6.0 ± 1.8 h. Both ketamine infusion rates provided similar and acceptable levels of sedation.

2.3. Etomidate

Etomidate is a carboxylated, imidazole-containing iv anesthetic agent that was first synthesized in 1964 and introduced into clinical anesthesia practice in 1972. Since the aqueous solution of etomidate is unstable at physiologic pH, it is available in a 0.2% (20 mg/mL) solution with 35% propylene glycol. The pH of 6.9 of this solution and the carrier vehicle—propylene glycol—account for the high incidence of pain and the development of thrombophlebitis with administration through peripheral iv sites. Although the propylene glycol is not an issue with single, short-term administration, toxicity from the carrier vehicle has been reported following long-term infusions (66).

Like the barbiturates, propofol, and benzodiazepines, it is postulated that etomidate provides its anesthetic effects by interactions with the GABA system and alterations of chloride conductance across the cell membrane (67). Unlike the barbiturates and propofol, etomidate has little effect on cardiovascular performance, even in patients with altered myocardial contractility (68,69).

Anesthetic induction doses ranging from 0.2–0.4 mg/kg provide a rapid onset of amnesia and sedation with a rapid emergence time following a single bolus dose. Following iv administration, etomidate undergoes ester hydrolysis by the liver with the formation of inactive water-soluble metabolites. The elimination half-life is prolonged in the setting of hepatic dysfunction. As etomidate possesses limited analgesic properties, it may not effectively blunt the hemodynamic response to endotracheal intubation in patients with normal cardiovascular function. Co-administration of an opioid such as fentanyl may provide a more stable hemodynamic profile.

Like the barbiturates and propofol, etomidate decreases the $CMRO_2$, resulting in cerebral vasoconstriction and a decrease in CBF and ICP. With its limited effects on cardiovascular function, CPP is maintained, making it a suitable induction agent for patients with altered myocardial contractility and increased ICP. Etomidate produces EEG changes similar to that seen with the barbiturates; however, it can also produce epileptic-like EEG potentials in patients with underlying seizure disorders. These potentials are produced without accompanying motor activity, making it a useful intra-operative agent to identify seizure foci during seizure surgery. Etomidate has also been used to treat status epilepticus (70).

To date, the vast majority of experience with etomidate centers around its use as a single dose for the induction of anesthesia in adults. Kay noted a rapid onset of anesthesia with etomidate and limited effects on cardiovascular function in 198 children ranging in age from 1 d to 15 yr (71). However, no data is given concerning the cardiovascular status of these patients. Tobias reported anecdotal experience with the use of etomidate for anesthetic induction in three children including a 33-mo-old with a dilated cardiomyopathy, a 9-yr-old trauma victim with hypovolemia and increased ICP, and a 10-yr-old with aortic stenosis and respiratory failure (72).

Because of its limited effects on cardiovascular function, there is a continuing interest in the use of etomidate for sedation during procedures outside of the operating room. Ford et al. compared incremental doses of thiopental at 50 mg or etomidate at 4 mg for sedation during cardioversion in 16 ASA (American Society of Anesthesiologists) class II or III adult males, age 55–66 yr *(73)*. Both drugs provided adequate levels of sedation. No significant difference was noted in heart rate and blood pressure. There was a statistically significant increase in respiratory rate with etomidate, and a decrease in respiratory rate with thiopental, and recovery times were similar. Mild myoclonus was noted with the use of etomidate.

Canessa et al. evaluated four anesthetic agents (thiopental 3 mg/kg, etomidate 0.15 mg/kg, midazolam 0.15 mg/kg, and propofol 1.5 mg/kg) during cardioversion in 45 adults *(74)*. All patients received 1.5 mcg/kg of fentanyl 3 min prior to the procedure. Etomidate produced mild pain on injection and myoclonus, but was the only one of the four agents that did not lower MAP. Propofol resulted in hypotension and a higher incidence of apnea. The duration of effect was similar with propofol, thiopental, and etomidate, but was prolonged with midazolam.

The information concerning the use of etomidate for sedation in children is more limited. McDowall et al. compared etomidate, propofol, and ketamine for sedation during procedures in pediatric oncology patients *(75)*. Ketamine was associated with vomiting (14.6%), agitation (15%), and tachycardia (19.5%). Etomidate was associated with vomiting (9.9%) and agitation (1.2%). Propofol resulted in hypoxemia in 15.7% of patients, which was usually managed by the administration of supplemental oxygen, but occasionally required bag-mask ventilation. Propofol resulted in a low incidence of vomiting (0.5%) and agitation (1.2%). Behrens et al. reported their experience with the use of etomidate for sedation during placement of percutaneous endoscopic gastrostomies in 139 patients *(76)*.

Etomidate has also been administered by the non-parenteral route. Streissand et al. evaluated the possible use of etomidate as a premedicant administered as a transmucosal lozenge in 10 adult volunteers *(77)*. The volunteers ingested transmucosal etomidate in doses of 25, 50, 75, and 100 mg on four study days. The peak plasma concentration was achieved at 20–30 min. Two volunteers experienced brief episodes of involuntary tremor after the 100-mg dose. Drowsiness and light sleep occurred in a dose-related manner. The authors concluded that this preparation might be effective when brief, mild to moderate sedation was needed.

Various adverse effects have been reported with etomidate (Table 2). Those related to the carrier vehicle include pain on injection, thrombophlebitis, and propylene glycol toxicity. The latter was reported only with pro-

Table 2
Adverse Effects Reported with Etomidate

Myoclonic movements
Nausea/vomiting
Pain on injection
Thrombophlebitis
Propylene glycol toxicity (with prolonged infusions)
Adrenal suppression (with prolonged infusions)

longed infusions. The most significant concern remains etomidate's effect on the endogenous production of corticosteroids. These effects limit its use for prolonged sedation in the ICU setting *(78)*. Etomidate inhibits the function of an enzyme system (11-beta hydroxylase), which is necessary for the production of cortisol, aldosterone, and corticosterone. Although inhibition is present after a single dose of etomidate *(79)*, this effect is not believed to be of clinical significance.

2.4. Barbiturates

The barbiturates are one of the oldest class of agents used in anesthesia practice. They can be classified according to their duration of activity. Short-acting agents include methohexital, thiopental, and thiamylal. Pentobarbital is considered an intermediate-acting agent, and phenobarbital is considered a long-acting agent. The short-acting agents have a duration of action of 5–10 min following a single bolus dose and are usually used by iv, bolus administration for brief procedures such as the induction of anesthesia and endotracheal intubation. When a more prolonged effect is needed, a continuous infusion may be used to maintain constant plasma levels. Thiopental and thiamylal are thiobarbiturates, and methohexital is an oxybarbiturate. Thiopental and thiamylal are commercially available as racemic mixtures of the two optical isomers. The L-isomers of both drugs are twice as potent as the D-isomers. Methohexital has two asymmetric centers, resulting in four isomers. Since the beta isomers produce excessive motor activity, methohexital is available as a mixture of the two alpha isomers. The three agents are reconstituted with sterile saline to solutions of 1–2.5%. Induction doses vary based on the potency of the agent. Methohexital is the most potent (2.5–3 times that of thiopental) and thiopental is the least potent. Induction doses are also higher in neonates and infants. Anesthetic induction doses for thiopental vary from 3–5 mg/kg in healthy adults, 5–6 mg/kg in children, and 6–8 mg/kg in neonates and infants. The barbiturates undergo predominant hepatic metabolism except for phenobarbital, which is also dependent on renal elimination. The rapid dissipation of anesthetic effect is not related to hepatic metabolism, but rather redistribution from the central compartment. During prolonged infusions, the peripheral compartments are saturated and a prolonged effect is seen.

Beneficial physiologic effects of the barbiturates include a decrease of the $CMRO_2$ with a reduction in CBF, cerebral vasoconstriction, and a decrease in ICP. They produce varying dose-dependent degrees of EEG suppression, and in sufficient does produce electrical silence. The barbiturates are potent anticonvulsants, and may be used to treat status epilepticus that is unresponsive to other agents. Although still controversial, it has also been suggested that the barbiturates may provide some degree of cerebral protection during periods of cerebral hypoxia or hypoperfusion. This effect has not been shown to occur if these agents are administered after the event. The CNS properties of the barbiturates are much the same as those described for the benzodiazepines, etomidate, and propofol.

As with many of the agents described, the barbiturates' effects on cardio-respiratory function are dose-dependent. In healthy patients, sedative doses have minimal effects on respiratory drive and airway protective reflexes, yet larger doses—especially in patients with cardiorespiratory compromise—can produce respiratory depression, apnea, or hypotension. The cardiorespiratory effects are additive when the barbiturates are used with other agents such as opioids. Hypotension results from both peripheral vasodilation with a decrease in preload/afterload and a direct negative inotropic effect.

Although the barbiturates are used most often in the operating room for the induction of anesthesia and in the ICU for their therapeutic effects (as anticonvulsants or to decrease ICP), these agents may play a role in providing sedation outside of the operating room. Sanderson et al. reported the use of iv pentobarbital to provide sedation during radiologic procedures in 149 children ranging in age from 3 mo to 7 yr *(80)*. One hundred forty-one of the patients received only pentobarbital, and eight also received midazolam and/ or fentanyl. The mean dose of pentobarbital was 4.6 mg/kg with a range of 2–10 mg/kg. The mean time from the start of sedation to the start of the scan was 7 min (range: 2–50 min). Sedation was successful in all cases. Adverse effects were noted in 22 of the 146 patients (14.7%), and included oxygen desaturation, vomiting, airway secretions, airway obstruction, coughing, and bronchospasm. No patient required endotracheal intubation or bag-mask ventilation. Similar success with iv pentobarbital for radiologic procedures has been reported by other investigators *(81,82)*. In addition to iv administration, rectal thiopental sodium has been successfully used in many centers for sedation for radiologic procedures *(83)*.

The barbiturate, pentobarbital, has also been used for sedation during mechanical ventilation in the pediatric ICU population. Tobias reported a retrospective evaluation of pentobarbital use in 50 children for pediatric ICU sedation *(84)*. The 50 patients ranged in age from 1 mo to 14 yr, and ranged in weight from 3.1 to 56 kg. Prior to switching to pentobarbital, the level of sedation was inadequate despite midazolam doses of 0.4 mg/kg/h with either fentanyl (10 mcg/kg/h) or morphine (100 mcg/kg/h). No significant adverse affects related to pentobarbital were noted.

One problem that may limit the use of barbiturates in the ICU setting is that the solution is alkaline, thereby making it incompatible with other medications and parenteral alimentation solutions. Therefore, the barbiturates should be administered separately from other medications. Local erythema and thrombophlebitis can occur with subcutaneous infiltration.

2.5. Nitrous Oxide

Nitrous oxide (N_2O) was first synthesized in 1776 by Priestley, and its anesthetic properties were first described by Humphrey Davy in 1799. Despite Davy's suggestion of the potential effects of this agent, it was not until 1844 that Gardner Colton used nitrous oxide as an anesthetic agent during a tooth extraction. Today, nitrous oxide remains one of the most widely used anesthetic agents.

Nitrous oxide possesses many of the characteristics of an ideal agent for sedation. It has a rapid onset of action, is relatively easy and inexpensive to use, its effects dissipate rapidly once discontinued, and it provides amnesia, sedation, and analgesia. Because of its low blood-gas partition coefficient (relative insolubility in blood), its alveolar concentration rises rapidly, resulting in a rapid onset of activity. Holst reported an astonishing experience of 3 million pediatric dental patients treated with 30–60% nitrous oxide without a single serious complication *(85)*. Griffin and colleagues describe its use in children in an emergency room setting for treating burns, suturing lacerations, and orthopedic reductions *(86)*.

Nitrous oxide is not a complete anesthetic. Its minimum alveolar concentration or MAC, (a measure of anesthetic potency, which describes the anesthetic concentration at which 50% of patients move in response to surgical incision), is 105%. The latter is impossible to achieve at normal barometric pressure. Even in concentrations of 70–80%, additional agents may be necessary.

Nitrous oxide can be administered by a face or nasal mask. Another option involves the use of a weighted mouthpiece that is held in place by the patient during administration. If the patient becomes too sleepy, the device falls from the patient, thereby stopping the administration of nitrous oxide. Safety issues mandate that nitrous oxide be administered with several safety features including standard monitoring. Additional monitors include: a monitor of the inspired oxygen concentration, a device that limits the ratio of the flow rates of oxygen to nitrous oxide (a proportioning system so that less than 30% oxygen cannot be administered), and a system that cuts off the nitrous oxide flow if the oxygen supply fails. Without this latter device, the nitrous oxide flow can continue without the addition of oxygen, leading to the delivery of a hypoxic mixture or 100% nitrous oxide.

In the operating room, nitrous oxide and oxygen are generally administered from the wall outlets connected to the hospital's central supply. In other areas when such a supply is not available, nitrous oxide can be administered from E cylinders and mixed with oxygen to provide the desired concentration. Alternatively, commercially available tanks are manufactured that contain a 50/50 oxygen and nitrous oxide mixture, thereby limiting the risk of a hypoxic mixture and the need for specialized equipment to mix oxygen and nitrous oxide from separate tanks.

A scavenger device attached to the delivery system is also required to remove waste gases and prevent environmental pollution. Repeated exposure of the patient or healthcare workers to nitrous oxide can lead to teratogenic effects, increased risk of spontaneous abortion, bone marrow suppression or megaloblastic anemia, and peripheral neuropathy as a result of its effects on B_{12} metabolism and protein synthesis. Because of the potential for abuse and/or illicit use, nitrous oxide tanks should be kept under close surveillance.

Despite its widespread use and long safety record, significant physiologic effects occur with nitrous oxide. Nitrous oxide exerts a dose-dependent negative depressant effect on myocardial contractility and increases pulmonary artery pressure. Like all sedative/analgesic agents, it also causes dose-dependent respiratory depression, resulting in an elevation of the resting P_aCO_2 level and blunting of the central respiratory response to hypercarbia and hypoxemia. Litman et al. evaluated the levels of sedation and respiratory effects of oral midazolam (0.5 mg/kg) combined with increasing concentrations of nitrous oxide in 20 children, age 1–3 yr *(87)*. Four concentrations of nitrous oxide were studied: 15%, 30%, 45%, and 60%. During nitrous oxide inhalation, 12 of the 20 patients developed an increasing end-tidal CO_2 with a decrease in the respiratory rate. At 30% nitrous oxide, one child met the American Academy of Pediatrics (AAP) criteria for deep sedation. With 60% nitrous oxide, six children were not clinically sedated, six met the AAP criteria for conscious sedation, six met the AAP criteria for deep sedation, and one child developed an even deeper level of sedation with no response to painful stimuli.

Table 3
Issues with Nitrous Oxide Administration

Potential for the administration of a hypoxic mixture
Contamination of tanks with nitrogen dioxide, nitric oxide
Healthcare worker exposure
Abuse potential
Megaloblastic anemia, bone marrow suppression
Teratogenesis
Myelopathy
Depressed myocardial contractility
Increased pulmonary artery pressure
Expansion of air-containing spaces
Increased cerebral blood flow, increased intracranial pressure

Additional issues/concerns with nitrous oxide are listed in Table 3. Nitrous oxide increases the incidence of postoperative nausea and vomiting. It diffuses into air-filled spaces, increasing the volume and pressure of the space. This can be an issue with any loculated collection of air, including bowel obstruction, intrathoracic injuries with the risk of pneumothorax, the middle ear, lung cysts, or in the presence of pneumocephalus. Nitrous oxide increases CBF/ICP, and is relatively contraindicated in patients with closed head injury and altered intracranial compliance.

Despite its relative insolubility in blood, during the administration of nitrous oxide, a large amount is taken up into the blood. This latter effect, known as the second gas effect of anesthesia, increases the alveolar PO_2, resulting in an added margin of safety during induction even if high concentrations of nitrous oxide (80–90%) are administered. Once the administration of nitrous oxide is discontinued, this effect occurs in the opposite direction, resulting in a lowering of the alveolar PO_2—which can result in hypoxemia unless supplemental oxygen is administered until the nitrous oxide is eliminated from the body.

2.6. Chloral Hydrate

In children, chloral hydrate remains one of the more commonly used agents for sedation. It was originally synthesized in 1832 and introduced into clinical practice in 1869 by Liebreich. For street and recreational use, chloral hydrate is the ingredient combined with alcohol in mixtures known as "knockout drops" and "Mickey Finns." It is available as capsules (250 mg, 500 mg), syrup (250 mg/5 mL and 500 mg/5 mL), and suppositories (325 mg, 500 mg, and 650 mg). Chloral hydrate tends to be a GI irritant, especially when administered on an empty stomach, and results in a relatively high incidence of nausea and vomiting. In younger children, these problems can be avoided with the use of suppositories. It has no analgesic properties; therefore, it should not be used to treat pain or during painful procedures unless combined with an analgesic agent such as an opioid.

Chloral hydrate is rapidly absorbed from the gastrointestinal tract with a bioavailability that approaches 100%. Its onset of action is within 20 min, with a peak effect at 30–60 min. Following absorption, it is metabolized in the liver by the enzyme alcohol dehydrogenase to the active ingredient, trichloroethanol (TCE). TCE is then further metabolized by either glucuronidation or oxidation to inactive metabolites. Less than 10% of chloral hydrate undergoes renal excretion. The plasma half-life of TCE is 8–12 h in children, but may be prolonged up to 24–36 h in neonates and infants *(88)*. These prolonged half-lives account for the prolonged effects that can occur in specific patient populations. Additive and prolonged effects are commonly seen following repeated administration over a period of days.

Chloral hydrate and its active metabolite TCE are CNS depressants. In therapeutic doses, there are minimal effects on cardiorespiratory function and airway control. Although apnea and hypotension can occur, these effects are generally only seen in an overdose situation. In the setting of an overdose, central respiratory depression with apnea and cardiovascular compromise is the leading cause of mortality. Cardiovascular effects relate to decreased myocardial contractility, a shortened refractory period, and an altered sensitivity of the myocardium to endogenous catecholamines *(89)*. The latter two effects account for the pro-arrythmogenic effects that are seen. These effects primarily relate to TCE—which is a halogenated hydrocarbon—and like halothane, shares the same myocardial effects. These properties suggest against the use of chloral hydrate as a sedative in patients with toxic ingestions that may predispose to arrhythmias such as tricyclic antidepressants *(90)*.

Several factors account for the continued use of chloral hydrate as a first-line agent for sedation in the pediatric population. These include physicians' familiarity with the agent, its wide therapeutic index, its cost, and a lack of significant effects on cardiorespiratory function. Dose recommendations vary widely, ranging from 25–30 mg/kg up to 80–100 mg/kg. The latter doses generally provide a greater degree of success when attempting to provide a motionless patient during radiographic imaging. Because of the possibility of a prolonged effect, extended post-procedure monitoring may be required. Despite a long record of safety with minimal effects on respiratory function in most patients, deaths from respiratory depression have occurred. Like all other sedative agents, respiratory depression can occur with chloral hydrate, and standard monitoring is mandatory. Additionally, the patient should be monitored until fully awake. More than one patient has been discharged before being fully awake, only to be found dead on arrival at home.

2.7. Benzodiazepines

The benzodiazepines used most commonly in the United States for sedation include diazepam, lorazepam, and midazolam. These agents bind to specific receptor sites that are part of the GABA receptor system, increasing the efficacy of the interaction between the GABA receptor and the chloride channel. Benzodiazepines provide several therapeutic effects including sedation, anxiolysis, amnesia, anticonvulsant properties, and spinally mediated muscle relaxation. It has been suggested that increasing the rate of occupancy of the benzodiazepine receptor results in an escalation of the benzodiazepine effect from anxiolysis to sedation to unconsciousness when 60% or more of the receptor sites are occupied.

Diazepam and lorazepam are insoluble in water, and are commercially available in a solution containing propylene glycol. The diluent, propylene glycol, can result in tissue irritation, pain on injection, and local thrombophlebitis. These problems are not seen with midazolam, which is water-soluble. Recently, diazepam has been made available in a lipid emulsion in an attempt to limit the issues of local tissue irritation and pain on injection.

Metabolism of the benzodiazepines occurs via hepatic oxidation and glucuronidation. Oxidative processes are primarily responsible for the metabolism of diazepam and midazolam, and glucuronidation pathways are responsible for lorazepam metabolism. Hepatic oxidative processes occurring via the P_{450} system are susceptible to hepatic dysfunction and the co-administration of medications, including cimetidine and anticonvulsants. Glucuronidation pathways are less influenced by hepatic dysfunction and are not altered by the co-administration of other medications. As such, lorazepam pharmacokinetics are not significantly altered, even in the setting of hepatic dysfunction, yet significant variability in the pharmacokinetics of midazolam and diazepam occur with hepatic disease processes. An additional issue of clinical importance concerning the metabolism of the benzodiazepines is the production of active metabolites. Hepatic oxidative metabolism of diazepam results in the active metabolites: desmethyl-diazepam and 3-hydroxy-diazepam, both of which have significantly prolonged half-lives when compared with the parent compound. Oxidation

Table 4
Dosing Guidelines for Midazolam

Route of delivery	Dose (mg/kg)
Intravenous	0.05–0.1
Oral	0.5–0.7
Rectal	0.7–1
Intranasal	0.2–0.4
Sublingual	0.2–0.4

of midazolam results in a hydroxy-metabolite, and following prolonged administration, such as the ICU setting, this can result in prolonged sedation.

Like the barbiturates, propofol, and etomidate, the benzodiazepines decrease the $CMRO_2$ CBF and ICP. They are also effective anticonvulsants. However, in contrast to these other agents, the benzodiazepines—even in high doses—do not produce electrical silence on the electroencephalogram (EEG). When used alone, especially in patients without underlying systemic illness, they have limited effects on cardiorespiratory function. However, when combined with opioids or other sedative agents or in patients with cardiorespiratory compromise, they may produce respiratory depression and apnea. Similar principles apply for the cardiovascular effects of these agents. In high doses and in compromised patients, the benzodiazepines decrease MAP by a direct negative inotropic effect as well as a decrease in vascular resistance.

In addition to iv administration, multiple options for route of delivery of midazolam have been investigated, especially in the pediatric population (Table 4). These options may be considered when faced with the anxious child in whom iv access has not yet been established. With oral administration, doses of 0.5 to 0.7 mg/kg will produce anxiolysis in 20–30 min. Oral midazolam is currently the preferred agent for premedication in many of the pediatric operating rooms across the country. The only significant disadvantage to oral administration is that the iv preparation, when used for oral administration, contains the preservative benzyl alcohol, which tastes bitter. Therefore, the medication must be delivered in a solution that conceals the bitter taste. One of the more popular alternatives currently used in many operating rooms is to dilute the medication in double- or quadruple-strength Kool-Aid or to mix it in Tylenol elixir, both of which are somewhat effective in hiding or masking the bitter taste. Additionally, Roche Pharmaceuticals has recently introduced an oral formulation of midazolam that may alleviate this issue.

Alternatives to oral administration include transmucosal routes (nasal or sublingual) *(91–93)*. One benefit when compared to oral administration is a relatively more rapid onset of action (10 min vs 25–30 min with oral administration). For nasal administration, the iv preparation (5 mg/mL) is used and a dose of 0.2 mg/kg is drawn up into a tuberculin syringe. The needle is removed and the medication is dripped into the nasopharynx. Because the iv preparation contains benzyl alcohol, a significant degree of discomfort and burning may occur when the medication contacts the nasal mucosa. An alternative in the cooperative child is to place the medication into the sublingual space, thereby avoiding the problems of burning that occur with nasal administration.

In contrast to the other sedative agents reviewed in this chapter, there is a specific reversal agent for the benzodiazepines—flumazenil. Flumazenil's chemical structure resembles that of the benzodiazepines, except that it has a carbonyl group instead of a phenyl group. It undergoes rapid hepatic metabolism with an elimination half-life of 1 h. When it is used to reverse the effects of longer-acting benzodiazepines, flumazenil may be metabolized more rapidly, resulting in a reappearance of the benzodiazepine's actions. Notable, with flumazenil, are reports of seizure activity following its administration to patients chronically treated with benzodiazepines or patients who have ingested other medications that lower the seizure threshold such as tricyclic antidepressants or phenothiazines. As such, it is intended only for the reversal of the clinical effect following the acute administration of benzodiazepines.

3. SUMMARY

There are several different sedative agents available to provide sedation during diagnostic and invasive procedures (Table 5). Aside from ketamine, these agents possess no analgesic properties, and should be combined with an analgesic agent as needed. Although the cardiorespiratory effects of these agents are limited in the patient with normal cardiorespiratory function, significant deleterious physiologic effects can occur. Each of the agents reviewed in this chapter have their specific advantages and disadvantages, and none represents the perfect agent. The choice of agent will depend on the clinical scenario, the specific procedure, its duration, the patient's underlying status, and one's own experience.

Table 5
Dosing Guidelines for Commonly Used Sedative Agents*

Agent	Bolus dose	Infusion range/comments
Propofol	1–3 mg/kg	25–100 mcg/kg/min
Ketamine	0.25–1 mg/kg	10–30 mcg/kg/min
Etomidate	0.2–0.4 mg/kg	No infusion because of potential for adrenal suppression
Thiopental	2.5 mg/kg	—
Pentobarbital	1–3 mg/kg	1–4 mg/kg/h
Midazolam	0.05–0.1 mg/kg	1–5 mcg/kg/min; larger doses needed for non-parenteral routs (*see* Table 4)
Chloral hydrate	80–100 mg/kg	Oral administration only, limited data regarding adult dose, limit maximum dose to 2.0 grams
Nitrous oxide	30–70% via inhalation route	

*These dosing guidelines are meant only as suggested ranges for the various agents. These medications should be administered only with the use of appropriate monitoring and ready availability of means to provide airway management and cardiovascular resuscitation. The actual dose should be decreased in patients with significant associated medical illnesses or with the extremes of age. With intravenous administration, the doses can be repeated and titrated to achieve the desired effect.

REFERENCES

1. Sebel, P. S. and Lowdon, J. D. (1989) Propofol: a new intravenous anesthetic. *Anesthesiology* 260–277.
2. Harris, C. E., Grounds, R. M., Murray, A. M., et al. (1990) Propofol for long-term sedation in the intensive care unit. A comparison with papaveretum and midazolam. *Anaesthesia* **45,** 366–372.
3. Beller, J. P., Pottecher, T., Lugnier, A., et al. (1988) Prolonged sedation with propofol in ICU patients: recovery and blood concentration changes during periodic interruption in infusion. *Br. J. Anaesth.* **61,** 583–588.
4. Ronan, K. P., Gallagher, T. J., George, B., and Hamby, B. (1995) Comparison of propofol and midazolam for sedation in intensive care unit patients. *Crit. Care Med.* **23,** 286–293.
5. Lebovic, S., Reich, D. L., Steinberg, G., et al. (1992) Comparison of propofol versus ketamine for anesthesia in pediatric patients undergoing cardiac catheterization. *Anesth. Analg.* **74,** 490–494.
6. Hemelrijck, J. V., Fitch, W., Mattheussen, M., Van Aken, H., Plets, C., and Lauwers, T. (1990) Effect of propofol on cerebral circulation and autoregulation in the baboon. *Anesth. Analg.* **71,** 49–54.

7. Nimkoff, L., Quinn, C., Silver, P., and Sagy, M. (1997) The effects of intravenous anesthetic agents on intracranial pressure and cerebral perfusion pressure in two feline models of brain edema. *J. Crit. Care* **12,** 132–136.

8. Watts ADJ, Eliasziw, M., and Gelb, A. W. (1998) Propofol and hyperventilation for the treatment of increased intracranial pressure in rabbits. *Anesth. Analg.* **87,** 564–568.

9. Herregods, L., Verbeke, J., Rolly, G., and Colardyn, F. (1988) Effect of propofol on elevated intracranial pressure. Preliminary results. *Anaesthesia* **43(Suppl),** 107–109.

10. Pinaud, M., Lelausque, J., Chetanneau, A., Fauchoux, N., Menegalli, D., and Souron, R. (1990) Effects of propofol on cerebral hemodynamics and metabolism in patients with brain trauma. *Anesthesiology* **73,** 404–409.

11. Mangez, J. F., Menguy, E., and Roux, P. (1987) Sedation par propofol a debit constant chez le traumatise cranien. Resultas preliminaires. *Ann. Fr. Anesth. Reanim* **6,** 336–337.

12. Ravussin, P., Guinard, J. P., Ralley, F., and Thorin, D. (1988) Effect of propofol on cerebrospinal fluid pressure and cerebral perfusion pressure in patients undergoing craniotomy. *Anaesthesia* **43(Suppl),** 107–109.

13. Farling, P. A., Johnston, J. R., and Coppel, D. L. (1989) Propofol infusion for sedation of patients with head injury in intensive care. *Anaesthesia* **44,** 222–226.

14. Spitzfadden, A. C., Jimenez, D. F., and , J. D. (1999) Propofol for sedation and control of intracranial pressure in children. *Pediatr. Neurosurg.* **31,** 194–200.

15. Yamaguchi, S., Midorikawa, Y., Okuda, Y., and Kitajima, T. (1999) Propofol prevents delayed neuronal death following transient forebrain ischemia in gerbils. *Can. J. Anaesth.* **46,** 593–598.

16. Young, Y., Menon, D. K., Tisavipat, N., et al. (1997) Propofol neuroprotection in a rat model of ischaemia reperfusion injury. *Eur. J. Anesth.* **14,** 320–326.

17. Pittman, J. E., Sheng, H., Pearlstein, R., et al. (1997) Comparison of the effects of propofol and pentobarbital on neurologic outcome and cerebral infarct size after temporary focal ischemia in the rat. *Anesthesiology* **87,** 1139–1144.

18. Brussel, T., Theissen, J. L., Vigfusson, G., et al. (1989) Hemodynamic and cardiodynamic effects of propofol and etomidate: Negative inotropic properties of propofol. *Anesth. Analg.* **69,** 35–40.

19. Tritapepe, L., Voci, P., Marino, P., et al. (1999) Calcium chloride minimizes the hemodynamic effects of propofol in patients undergoing coronary artery bypass grafting. *J. Cardiothor. Vasc. Anes.* **13,** 150–153.

20. Sochala, C., Van Deenen, D., De Ville, A., and Govaerts, M. J. M. (1999) Heart block following propofol in a child. *Paediatr. Anaes.* **9,** 349–351.

21. Egan, T. D., and Brock-Utne, J. G. (1991) Asystole and anesthesia induction with a fentanyl, propofol, and succinylcholine sequence. *Anesth. Analg.* **73,** 818–820.

22. Trotter, C. and Serpell, M. G. (1992) Neurological sequelae in children after prolonged propofol infusions. *Anaesthesia* **47,** 340–342.

23. Saunders, P. R. I. and Harris, M. N. E. (1992) Opisthotonic posturing and other unusual neurological sequelae after outpatient anesthesia. *Anaesthesia* **47,** 552–557.

24. Collier, C. and Kelly, K. (1991) Propofol and convulsions—The evidence mounts. *Anaesthesiol. Intensive Care* **19,** 573–575.

25. Finley, G. A., MacManus, B., Sampson, S. E., Fernandez, C. V., and Retallick, I. (1993) Delayed seizures following sedation with propofol. *Can. J. Anaesth.* **40,** 863–865.

26. Lowenstein, D. H. and Alldredge, B. K. (1998) Status epilepticus. *N. Engl. J. Med.* **338,** 970–976.

27. Hertzog, J. H., Campbell, J. K., Dalton, H. J., and Hauser, G. J. (1999) Propofol anesthesia for invasive procedures in ambulatory and hospitalized children: experience in the Pediatric Intensive Care Unit. *Pediatrics* **103,** e30.

28. Chih-Chung, L., Ming-Hwang, S., and Tan, P. P. C., et al. (1999) Mechanisms underlying the inhibitory effect of propofol on the contraction of canine airway smooth muscle. *Anesthesiology* **91,** 750–759.

29. Parke, T. J., Stevens, J. E., Rice, A. S. C., et al. (1992) Metabolic acidosis and fatal myocardial failure after propofol infusion in children: five case reports. *Br. Med. J.* **305,** 613–616.

30. Strickland, R. A. and Murray, M. J. (1995) Fatal metabolic acidosis in a pediatric patient receiving an infusion of propofol in the intensive care unit: is there a relationship? *Crit. Care Med.* **23,** 405–409.

31. Bray, R. J. (1998) Propofol infusion syndrome in children. *Paediatr. Anaes.* **8,** 491–499.

32. Hanna, J. P. and Ramundo, M. L. (1998) Rhabdomyolysis and hypoxia associated with prolonged propofol infusion. *Neurology* **50,** 301–303.

33. Laxenaire, M. C., Mata-Bermejo, E., Moneret-Vautrin, D. A., and Gueant, J. L. (1992) Life-threatening anaphylactoid reactions to propofol. *Anesthesiology* **77,** 275–280.

34. Haugen, R. D., Vaghadia, H., Waters, T., and Merrick, P. M. (1995) Thiopentone pretreatment for propofol injection pain in ambulatory patients. *Can. J. Anaesth.* **42,** 1108–1112.

35. Mangar, D. and Holak, E. J. (1992) Tourniquet at 50 mmHg followed by intravenous lidocaine diminishes hand pain associated with propofol injection. *Anesth. Analg.* **74,** 250–252.

36. Tobias, J. D. (1996) Prevention of pain associated with the administration of propofol in children: lidocaine versus ketamine. *Am. J. Anesthesiol.* **23,** 231–232.

37. Sosis, M. B. and Braverman, B. (1993) Growth of Staphylococcus aureus in four intravenous anesthetics. *Anesth. Analg.* **77,** 766–768.

38. Postsurgical infections associated with extrinsically contaminated intravenous anesthetic agent—California, Illinois, Maine, and Michigan, 1990. (1990) *MMWR* **39,** 426–427, 433.

39. Gottardis, M., Khunl-Brady, K. S., Koller, W., et al. (1989) Effect of prolonged sedation with propofol on serum triglyceride and cholesterol concentrations. *Br. J. Anaesth.* **62,** 393–396.

40. Valente, J. F., Anderson, G. L., Branson, R. D., et al. (1994) Disadvantages of propofol sedation in the critical care unit. *Crit. Care Med.* **22,** 710–712.

41. Domino, E. F., Chodoff, P., and Corssen, G. (1965) Pharmacologic effects of CI-581, a new dissociative anesthetic in man. *Clin. Pharmacol. Ther.* **6,** 279–291.

42. White, P. F., Ham, J., Way, W. L., et al. (1980) Pharmacology of ketamine isomers in surgical patients. *Anesthesiology* **52,** 231–239.

43. Tobias, J. D. (1999) End-tidal carbon dioxide monitoring during sedation with a combination of midazolam and ketamine for children undergoing painful, invasive procedures. *Pediatr. Emerg. Care* **15,** 173–175.

44. Chernow, B., Laker, R., Creuss, D., et al. (1982) Plasma, urine, and cerebrospinal fluid catecholamine concentrations during and after ketamine sedation. *Crit. Care Med.* **10,** 600–603.

45. Wayman, K., Shoemaker, W. C., Lippmann, M. (1980) Cardiovascular effects of anesthetic induction with ketamine. *Anesth. Analg.* **59,** 355–358.

46. Spotoft, H., Korshin, J. D., Sorensen, M. B., et al. (1979) The cardiovascular effects of ketamine used for induction of anesthesia in patients with valvular heart disease. *Can Anaesth Soc J* **26,** 463–467.

47. Gooding, J. M., Dimick, A. R., Travakoli, M., et al. (1977) A Physiologic analysis of cardiopulmonary responses to ketamine anesthesia in non-cardiac patients. *Anesth. Analg.* **56,** 813–816.

48. Morray, J. P., Lynn, A. M., Stamm, S. J., et al. (1984) Hemodynamic effects of ketamine in children with congenital heart disease. *Anesth. Analg.* **63,** 895–899.

49. Hickey, P. R., Hansen, D. D., Cramolini, G. M., et al. (1985) Pulmonary and systemic hemodynamic responses to ketamine in infants with normal and elevated pulmonary vascular resistance. *Anesthesiology* **62,** 287–293.

50. Fleischer, F., Polarz, H., Lang, J., and Bohrer, H. (1991) Changes in oxygen saturation following low-dose intramuscular ketamine in pediatric cardiac surgical patients. *Paediatric Anaesthesia* **1,** 33–36.

51. Mankikian, B., Cantineau, J. P., Sartene, R., et al. (1986) Ventilatory and chest wall mechanics during ketamine anesthesia in humans. *Anesthesiology* **65,** 492–499.

52. Hirshman, C. A., Downes, H., Farbood, A., and Bergman, N. A. (1979) Ketamine block of bronchospasm in experimental canine asthma. *Br. J. Anaesth.* **51,** 713–718.

53. Bourke, D. L., Malit, L. A., and Smith, T. C. (1987) Respiratory interactions of ketamine and morphine. *Anesthesiology* **66,** 153–156.

54. Lanning, C. F., Harmel, M. H. (1975) Ketamine anesthesia. *Annu. Rev. Med.* **26,** 137–141.

55. Taylor, P. A. and Towey, R. M. (1971) Depression of laryngeal reflexes during ketamine administration. *Br. Med. J.* **2,** 688–689.

56. Shapiro, H. M., Wyte, S. R., and Harris, A. B. (1972) Ketamine anesthesia in patients with intracranial pathology. *Br. J. Anaesth.* **44,** 1200–1204.

57. Gardner, A. E., Dannemiller, F. J., and Dean D. (1972) Intracranial cerebrospinal fluid pressure in man during ketamine anesthesia. *Anesth. Analg.* **51,** 741–745.

58. Reicher, D., Bhalla, P., and Rubinstein, E. H. (1987) Cholinergic cerebral vasodilator effects of ketamine in rabbits. *Stroke* **18,** 445–449.

59. Oren, R. E., Rasool, N. A., and Rubinstein, E. H. (1987) Effect of ketamine on cerebral cortical blood flow and metabolism in rabbits. *Stroke* **18,** 445–444.

60. White, P. F., Way, W. L., and Trevor, A. J. (1982) Ketamine—its pharmacology and therapeutic uses. *Anesthesiology* **56,** 119–136.

61. Weksler, N., Ovadia, L., Muati, G., and Stav, A. (1993) Nasal ketamine for paediatric premedication. *Can. J. Anaesth.* **40,** 119–121.

62. Qureshi, F. A., Mellis, P. T., and McFadden, M. A. (1995) Efficacy of oral ketamine for providing sedation and analgesia to children requiring laceration repair. *Pediatr. Emerg. Care* **11,** 93–97.

63. Tobias, J. D., Phipps, S., Smith, B., and Mulhern, R. K. (1992) Oral ketamine premedication to alleviate the distress of invasive procedures in pediatric oncology patients. *Pediatrics* **90,** 537–541.

64. Tobias, J. D., Martin, L. D., and Wetzel, R. C. (1990) Ketamine by continuous infusion for sedation in the pediatric intensive care unit. *Crit. Care Med.* **18,** 819–821.

65. Hartvig, P., Larsson, E., and Joachimsson, P. O. (1993) Postoperative analgesia and sedation following pediatric cardiac surgery using a constant infusion of ketamine. *J. Cardiothor. Vasc. Anes.* **7,** 148–153.

66. Van de Wiele, B., Rubinstein, E., Peacock, W., and Martin, N. (1995) Propylene glycol toxicity caused by prolonged etomidate infusion. *J. Neurosurg. Anesth.* **7,** 259–262.

67. Belelli, D., Pistis, M., Peters, J. A., and Lambert, J. J. (1999) The interaction of general anesthetics and neurosteroids with GABA$_A$ and glycine receptors. *Neurochem. Int.* **34,** 447–452.

68. Giese, J. L., Stockham, R. J., Stanley, T. H., et al. (1985) Etomidate versus thiopental for induction of anesthesia. *Anesth. Analg.* **64,** 871–876.

69. Brussel, T., Theissen, J. L., Vigfusson, G., et al. (1989) Hemodynamic and cardiodynamic effects of propofol and etomidate: negative inotropic properties of propofol. *Anesth. Analg.* **69,** 35–40.

70. Modica, P. A., Tempelhoff, R., and White, P. F. (1990) Pro- and anticonvulsant effects of anesthetics (part 2). *Anesth. Analg.* **70,** 433–439.

71. Kay, B. (1976) A clinical assessment of the use of etomidate in children. *Br. J. Anaesth.* **48,** 207–210.

72. Tobias, J. D. (1997) Etomidate: applications in pediatric anesthesia and critical care. *J. Intensive Care Med.* **12,** 324–326.

73. Ford, S. R., Maze, M., and Gaba, D. M. (1991) A comparison of etomidate and thiopental anesthesia for cardioversion. *J. Cardiothor. Vasc. Anes.* **5,** 563–565.

74. Canessa, R., Lema, G., Urzua, J., et al. (1991) Anesthesia for elective cardioversion: a comparison of four anesthetic agents. *J. Cardiothor. Vasc. Anes.* **5,** 566–568.

75. McDowall, R. H., Scher, C. S., and Barst, S. M. (1995) Total intravenous anesthesia for children undergoing brief diagnostic or therapeutic procedures. *J. Clin. Anesth.* **7,** 273–280.

76. Behrens, R., Lang, T., Muschweck, H., Richter, T., and Hofbeck, M. (1997) Percutaneous endoscopic gastrostomy in children and adolescents. *J. Pediatr. Gasterenterol. Nut.* **25,** 487–491.

77. Streissand, J. B., Jaarsma, R. L., Gay, M. A., et al. (1998) Oral transmucosal etomidate in volunteers. *Anesthesiology* **88,** 89–95.

78. Wagner, R. L., White, P. F., Kan, P. B., et al. (1984) Inhibition of adrenal steroidogenesis by the anesthetic etomidate. *N. Engl. J. Med.* **310,** 1415–1418.

79. Absalom, A., Pledger, D., and Kong, A. (1999) Adrenocortical function in critically ill patients 24 hour after a single dose of etomidate. *Anaesthesia* 54, 861–867.

80. Sanderson, P. M. (1997) A survey of pentobarbital sedation for children undergoing abdominal CT scans after oral contrast medium. *Paediatr. Anaesth.* **7,** 309–315.

81. Pereira, J. K., Burrows, P. E., Richards, H. M., et al. (1993) Comparison of sedative regimens for pediatric outpatient CT. *Pediatr. Radiol.* **23,** 341–344.

82. Strain, J. D., Harvey, L. A., Foley, L. C., et al. (1986) Intravenously administered pentobarbital for sedation in paediatric CT. *Radiology* **161,** 105–108.

83. Glasier, C. M., Stark, J. E., Brown R., et al. (1995) Rectal thiopental sodium for sedation of pediatric patients undergoing MR and other imaging studies. *Am. J. Neuroradiol.* **16,** 111–114.

84. Tobias, J. D. (2000) Pentobarbital for sedation during mechanical ventilation in the Pediatric ICU patient. *J. Intens. Care Med.* **15,** 115–120.

85. Holst, J. J. (1962) Use of nitrous oxide-oxygen analgesia in dentistry. *Int. Dent. J.* **12,** 47–51.

86. Griffin, G. C., Campbell, V. D., and Joni, R. (1981) Nitrous oxide-oxygen sedation for minor surgery: experience in a pediatric setting. *JAMA* **245,** 2411–2414.

87. Litman, R. S., Berkowitz, R. J., and Ward, D. S. (1996) Levels of consciousness and ventilatory parameters in young children during sedation with oral midazolam and nitrous oxide. *Arch. Pediatr. Adolesc. Med.* **150,** 671–675.

88. Mayers, D. J., Hindmarsh, K. W., Sankaran, K., et al. (1992) Chloral hydrate disposition following single-dose administration to critically ill neonates and children. *Dev. Pharmacol. Ther.* **19,** 141–146.

89. Graham, S. R., Day, R. O., Lee, R., et al. (1988) Overdose with chloral hydrate: A pharmacological and therapeutic review. *Med. J. Aust.* **149,** 686–688.

90. Seger, D. and Schwartz, G. (1994) Chloral hydrate: a dangerous sedative for overdose patients. *Pediatr. Emerg Care* **10,** 349–350.

91. Theroux, M. C., West, D. W., Cordry, D. H., et al. (1993) Efficacy of midazolam in facilitating suturing of lacerations in preschool children in the emergency department. *Pediatrics* **91,** 624–627.

92. Zedie, N., Amory, D. W., Wagner, B. K. J., et al. (1996) Comparison of intranasal midazolam and sufentanil premedication in pediatric outpatients. *Clin. Pharmacol. Ther.* **59,** 341–348.

93. Geldner, G., Hubmann, M., Knoll, R., and Jacobi, K. (1997) Comparison between three transmucosal routes of administration of midazolam in children. *Paediatr. Anaes.* **7,** 103–109.

7

Opioids in the Management of Acute Pediatric Pain

Myron Yaster, MD, Lynne G. Maxwell, MD, and Sabine Kost-Byerly, MD

1. INTRODUCTION

The treatment and alleviation of pain is a basic human right that exists regardless of age (1–4). Unfortunately, even when their pain is obvious, children frequently receive no treatment, or inadequate treatment, for pain and for painful procedures (5). The newborn and the critically ill child are especially vulnerable to no treatment or undertreatment (6–10). The conventional "wisdom" that children do not respond to nor remember painful experiences to the same degree as adults is simply untrue (11,12). Indeed, all of the nerve pathways essential for the transmission and perception of pain are present and functioning by 24 wk of gestation (13). Recent research in newborn animals has revealed that the failure to provide analgesia for pain results in "rewiring" the nerve pathways responsible for pain transmission in the dorsal horn of the spinal cord and results in increased pain perception for *future* painful insults (12–17). This confirms human newborn research, in which the failure to provide anesthesia or analgesia for newborn circumcision resulted in short-term physiologic perturbations as well as in longer-term behavioral changes, particularly during immunization (18).

Nurses are taught to be wary of physicians' orders (and patients' requests) as well. The most common prescription order for potent analgesics, "to give as needed" (pro re nata, "PRN"), in reality means "to give as infrequently as possible." The "PRN" order also means that either the patient must know or remember to ask for pain medication, or the nurse must identify when a patient is in pain. Neither of these requirements can be met by children who are in pain. Children less than 3 yr of age or critically ill children may be unable to adequately verbalize when or where they hurt. Alternatively, they may be afraid to report their pain. Many children will withdraw or deny

From: *Contemporary Clinical Neuroscience: Sedation and Analgesia for Diagnostic and Therapeutic Procedures*
Edited by: S. Malviya, N. N. Naughton, and K. K. Tremper © Humana Press Inc., Totowa, NJ

their pain in an attempt to avoid yet another terrifying and painful experience—the intramuscular (im) injection or "shot." Finally, several studies have documented the inability of nurses, physicians, and parents to correctly identify and treat pain even in postoperative pediatric patients *(19–21)*.

Fortunately, the past 10 years have seen an explosion in research and interest in pediatric pain management. Pain management for pediatric patients with acute, postoperative, terminal, neuropathic, and chronic pain has become commonplace. Procedure-related pain requires special attention *(22–26)*. This is pain that is deliberately inflicted on patients by nurses and physicians in the course of performing medical procedures and tests. Examples include immunization, bone-marrow aspirations and lumbar punctures, blood sampling from a vein or artery, and suturing traumatic lacerations. Although procedure-related pain is one of the most common forms of pain that children experience when dealing with health care professionals, it is also among the most difficult to manage, both by the patient experiencing it and by the health care professionals who must inflict it. Indeed, the most common response by nurses and physicians to procedure-related pain is denial, which is made easy because children can be physically restrained, are not routinely asked whether they are in pain, and are unable to withdraw consent to stop a procedure. It is our belief that much of this pain can be abolished, and is best treated with the proper administration of local anesthetics. In fact, opioids, the subject of this chapter, are really only adjuvants to good regional blockade in the management of procedure-related pain. The use of local anesthetics in the treatment of pediatric pain has been the subject of several reviews *(27,28)*. In this chapter, we have attempted to comprehensively consolidate the recent advances in opioid pharmacology and the various modalities available that are useful in the treatment of acute procedure-related, post-procedure, and childhood pain.

2. PHARMACOKINETICS

Drugs are fundamental in the treatment of pain. A thorough understanding of the history, chemical and physical properties, physiological effects, disposition, mechanisms of action, and therapeutic uses of the drugs used in the treatment of pain is essential for clinicians who treat pain in infants, children, and adolescents. When physicians administer drugs to their patients, they do so with the expectation that an anticipated therapeutic effect will occur. Unfortunately, other less desirable results can also occur—namely, the patient may derive inadequate or no therapeutic benefit from the administered drug, or worse yet, they may develop a toxic reaction. The aim of modern clinical pharmacology is to take the guess work out of this process and to establish the relationship between the dose of a drug given and the response elicited. To attain this goal, clinicians need a working knowledge of the principles of drug absorption, distribution, and elimination, and how these processes are related to the intensity and duration of drug action.

Unfortunately, it is also important to understand that the science of clinical pharmacology is not always predictable and exact. The relationship between the concentration of drug in the blood and the clinical response to that plasma drug level is not always predictable. Individuals vary widely in their response to drugs, and this may be a result of differences in the concentration of drug available at the drug's site of action or differences in the individual's inherent sensitivity to the drug. Clearly, the end point of drug therapy is clinical efficacy, not simply attaining a certain blood level of drug. "Best practice" requires an attempt by the physician to define the optimal dose-response relationship in each individual patient based on history, diagnosis, and clinical judgement.

2.1. Physiologic Changes Affecting Pharmacokinetics in Infants, Children, and Adolescents

Unfortunately, very few studies have evaluated the pharmacokinetic and pharmacodynamic properties of drugs in children. Most pharmacokinetic studies are performed using healthy adult volunteers, adult patients who are only minimally ill, or adult patients in the stable phase of a chronic disease. These data are then extrapolated to infants, children, adolescents, and to the critically ill (both adult and pediatric). Drug manufacturers simply do not perform these studies in children. In fact, so little pharmacokinetic and dynamic testing has been performed in children that they are often considered "therapeutic orphans." *(29)* Indeed, more than 70% of all the drugs used to treat children have never been formally tested or approved for use in children. Occasionally, this has resulted in catastrophe, as in the development of "gray baby syndrome" in neonates treated with chloramphenicol *(30,31)*. Why children are different is obvious. Newborns, children less than 2–3 yr of age, and unstable, critically ill pediatric patients of any age often present significant hemodynamic alterations and organ dysfunction, which may significantly alter drug absorption and the transport, metabolism, and excretion of drugs. Studies performed in healthy older children or adult patients may offer little insight into how these drugs perform in these other patient populations *(32–35)*. To help remedy this situation, the Food and Drug Administration (FDA) has mandated pediatric pharmacokinetic and dynamic studies in all new drugs that enter the American marketplace *(36–38)*. Unfortunately, despite these new regulations, the pharmaceutical industry has, with very few exceptions, delayed, evaded, and "stone-walled" the process, leaving children with very little protection.

2.2. Opioid Pharmacokinetics

To relieve or prevent pain, a drug must reach the receptors that alleviate pain within the central nervous system (CNS). Drugs that bind to a receptor to produce a positive effect (the diminution or elimination of pain) are called *agonists*. There are essentially two ways that an agonist gets inside the brain; it is either transported into the brain via the bloodstream (following intravenous (iv), im, oral, nasal, transdermal, or mucosal administration), or it is directly deposited (intrathecal or epidural) into the cerebrospinal fluid (CSF) *(39–41)*. Agonists administered via the bloodstream must cross the blood-brain barrier—a lipid membrane interface between the endothelial cells of the brain vasculature and the extracellular fluid of the brain—to reach the receptor. Normally, highly lipid-soluble agonists, such as fentanyl, rapidly diffuse across the blood-brain barrier, whereas agonists with limited lipid solubility, such as morphine, have limited brain uptake *(42–46)*. The blood-brain barrier may be immature at birth, and is known to be more permeable to morphine. Indeed, Way et al. demonstrated that morphine concentrations were 2–4 times greater in the brains of younger rats than in older rats, despite equal blood concentrations *(47)*. Obviously, the immaturity of the blood-brain barrier will have less of an effect on highly lipid-soluble agents such as fentanyl *(48)*.

Spinal administration, either intrathecally or epidurally, bypasses the blood and directly places an agonist into the CSF, which bathes the receptor sites in the spinal cord (substantia gelatinosa) and brain. This "back door" to the receptor significantly reduces the amount of agonist needed to relieve pain *(49)*. After spinal administration, opioids are absorbed by the epidural veins and redistributed to the systemic circulation, where they are metabolized and excreted. Hydrophilic agents, such as morphine, cross the dura more slowly than more lipid-soluble agents such as fentanyl or meperidine *(50)*. This physico-chemical property is responsible for the more prolonged duration of action of spinal morphine, and its very slow onset of action following epidural administration *(41,51,52)*.

Although it would be desirable to adjust opioid dosage based on the concentration of drug achieved at the receptor site, this is rarely feasible. The alternative is to measure blood or plasma concentrations and model how the body handles a drug. Pharmacokinetic studies thereby help the clinician select suitable routes, timing, and dosing of drugs to maximize a drug's dynamic effects.

Following administration, the disposition of a drug is dependent on distribution ($t_{1/2}\alpha$) and elimination. The terminal half-life of elimination ($t_{1/2}\beta$) is directly proportional to the volume of distribution (Vd) and inversely proportional to the total body clearance by the following formula:

$$t_{1/2}\beta = 0.693 \times (Vd/Cl)$$

Thus, a prolongation of the $t_{1/2}\beta$ may be caused by either an increase in a drug's volume of distribution or by a decrease in its clearance.

The liver is the major site of biotransformation for most opioids. The major metabolic pathway for most opioids is oxidation. The exceptions are morphine and buprenorphine, which primarily undergo glucuronidation, and remifentanil, which is cleared by ester hydrolysis *(53–55)*. Many of these reactions are catalyzed in the liver by microsomal mixed-function oxidases that require the cytochrome P_{450} system, NADPH, and oxygen. The cytochrome P_{450} system is very immature at birth and does not reach adult levels until the first month or two of life *(56,57)*. This immaturity of this hepatic enzyme system may explain the prolonged clearance or elimination of some opioids in the first few days to the first few weeks of life. On the other hand, the P_{450} system can be induced by various drugs (phenobarbital) and substrates, and matures regardless of gestational age. Thus, it may be the age from birth, and not the duration of gestation, that determines how premature and full-term infants metabolize drugs. Indeed, Greeley et al. have demonstrated that sufentanil is more rapidly metabolized and eliminated in 2–3-wk-old infants than newborns less than 1 wk of age *(58)*.

Morphine is primarily glucuronidated into two forms—an inactive form, morphine-3-glucuronide and an active form, morphine-6-glucuronide. Both glucuronides are excreted by the kidneys. In patients with renal failure or with reduced glomerular filtration rates (e.g., neonates), the morphine 6-glucuronide can accumulate and cause toxic side effects, such as respiratory depression. This is an important consideration when prescribing morphine and when administering other opioids that are metabolized into morphine, such as methadone and codeine.

The pharmacokinetics of opioids in patients with liver disease requires special attention. Oxidation of opioids is reduced in patients with hepatic cirrhosis, resulting in decreased drug clearance (meperidine, dextropropoxyphene, pentazocine, tramadol, and alfentanil) and/or increased oral bioavailability caused by a reduced first-pass metabolism (meperidine, pentazocine, and dihydrocodeine). Although glucuronidation is believed to be less affected in liver cirrhosis, the clearance of morphine is decreased and oral bioavailability is increased. The result of reduced drug metabolism is the risk of accumulation in the body, especially with repeated administration. Lower doses or longer administration intervals should be used to minimize this risk. Meperidine poses a special concern because it is metabolized into normeperidine, a toxic metabolite that causes seizures and accumulates in liver disease *(59,60)*. On the other hand, drugs that are inactive but are metabolized in the liver into active forms such as codeine may be ineffective in patients with liver disease. Finally, the disposition of a few opioids—such as fentanyl, sufentanil and remifentanil—appears to be unaffected in liver disease, and are the drugs we use preferentially in managing pain in patients with liver disease *(61)*.

The pharmacokinetics of morphine have been extensively studied in adults, older children, and in the premature and full-term newborn *(62–68)*. Following an iv bolus, 30% of morphine is protein bound in the adult vs only 20% in the newborn. This increase in unbound ("free") morphine allows a greater proportion of active drug to penetrate the brain. This may explain, in part, the observation of Way et al. of increased brain levels of morphine in the newborn and its more profound respiratory depressant effects *(47,69)*. The elimination half-life of morphine in adults and older children is 3–4 h and is consistent with its duration of analgesic action (Table 1). The $t_{1/2}\beta$ is more than twice as long in newborns less than 1 wk of age than older children and adults, and is even longer in premature infants and children requiring pressor support *(63,70–72)*. Clearance is similarly decreased, in the newborn compared to the older child and adult. Thus, infants less than 1 mo of age will attain higher serum levels that will decline more slowly than older children and adults. This may also account for the increased respiratory depression associated with morphine in this age group *(73)*.

Interestingly, the half-life of elimination and clearance of morphine in children older than 1–2 mo of age is similar to adult values. Thus the hesitancy in prescribing and administering morphine in children less than 1 yr of age may not be warranted. However, the use of any opioid in children less than 2 mo of age, particularly those born prematurely, must be limited to a monitored, intensive care unit (ICU) setting, not only because of pharmacokinetic and dynamic reasons but because of immature ventilatory responses to hypoxemia, hypercarbia, and airway obstruction in the neonate *(74–77)*.

3. OPIOIDS OVERVIEW

Historically, opium and its derivatives (e.g., paregoric and morphine) were used for the treatment of diarrhea (dysentery) and pain. Indeed, the beneficial psychological and physiological effects of opium, as well as its toxicity and potential for abuse, have been well-known to physicians and

Table 1
Commonly Used Mu-Agonist Drugs

Agonist	Equipotent IV dose (mg/kg)	Duration (h)	Bioavailability (%)	Comments
Morphine	0.1	3–4	20–40	• Seizures in newborns; also in all patients at high doses • Histamine release, vasodilation →→ avoid in asthmatics and in circulatory compromise • MS-contin® 8–12-h duration
Meperidine	1.0	3–4	40–60	• Catastrophic interactions with MAO inhibitors • Tachycardia; negative inotrope • Metabolite produces seizures; not recommended for chronic use
Methadone	0.1	6–24	70–100	• Can be given intravenously even though the package insert says SQ or intramuscularly
Fentanyl	0.001	0.5–1		• Bradycardia; minimal hemodynamic alterations • Chest wall rigidity(>5 μg/kg rapid IV bolus), prescription with either naloxone or paralyze with succinylcholine or pancuronium • Transdermal patch available for chronic pain, contra-indicated in acute pain
Codeine	1.2	3–4	40–70	• Oral route only • Prescribe with acetaminophen
Hydromorphone (Dialaudid)	0.015–0.02	3–4	40–60	• < CNS depression than morphine • < Itching, nausea than morphine • Can be used in iv and epidural PCA
Oxycodone (Component opioid in Tylox)	0.15	3–4	50	• One-third less than morphine but with better oral bioavailability, it is often used when weaning from iv to oral medication • Available as a continuous release preparation

the public for centuries *(78,79)*. In 1680, Sydenham wrote, "Among the remedies which it has pleased Almighty God to give man to relieve his sufferings, none is so universal and so efficacious as opium." On the other hand, many physicians through the ages have underutilized the use of opium when treating patients in pain because of their fear that their patients would be harmed by its use. In the present era, addiction is particularly feared. Opium's easy availability, despite every effort by the government to control it, has resulted in a scourge of addiction that has devastated large segments of our population. Until and unless we can separate opium's dark consequences (yin) from its benefits (yang), innumerable numbers of patients will suffer unnecessarily. The purpose of this chapter is to delineate the role of opioid receptors in the mechanism of opioid analgesia, to highlight recent advances in opioid pharmacology and therapeutic interventions, and to provide a pharmacokinetic and pharmacodynamic framework regarding the use of opioids in the treatment of childhood pain.

3.1. Terminology

The terminology used to describe potent analgesic drugs is constantly changing *(79–81)*. They are commonly referred to as "narcotics" (from the Greek "narco"—to deaden), "opiates" (from the Greek "opion"—poppy juice, for drugs derived from the poppy plant), "opioids" (for all drugs with morphine-like effects, whether synthetic or naturally occurring), or euphemistically as "strong analgesics" (when the physician is reluctant to tell the patient or the patient's family that narcotics are being used) *(79,82,83)*. Furthermore, the discovery of endogenous endorphins and opioid receptors has necessitated the reclassification of these drugs into agonists, antagonists, and mixed agonist-antagonists based on their receptor-binding properties *(79,83–87)*.

3.2. Opioid Receptors

Over the past twenty years, multiple opioid receptors and subtypes have been identified and classified *(79,83–88)*. An understanding of the complex nature and organization of these multiple opioid receptors is essential for an adequate understanding of the response to, and control of, pain *(41)*. In the CNS, there are four primary opioid-receptor types, designated mu (μ) (for morphine), kappa (κ), delta (δ), and sigma (σ). Recently, the μ, κ, and δ receptors have been cloned and have yielded invaluable information of receptor structure and function *(89–92)*.

The μ receptor is further subdivided into μ_1 (supraspinal analgesia) and μ_2 (respiratory depression, inhibition of gastrointestinal motility, and spinal analgesia) subtypes *(84,93,94)*. When morphine and other mu agonists are given systemically, it acts predominantly through supraspinal μ_1 receptors. The kappa and delta receptors have been subtyped as well, and other receptors and subtypes will surely be discovered as research in this area progress (95).

The differentiation of agonists and antagonists is fundamental to pharmacology. A neurotransmitter is defined as having agonist activity, and a drug that blocks the action of a neurotransmitter is an antagonist (96–100). By definition, receptor recognition of an agonist is "translated" into other cellular alterations (the agonist initiates a pharmacologic effect), whereas an antagonist occupies the receptor without initiating the transduction step (it has no intrinsic activity or efficacy) (101). The intrinsic activity of a drug defines the ability of the drug-receptor complex to initiate a pharmacologic effect. Drugs that produce less than a maximal response have a lowered intrinsic activity and are called partial agonists. Partial agonists also have antagonistic properties, because by binding the receptor site, they block access of full agonists to the receptor site. Morphine and related opiates are μ agonists, and drugs that block the effects of opiates at the μ receptor, such as naloxone, are designated as antagonists. The opioids most commonly used in the management of pain are μ agonists and include morphine, meperidine, methadone, codeine, oxycodone, and the fentanyls. Mixed agonist-antagonist drugs act as agonists or partial agonists at one receptor and antagonists at another receptor. Mixed (opioid) agonist-antagonist drugs include pentazocine (Talwin®), butorphanol (Stadol®), nalorphine, dezocine (Dalgan®), and nalbuphine (Nubain®). Most of these drugs are agonists or partial agonists at the κ and δ receptors and antagonists or partial agonists at the μ receptor. Thus, these drugs will produce antinociception alone, and will dose-dependently antagonize the effects of morphine.

The μ receptor and its subspecies and the δ receptor produce analgesia, respiratory depression, euphoria, and physical dependence. Morphine is fifty to one hundred times weaker at the δ receptor than at the μ receptor. By contrast, the endogenous opiate-like neurotransmitter peptides known as the enkephalins tend to be more potent at δ and κ than μ receptors. The κ receptor, located primarily in the spinal cord, produces spinal analgesia, miosis, and sedation with minimal associated respiratory depression. A number of studies suggest that the respiratory depression and analgesia produced by μ agonists involve different receptor subtypes (102–104). Other studies have disputed these findings (95,105). These receptors change in number in an age-related fashion and can be blocked by naloxone. Pasternak et al., working with newborn rats, showed that 14-d-old rats are 40 times more sensitive to morphine analgesia than 2-d-old rats (102,103). Nevertheless, morphine depresses the respiratory rate in 2-d-old rats to a greater degree than in 14-d-old rats. Thus, the newborn may be particularly sensitive to the respiratory depressant effects of the commonly administered opioids in what may be an age-related receptor phenomenon *(73)*. Obviously, this has important clinical implications for the use of opioids in the newborn.

4. OPIOID DRUG SELECTION

Many factors are considered in the selection of the appropriate opioid analgesic to administer to a patient in pain. These include pain intensity, patient age, co-existing disease, potential drug interactions, prior treatment history, physician preference, patient preference, and route of administration. The idea that some opioids are "weak" (e.g., codeine) and others "strong" (e.g., morphine) is outdated. All are capable of treating pain regardless of its intensity if the dose is adjusted appropriately. And at equipotent doses, most opioids have similar effects and side effects (Table 1).

4.1. Morphine

Morphine (from Morpheus, the Greek God of Sleep) is the gold standard for analgesia against which all other opioids are compared. When small doses, 0.1 mg·kg^{-1} (iv, im), are administered to otherwise unmedicated patients in pain, analgesia usually occurs without loss of consciousness. The relief of tension, anxiety, and pain usually results in drowsiness and sleep as well. Older patients suffering from discomfort and pain usually develop a sense of well-being and/or euphoria following morphine administration. Interestingly, when morphine is given to pain-free adults, they may show the opposite effect—namely, dysphoria and increased fear and anxiety. Mental clouding, drowsiness, lethargy, an inability to concentrate, and sleep may occur following morphine administration, even in the absence of pain. Less advantageous CNS effects of morphine include nausea and vomiting, pruritus, especially around the nose, miosis, and seizures at high doses *(106)*. Seizures are a particular problem in the newborn because they may occur at commonly prescribed doses (0.1 mg/kg) *(63,66,67,107)*.

Although morphine produces peripheral vasodilation and venous pooling, it has minimal hemodynamic effects (e.g., cardiac output, left ventricular stroke work index, and pulmonary artery pressure) in normal, euvolemic, supine patients. The vasodilation associated with morphine is primarily a result of its histamine-releasing effects. The magnitude of morphine-induced histamine release can be minimized by limiting the rate of morphine infusion to 0.025–0.05 mg/kg/min, by keeping the patient in a supine to a slightly head down (Trendelenburg's) position, and by optimizing intravascular volume. Significant hypotension may occur if sedatives such as diazepam are concurrently administered with morphine or if a patient suddenly changes from a supine to a standing position. Otherwise, it produces virtually no

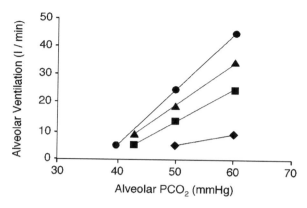

Fig. 1. Relationship between ventilation and carbon dioxide is represented by a family of curves. Each curve has two parameters: intercept and slope. Sedatives and opioids increase intercept and decrease ventilation-carbon dioxide response curve slope. The combination of sedatives and opioids produces the most profound effect *(109)*.

cardiovascular effects when used alone. *It will cause significant hypotension in hypovolemic patients, and its use in trauma patients is therefore limited.*

Morphine (and all other opioids at equipotent doses) produces a dose-dependent depression of ventilation, primarily by reducing the sensitivity of the brainstem respiratory centers to hypercarbia and hypoxia. Opioid agonists also interfere with pontine and medullary ventilatory centers that regulate the rhythm of breathing. This results in prolonged pauses between breaths and periodic breathing patterns. This process explains the classic clinical picture of opioid-induced respiratory depression. Initially, the respiratory rate is affected more than tidal volume, but as the dose of morphine is increased, tidal volume becomes affected as well. Increasing the dose further results in apnea.

One of the most sensitive methods of measuring the respiratory depression produced by any drug is by measuring the reduction in the slope of the carbon dioxide response curve and by the depression of minute ventilation (mL/kg) that occurs at $pCO_2 = 60$ mmHg. Morphine shifts the carbon dioxide response curve to the right and also reduces its slope. This is demonstrated in Fig. 1. The combination of any opioid agonist with any sedative produces more respiratory depression than when either drug is administered alone *(108,109)* (Fig. 1). Clinical signs that predict impending respiratory depression include somnolence, small pupils, and small tidal volumes. Aside from newborns (and the elderly) who have liver or kidney disease, patients who are at particular risk to opioid-induced respiratory depression include those who have an altered mental status, are hemodynamically unstable, have a history of apnea or disordered control of ventilation, or who have liver or kidney disease, a known airway problem. Morphine also depresses the cough reflex by its direct effect on the cough center in the medulla, and is not related to its effects on ventilation. It also depresses the sense of air hunger that occurs when arterial carbon dioxide levels rise. This explains morphine's use as a sedative in terminally ill patients and in critically ill patients who are "fighting the ventilator."

Morphine (and all other opioids at equipotent doses) inhibits intestinal smooth-muscle motility. This decrease in peristalsis of the small and large intestine and increase in the tone of the pyloric sphincter, ileocecal valve, and anal sphincter explains the historic use of opioids in the treatment of diarrhea as well as its "side effect" when treating chronic pain—namely, constipation. Indeed, the use of opium to treat dysentery (diarrhea) preceded its use in Western medicine for analgesia. The gastrointestinal tract is very sensitive to opioids, even at low doses. In the rat, 4 times more morphine is needed to produce analgesia than is needed to slow GI motility *(110)*. Opioids affect the bowel centrally and by direct action on gut mu and delta opioid-receptor sites. In fact, loperamide—an opioid receptor agonist with limited ability to cross the blood-brain barrier—is used clinically to treat diarrhea, suggesting that direct, local gut action is present in the opioid-constipating effect in diarrhea. Tolerance to the constipating effects of morphine is minimal. Because of this, we routinely prescribe laxatives or stool softeners for patients who are expected to be treated with morphine (and all other opioids) for more than 2–3 d. Alternatively, naloxone, a nonselective opioid antagonist can prevent or treat opioid-induced constipation. Unfortunately, it also antagonizes opioid-induced analgesia.

Morphine will potentiate biliary colic by causing spasm of the sphincter of Oddi, and should be used with caution in patients with, or at risk for, cholelithiasis (e.g., sickle-cell disease). This effect is antagonized by naloxone and glucagon (2 mg iv in adult patients). Biliary colic can be avoided by using mixed agonist-antagonist opioids such as pentazocine. Whether other pure μ agonists such as meperidine or fentanyl produce less biliary spasm than morphine is disputed in the literature. Some studies show that meperidine produces less biliary spasm than morphine, and others show that at equi-analgesic doses it produces virtually identical increases in common bile-duct pressure.

The nausea and vomiting that are seen with morphine administration are caused by stimulation of the chemo-receptor trigger zone in the brainstem *(111)*. This may reflect the role of opioids as partial dopamine agonists at dopamine receptors in the chemoreceptor trigger zone and the use of dopamine antagonists such as droperidol, a butyrophenone, or chlorpromazine, a phenothiazine, in the treatment of opioid-induced nausea and vomiting. Morphine increases tone and contractions in the ureters, bladder, and in the detrusor muscles of the bladder, which may make urination difficult. This may also explain the increased occurrence of bladder spasm and pain that occur when morphine is used to treat postoperative bladder surgery patients.

Regardless of its route of administration, morphine (and fentanyl) commonly produce pruritus, which can be maddening and impossible to treat. Indeed, some patients refuse opioid analgesics because they would rather hurt than itch. Opioid-induced itching is caused either by the release of histamine and histamine's effects on the peripheral nociceptors or via central mu receptor activity *(112,113)*. Traditional antihistamines such as diphenhydramine and hydroxyzine are commonly used to treat this side effect. Additionally, there is an increasing use of low-dose mu antagonists (naloxone and nalmefene) and mixed-agonist antagonists (butorphanol) in the treatment of opioid-induced pruritus *(114–116)*. Interestingly, these latter agents may also be effective for non-opioid-induced pruritus, such as the itching that accompanies end-stage liver and kidney disease *(117)*.

4.2. Suggested Morphine Dosage

The "unit" dose of intravenously administered morphine is 0.1 mg/kg, and is modified based on patient age and disease state (Table 1). Indeed, in order to minimize the complications associated with iv morphine (or any opioid) administration, we always recommend *titration of the dose at the bedside* until the desired level of analgesia is achieved. Based on its relatively short half-life (3–4 h), one would expect older children and adults to require morphine supplementation every 2–3 h when being treated for pain, particularly if the morphine is administered intravenously *(80,118)*. This has led to the recent use of continuous-infusion regimens of morphine (0.02–0.03 mg/kg/h) and patient-controlled analgesia, which maximize pain-free periods *(119–124)*. Alternatively, longer-acting agonists such as methadone may be used *(125–129)*. Finally, only about 20–30% of an orally administered dose of morphine reaches the systemic circulation *(130,131)*. When converting a patient's iv morphine requirements to oral maintenance, one needs to multiply the iv dose by 3–5 times. Oral morphine is available as liquid, tablet, and sustained-release preparations (MS-contin®). Unfortunately, not all sustained-release products are the same. There are a number of modified-release formulations of morphine with recommended dosage intervals of either 12 or 24 h, including tablets (MS Contin, Oramorph SR), capsules (Kapanol, Skenan), suspension, and suppositories. Orally administered solid dosage forms are most popular, but significant differences exist in the resultant pharmacokinetics and bioequivalence status of morphine after both single doses and at steady state *(132)*. Rectal administration is not recommended because of the extremely irregular absorption (6–93% bioavailability) *(133)*.

5. FENTANYL(S)

Because of its rapid onset (usually less than 1 min) and brief duration of action (30–45 min), fentanyl has become a favored analgesic for short procedures, such as bone marrow aspirations, fracture reductions, suturing lacerations, endoscopy, and dental procedures. Fentanyl is approx 100 *(50–100)* times more potent than morphine (the equi-analgesic dose is 0.001 mg·kg^{-1}), and is largely devoid of hypnotic or sedative activity. Sufentanil is a potent fentanyl derivative and is approx 10 times more potent than fentanyl. It is most commonly used as the principal component of cardiac anesthesia, and is administered in doses of 15–30 µg/kg. It can be given intranasally for short procedures *(134,135)*. Alfentanil is approx 5–10 times less potent than fentanyl and has an extremely short duration of action, usually less than 15–20 min. Remifentanil (Ultiva®) is a new µ-opioid receptor agonist with unique pharmacokinetic properties. It is approx 10 times more potent than fentanyl and must be given by continuous iv infusion because it has an extremely short half-life *(136,137)*.

Fentanyl's ability to block nociceptive stimuli with concomitant hemodynamic stability is excellent, and this makes it the drug of choice for trauma, cardiac, or ICU patients. Furthermore, in addition to its ability to block the systemic and pulmonary hemodynamic responses to pain, fentanyl also prevents the biochemical and endocrine stress (catabolic) response to painful stimuli that may be so harmful in the seriously ill patient. Fentanyl does have some serious side effects—namely, the development of glottic and chest-wall rigidity following rapid infusions of 0.005 mg·kg^{-1} or greater and the development of bradycardia. The etiology of the glottic and chest-wall rigidity is unclear, but its implications are not because it may make ventilation difficult or impossible. Chest-wall rigidity can be treated with muscle relaxants such as succinylcholine or pancuronium, or with naloxone.

5.1. Pharmacokinetics

Fentanyl like morphine, is primarily glucuronidated into inactive forms that are excreted by the kidneys. It is highly lipid-soluble and is rapidly distributed to tissues that are well-perfused, such as the brain and the heart. Normally, the effect of a single dose of fentanyl is terminated by rapid redistribution to inactive tissue sites such as fat, skeletal muscles, and lung, rather than by elimination. This rapid redistribution produces a dramatic decline in the plasma concentration of the drug. In this manner, its very short duration of action is very much akin to other drugs whose action is terminated by redistribution such as thiopental. However, following multiple or large doses of fentanyl (e.g., when it is used as a primary anesthetic agent or when used in high-dose or lengthy continuous infusions), prolongation of effect will occur, because elimination and not distribution will determine the duration of effect. Indeed, it is now clear that the duration of drug action for many drugs is not solely the function of clearance or terminal elimination half-life, but rather reflects the complex interaction of drug elimination, drug absorption, and rate constants for drug transfer to and from sites of action ("effect sites"). The term "context sensitive half time" refers to the time for drug concentration at idealized effect sites to decrease in half *(138)*. The context sensitive half time for fentanyl increases dramatically when it is administered by continuous infusion *(138,139)*. In newborns receiving fentanyl infusions for more than 36 h, the context sensitive half life was greater than 9 h following cessation of the infusion *(140)*. Even single doses of fentanyl may have prolonged effects in the newborn, particularly those neonates with abnormal or decreased liver blood flow following acute illness or abdominal surgery *(141–144)*. Additionally, certain conditions that may raise intra-abdominal pressure may further decrease liver blood flow by shunting blood away from the liver via the still patent ductus venosus *(144–147)*.

Fentanyl and its structurally related relatives—sufentanil, alfentanil, and remifentanil—are highly lipophilic drugs that rapidly penetrate all membranes including the blood-brain barrier. Following an iv bolus, fentanyl is rapidly eliminated from plasma as the result of its extensive uptake by body tissues. The fentanyls are highly bound to α-1 acid glycoproteins in the plasma, which are reduced in the newborn *(148,149)*. The fraction of free unbound sufentanil is significantly increased in neonates and children less than 1 yr of age (19.5 ± 2.7 and 11.5 ± 3.2 percent respectively) compared to older children and adults (8.1 ± 1.4 and 7.8 ± 1.5 percent respectively), and this correlates to levels of α-1 acid glycoproteins in the blood.

Fentanyl pharmacokinetics differ between newborn infants, children, and adults. The total body clearance of fentanyl is greater in infants 3–12 mo of age than in children older than 1 yr of age or adults (18.1 ± 1.4, 11.5 ± 4.2, and 10.0 ± 1.7 mL·kg^{-1}·min^{-1}, respectively) and the half-life of elimination is longer (233 ± 137, 244 ± 79, and 129 ± 42 min, respectively) *(150)*. The prolonged elimination half-life of fentanyl from plasma has important clinical implications. Repeated doses of fentanyl for maintenance of analgesic effects will lead to accumulation of fentanyl and its ventilatory depressant effects

(150–153). Very large doses (0.05–0.10 mg·kg^{-1}, as used in anesthesia) may be expected to induce long-lasting effects because plasma fentanyl levels will not fall below the threshold level at which spontaneous ventilation occurs during the distribution phases. On the other hand, the greater clearance of fentanyl in infants greater than 3 mo of age produces lower plasma concentrations of the drug and may allow these children to tolerate a greater dose without respiratory depression *(142,150)*. In adult studies, the mean plasma concentration of fentanyl needed to produce analgesia varies between 0.5 and 1.5 ng/mL *(154,155)*.

Alfentanil has a shorter half-life of elimination and redistribution than fentanyl. It may cause less postoperative respiratory depression than either morphine or fentanyl and is often given by infusion. Following a bolus dose, Gronert et al. observed very little respiratory depression when alfentanil was used intra-operatively, even in very young infants *(156)*. The pharmacokinetics of alfentanil differ in the neonate compared to older children. Compared with older children, premature infants demonstrated a significantly larger apparent volume of distribution (1.0 ± 0.39 vs. 0.48 ± 0.19 l/kg), a smaller clearance (2.2 ± 2.4 vs 5.6 ± 2.4 mL/kg/min) and a markedly prolonged elimination half-life (525 ± 305 vs 60 ± 11 min) *(157)*.

The pharmacokinetics of remifentanil are characterized by small volumes of distribution, rapid clearances, and low variability compared to other iv anesthetic drugs *(53–55,136,137,158)*. The drug has a rapid onset of action (half-time for equilibration between blood and the effect compartment = 1.3 min) and a short context-sensitive half-life (3–5 min). The latter property is attributable to hydrolytic metabolism of the compound by nonspecific tissue and plasma esterases. Virtually all (99.8%) of an administered remifentanil dose is eliminated during the α half-life (0.9 min) and β half-life (6.3 min). The pharmacokinetics of remifentanil suggest that within 10 min of starting an infusion, remifentanil will nearly reach steady state. Thus, changing the infusion rate of remifentanil will produce rapid changes in drug effect. The rapid metabolism of remifentanil and its small volume of distribution mean that remifentanil will not accumulate. Discontinuing the drug rapidly terminates its effects, regardless of how long it was being administered *(138,139)*. Finally, the primary metabolite has little biologic activity, making it safe even in patients with renal disease.

5.2. Suggested Dosage

When used to provide analgesia for short procedures, fentanyl is often administered intravenously in doses of 1–3 µg/kg. However, if any sedative (e.g., midazolam or chloral hydrate) is administered concomitantly, respiratory depression is potentiated, and the dose of both drugs must be reduced *(108)* (Fig. 1). Fentanyl can also be used in the ICU or the operating room to provide virtually complete anesthesia in doses of 10–50 µg/kg *(159,160)*.

The lower dose is often used to provide anesthesia for intubation, particularly in the newborn and in head trauma, cardiac, and hemodynamically unstable patients. Continuous infusions of fentanyl are often used to provide analgesia and sedation in intubated and mechanically ventilated patients. Following a loading dose of 10 μg/kg, an infusion is begun of 2–5 μg/kg/h. Rapid tolerance develops, and an increasing dose of fentanyl is required to provide satisfactory analgesia and sedation. It can also be administered via patient-controlled analgesia pumps, usually in doses of 0.5 mcg/kg/bolus dose. Remifentanil is increasingly being used as an intra-operative analgesic, and may also play a role in postoperative pain and sedation management. In the operating room, it is administered via a bolus (0.5–1 mcg/kg) followed by an infusion that ranges between 0.1 and 1 mcg/kg/min.

Sufentanil, which is 5–10 times more potent than fentanyl, can be administered intranasally in doses of 1.5–3.0 μg/kg to produce effective analgesia and sedation within 10 min of administration *(134)*. Higher doses (4.5 μg/kg) produce undesirable side effects including chest-wall rigidity, convulsions, respiratory depression, and increased postoperative vomiting *(134)*.

Another exciting alternative to iv or im injection is the fentanyl lollipop or "oral transmucosal fentanyl citrate" (OTFC) *(161–163)*. In doses of 15–20 μg/kg, this is an effective, nontraumatic method of premedication that is self-administered and extremely well-tolerated by children *(164)*. Side effects include facial pruritus *(90%)*, slow onset time (25–45 min to peak effect), and an increase in gastric volume compared to umpremedicated patients (15.9 ± 10.8 mL compared to 9.0 ± 6.2 mL [mean ± SD]). Finally, transdermal fentanyl preparations are now available to provide sustained plasma fentanyl concentrations. This has great potential use in the treatment of cancer and postoperative pain, but is **contra-indicated** for procedure or acute pain management.

6. HYDROMORPHONE

Hydromorphone (Dilaudid®), a derivative of morphine, is an opioid with appreciable selectivity for mu opioid receptors. It is noted for its rapid onset and 4–6 h duration of action. It differs from its parent compound (morphine) in that it is 5 times more potent and 10 times more lipid-soluble, and does not have an active metabolite *(120,165)*. Its half-life of elimination is 3–4 h, and like morphine and meperidine, shows very wide intrasubject pharmacokinetic variability. Hydromorphone is far less sedating than morphine, and is believed by many to be associated with fewer systemic side effects. Indeed, it is often used as an alternative to morphine in patient controlled Analgesia (PCA) or when the latter produces too much sedation or nausea. Additionally, hydromorphone is receiving renewed attention as an alternative to morphine for treatment of prolonged cancer-related pain because it can be prepared in more concentrated aqueous solutions than morphine.

Hydromorphone is effective when administered intravenously, subcutaneously, epidurally, and orally *(120,166)*. The iv route of administration is the most commonly used technique in hospitalized patients. Following a loading dose of 0.005–0.015 mg/kg, a continuous infusion ranging between 0.003 and 0.005 mg/kg/h is started. Supplemental boluses of 0.003–0.005 mg/kg are administered either by the nurse or by the patient as needed.

7. CODEINE

Codeine is a mu opioid agonist, which is most frequently used as an antitussive as well as an agent to treat mild to moderate pain in children and adults. It is a phenanthrene alkaloid, derived from morphine. Although effective when administered either orally or parenterally, it is most commonly administered in the oral form, usually in combination with acetaminophen (or aspirin). In equipotent doses, codeine's efficacy as an analgesic and respiratory depressant approaches that of morphine. In addition, codeine shares with morphine and the other opioid agonists common effects on the CNS including sedation, respiratory depression, and stimulation of the chemoreceptor trigger zone in the brainstem. It also delays gastric emptying and can increase biliary tract pressure. Codeine is very nauseating; many patients claim they are "allergic" to it because it so often induces vomiting. There are much fewer nausea and vomiting problems with oxycodone. Indeed, because of this, oxycodone or hydrocodone are now preferred oral opioids. Finally, codeine has potent antitussive properties that are similar to most other opioids and is most commonly prescribed for this effect.

Codeine has a bioavailability of approx 60% following oral ingestion. The analgesic effects occur as early as 20 min following ingestion and reach a maximum at 60–120 min. The plasma half-life of elimination is 2.5–3 h. Codeine undergoes nearly complete metabolism in the liver prior to its final excretion in urine. Interestingly, the analgesic effects of codeine are not caused by codeine itself; it must be first metabolized via O-demethylation into morphine through a pathway dependent on p450 subtype 2D6 (CYP2D6). Only about 5–10% of an administered codeine dose is demethylated in the liver into morphine *(167,168)*. A significant portion of the population (ranging between 4% and 10%) depending on ethnic group (e.g., Chinese) or age (e.g., newborns) lacks CYP2D6, and these patients achieve very little analgesia (or respiratory depression) when they receive codeine *(167,168)*.

Oral codeine is almost always prescribed in combination with either acetaminophen or aspirin. It is available as a liquid or tablet *(169)*. If prescribing codeine, we recommend the premixed combination compound for most children because when prescribed as a single agent, codeine is not readily available in liquid form at most pharmacies, and is almost twice as expensive as the combined form. Furthermore, acetaminophen potentiates the analgesia produced by codeine and allows the practitioner to use less opioid and yet achieve satisfactory analgesia. Nevertheless, it is important to understand that all "combination preparations" of acetaminophen may result in inadvertent administration of a hepatotoxic acetaminophen dose when increasing doses are given for uncontrolled pain *(169–172)*. Acetaminophen toxicity may result from a single toxic dose, from repeated ingestion of large doses of acetaminophen (e.g., in adults, 7.5–10 g daily for 1–2 d, children 60–420 mg/kg/d for 1–42 d) or from chronic ingestion *(170–172)*.

Codeine and acetaminophen are available as an elixir (120 mg acetaminophen and 12 mg codeine) and as "numbered" tablets, e.g., Tylenol® number 1, 2, 3, or 4. The number refers to how much codeine is in each tablet. Tylenol® number 4 has 60 mg codeine, number 3 has 30 mg, number 2 has 15 mg, and number 1 has 7.5 mg. Progressive increases in dose are associated with a similar degree of respiratory depression, delayed gastric emptying, nausea, and constipation as with other opioid drugs. Although it is an effective analgesic when administered parenterally, im codeine has no advantage over morphine or meperidine (despite 100 years of neurosurgical gospel). Intravenous administration of codeine is associated with serious complications, including apnea and severe hypotension, probably secondary to histamine release. Therefore, we do not recommend the iv administration of this drug in children. Codeine is used for the treatment of mild to moderate pain (or cough), usually in an outpatient setting. Typically, it is prescribed in a dose of 0.5–1 mg·kg^{-1} with a concurrently administered dose of acetaminophen (10 mg·kg^{-1}). Only about half of the analgesic dose is needed to treat a cough.

8. OXYCODONE AND HYDROCODONE

Oxycodone (the opioid in Tylox® and Percocet®) and hydrocodone (the opioid in Vicodin® and Lortab®) are opiates that are frequently used to treat pain in children and adults, particularly for less severe pain or when patients are being converted from parenteral opioids to enteral ones *(123)*. Like codeine, oxycodone and hydrocodone are administered in the oral form, usually in combination with acetaminophen (Tylox®, Percocet®, Vicodin®, Lortab®) or aspirin *(169)*.

In equipotent doses, oxycodone, hydrocodone, and morphine are equal both as analgesics and respiratory depressants. These drugs also share with other opioids common effects on the CNS including sedation, respiratory depression, and stimulation of the chemoreceptor trigger zone in the brain stem. Hydrocodone and oxycodone have a bioavailability of approx 60% following oral ingestion. Oxycodone is metabolized in the liver into oxymorphone, an active metabolite, both of which may accumulate in patients with renal failure *(173)*. The analgesic effects occur as early as 20 min following ingestion and reach a maximum at 60–120 min. The plasma half-life of elimination is 2.5–4 h. Like oral codeine, hydrocodone and oxycodone are usually prescribed in combination with either acetaminophen or aspirin (Tylenol and codeine elixir, Percocet, Tylox, Vicodin, Lortab), and the same risk of acetaminophen-induced hepatotoxicity exists.

Hydrocodone is prescribed in a dose of 0.05–0.1 mg/kg. The elixir is available as 2.5 mg/5 mL combined with acetaminophen 167 mg/5 mL. As a tablet, it is available in hydrocodone doses between 2.5 and 10 mg, combined with 500–650 mg acetaminophen. Oxycodone is prescribed in a dose of 0.05–0.1 mg/kg. Unfortunately, the elixir is not available in most pharmacies. When it is, it comes in two forms, either 1 mg/mL or 20 mg/mL. Obviously, this has enormous implications, and can easily lead to a catastrophic overdose. In tablet form, oxycodone is commonly available as Tylox (500 mg acetaminophen and 5.0 mg oxycodone) and as Percocet (325 mg acetaminophen and 5 mg oxycodone.) Oxycodone is also available without acetaminophen in a sustained-release tablet for use in chronic pain. Like all time-release tablets, it must *not* be ground up, and therefore cannot be administered through a gastric tube. Crushing the tablet releases large amounts of oxycodone, a fact that has led to its abuse by drug addicts. Like sustained-release morphine, sustained-release oxycodone is intended for use only in opioid-tolerant patients with chronic pain, *not* for acute pain management. Also note that in patients with rapid GI transit, sustained-release preparations may not be absorbed at all (liquid methadone may be an alternative) *(169)*. Finally, oxycodone is very well-absorbed rectally *(174)*. Unfortunately, a rectal suppository is not commercially available, but the oral form can be given rectally to good effect.

9. NOVEL ROUTES OF OPIOID ADMINISTRATION

Although opioids are traditionally administered parenterally (iv, im), spinally (intrathecal, epidural), and enterally (oral, rectal) the need for alternatives, particularly when treating children with either acute or chronic pain has resulted in the development of novel routes of opioid administration. Some, such as transdermal and transmucosal administration, have achieved widespread use. Others such as intranasal, inhalational, and iontophoretic administration have not. All of these modes of delivery can now be considered as conventional, although few have been specifically tested or approved for use in children.

9.1. Transdermal and Transmucosal Fentanyl

Because fentanyl is extremely lipophilic, it can be readily absorbed across any biologic membrane, including the skin. Thus, it can be given painlessly by new, non-intravenous routes of drug administration, including the transmucosal (nose and mouth) and transdermal routes. The transdermal route is frequently used to administer many drugs chronically, including scopolamine, clonidine, and nitroglycerin. A selective semi-permeable membrane patch with a reservoir of drug allows for the slow, steady-state absorption of drug across the skin. The patch is attached to the skin by a contact adhesive, which often causes skin irritation. Many factors, including body site, skin temperature, skin damage, ethnic group, or age will affect the absorption of fentanyl across the skin.

As fentanyl is painlessly absorbed across the skin, a substantial amount is stored in the upper skin layers, which then act as a secondary reservoir. The presence of skin depot has several implications: It dampens the fluctuations of fentanyl effect, must be reasonably filled before significant vascular absorption occurs, and contributes to a prolonged residual fentanyl plasma concentration after patch removal. Indeed, the amount of fentanyl remaining within the system and skin depot after removal of the patch is substantial: At the end of a 24-h period a fentanyl patch releasing drug at the rate of 100 (μg/h, 1.07 ± 0.43 mg fentanyl (approx 30% of the total delivered dose mfrom the patch) remains in the skin depot. Thus removing the patch does not stop the continued absorption of fentanyl into the body *(175)*.

Because of its long onset time, inability to rapidly adjust drug delivery, and long elimination half-life, *transdermal fentanyl is contraindicated for acute pain management.* And as stated previously, the safety of this drug delivery system is compromised even further, because fentanyl will continue to be absorbed from the subcutaneous fat for almost 24 h after the patch is removed. In fact, the use of this drug delivery system for acute pain has resulted in the death of an otherwise healthy patient. Transdermal fentanyl is applicable only for patients with chronic pain (e.g., cancer) or in opioid-tolerant patients. Even when transdermal fentanyl is appropriate, the vehicle imposes its own constraints: the smallest "denomination" of fentanyl "patch" delivers 25 μg of fentanyl per h; the others deliver 50, 75, and 100 μg of fentanyl per h. Patches **cannot** be physically cut in smaller pieces to deliver less fentanyl. This often limits usefulness in smaller patients.

On the other hand, the transmucosal route of fentanyl administration is extremely effective for acute pain relief and heralds a new era in the management of acute pain management in children. In this novel delivery technique, fentanyl is manufactured in a candy matrix (Fentanyl Actiq®) attached to a plastic applicator (it looks like a lollipop); as the child sucks on the candy, fentanyl is absorbed across the buccal mucosa and is rapidly (10–20 min) absorbed into the systemic circulation *(24,162,176–179)*. If excessive sedation occurs, the fentanyl is removed from the child's mouth by the applicator. It is more efficient than ordinary oral-gastric intestinal administration because transmucosal absorption bypasses the efficient first-pass hepatic metabolism of fentanyl that occurs following enteral absorption into the portal circulation. Actiq® has been approved by the FDA for use in children for premedication prior to surgery and for procedure-related pain (e.g., lumbar puncture, bone marrow aspiration) *(180)*. It is also useful in the treatment of cancer pain and as a supplement to transdermal fentanyl *(181)*. When administered transmucosally, fentanyl is given in doses of 10–15 µg/kg, is effective within 20 min, and lasts approx 2 h. Approximately 25–33% of the given dose is absorbed. Thus, when administered in doses of 10–15 µg/kg, blood levels equivalent to 3–5 µg/kg iv fentanyl are achieved. The major side effect, nausea and vomiting, occurs in approx 20–33% of patients who receive it *(182)*. This product is only available in hospital (and Surgicenter) pharmacies, and will— like all sedative/analgesics—require vigilant patient monitoring.

9.2. Intranasal

The intranasal route of opioid administration has long been favored by drug abusers and has only recently been used therapeutically. Rapid, painless, and safe, it is a reliable method of giving opioids to patients in whom there is no iv access or who cannot tolerate the parenteral route of drug administration. Fentanyl, sufentanil, and butorphanol are the most commonly administered intranasal opioids, although there are also reports of using oxycodone and meperidine by this route. Absorption of drug across the nasal mucosa depends on lipid solubility and has the advantage of avoiding first-pass metabolism. Unfortunately, there have been few pharmacokinetic studies involving intranasal opioids in children. In practice, fentanyl, sufentanil, and butorphanol produce analgesia within 10–30 min of intranasal administration.

Intranasal opioids can be administered as a dry powder or dissolved in water or saline. Sufentanil has been given with a 1- or 3-mL syringe, nasal spray, or nasal dropper, and butorphanol has been formulated in an intranasal metered-dose spray (0.25 mg). Butorphanol has been used in the treatment of acute migraine headache, for postoperative pain relief following myringotomy and tube surgery, and for musculo-skeletal pain *(134,183–185)*. There are few reported side effects related specifically to the intranasal route of administration, presumably because (unlike midazolam) none of the opioids are particularly irritating. For example, 85% of children cried after intranasal midazolam compared with 28% of those receiving sufentanil as premedication for day-care anesthesia *(186,187)*.

9.3. Inhalation

Nebulized or inhaled opioids are most commonly used in the palliative care of terminally ill patients who are suffering from dyspnea *(188)*. Although it is unclear whether inhaled opioids provide superior relief to patients suffering from air hunger, anecdotal evidence and some studies with adults have suggested that inhalation administration of opioids is not just another method of systemic administration of opioids, but specifically targets opioid receptors in the lungs. Using immmunoreactive techniques, opioid peptides have been detected in bronchial mucosal cells, and doses as low as 5 mg of nebulized morphine have been reported to significantly reduce the sensation of breathlessness in patients with chronic lung disease *(189)*.

Wide dosing ranges, concentrations, and volumes to be administered have been used in the treatment of dyspnea. Chandler suggests starting opioid-naive adults with 5–10 mg morphine q 4-h, and opioid-tolerant adults with 10–20 mg *(188)*. Theoretically, there should be near-total transmucosal absorption, but much of the dose is deposited in the nebulizer apparatus, with a bioavailability of only 5–30% *(188)*. There are almost no studies using this technique in children. Based on extrapolation from adult studies, in our practice, we start with 4 h of the child's usual iv opioid dose. This can be administered as the parenteral solution mixed with a few mL of saline, delivered via a portable oxygen tank and simple "neb mask" (such as that used to deliver albuterol). Opioid-naive caregivers must not inhale the opioid aerosol. Nebulized morphine has been reported to cause bronchospasm in individuals with underlying reactive airway disease. Nebulized fentanyl may cause fewer problems because it releases less histamine. Independent of special relief of dyspnea, using the nebulized route may satisfy the family and nurses that we are "doing something different" at a time when little can be done. Other studies suggest that simple nebulized saline may be as helpful as nebulized opioids. Finally, some work suggests that blow-by air can be as effective as blow-by oxygen *(190)*.

9.4. Iontophoresis

Iontophoresis is a method of transdermal administration of ionizable drugs, in which the electrically charged components are propelled through the skin by an external electric field. Several drugs, such as lidocaine, corticosteroids, morphine, and fentanyl can be delivered iontophoretically *(191–194)*. This technique is not completely painless, and some younger children object to its use.

10. TOLERANCE, PHYSICAL DEPENDENCE, AND ADDICTION

Finally, *tolerance* and *physical dependence* with repeated opioid administration are characteristics common to all opioid agonists. *Tolerance* is the development of a need to increase the dose of opioid agonist to achieve the same analgesic effect previously achieved with a lower dose. Tolerance usually develops following 10–21 d of morphine administration, although the constipating and miotic actions of morphine may persist. Additionally, cross-tolerance develops between all of the μ opioid agonists. *Physical dependence*, sometimes referred to as "neuroadaptation," is caused by repeated administration of an opioid, which necessitates the continued administration of the drug to prevent the appearance of a withdrawal or abstinence syndrome that is characteristic for that particular drug. It usually occurs after 2–3 wk of morphine administration, but may occur after even a few days of therapy. Very young infants treated with very high-dose fentanyl infusions following surgical repair of congenital heart disease and/or who required extra-corporeal membrane oxygenation (ECMO) have been identified to be at particular risk *(71,195–197)*. Several studies have suggested that the intrinsic efficacy of an opioid analgesic can determine, in part, the degree of tolerance to that agent. Specifically, animal and human studies have demonstrated that the tolerance that develops to equi-effective doses of opioid analgesics with high intrinsic efficacy is less than the tolerance that develops to lower-intrinsic-efficacy compounds *(198,199)*. Additionally, these effects occur more rapidly after continuous infusion compared to intermittent dosing *(200)*.

Tolerance develops to some drug effects much more rapidly than to other effects of the same drug. For example, tolerance develops rapidly to opioid-induced euphoria and respiratory depression, but much more slowly to the gastrointestinal effects. Opioids given acutely or chronically induce the downregulation, internalization, and desensitization of opioid receptors *(201)*. When physical dependence has been established, discontinuation of an opioid agonist produces a *withdrawal* syndrome within 24 h of drug cessation.

Physical dependence must be differentiated from *addiction*. *Addiction* is a term used to connote a severe degree of drug abuse and dependence that is an extreme of behavior, in which drug use pervades the total life activity of the user and of the range of circumstances in which drug use controls the user's behavior. Patients who are addicted to opioids often spend large amounts of time acquiring or using the drug, abandon social or occupational activities because of drug use, and continue to use the drug despite adverse psychological or physical effects. In a sense, addiction is a subset of physical dependence. Anyone who is addicted to an opioid is physically dependent; however, not everyone who is physically dependent is addicted. Patients who are appropriately treated with morphine and other opioid agonists for pain can become tolerant and physically dependent. They rarely, if ever, become addicted.

11. CONCLUSION

Opioids are essential only in the management of acute and chronic pain. In this chapter, we have provided a pharmacokinetic and pharmacologic framework regarding the use of these drugs in the management of childhood pain.

REFERENCES

1. Schechter, N. L., Berde, C. B., and Yaster, M. (1993) *Pain in infants, children, and adolescents.* Williams and Wilkins, Baltimore, MD.
2. Yaster, M., Krane, E. J., Kaplan, R. F., Cote', C. J., and Lappe, D. G. (1997) *Pediatric Pain Management and Sedation Handbook.* Mosby Year Book, Inc., St. Louis, MO.
3. Agency for Health Care Policy and Research. (1992) *Clinical Practice Guidelines: Acute Pain Management in Infants, Children, and Adolescents: Operative and Medical Procedures.* US Department of Health and Human Services, Rockville, MD.
4. Agency for Health Care Policy and Research. (1992) Clinical Practice Guideline: Acute Pain Management: Operative or Medical Procedures and Trauma. US Department of Health and Human Resources, Rockville, MD.
5. Schechter, N. L. (1989) The undertreatment of pain in children: an overview. *Pediatr. Clin. N. Am.* **36(4),** 781–794.
6. Anand, K. J., Sippell, W. G., and Aynsley-Green, A. (1987) Randomised trial of fentanyl anaesthesia in preterm babies undergoing surgery: effects on the stress. *Lancet* **1(8524),** 62–66.
7. Anand, K. J. and Hickey, P. R. (1987) Pain and its effects in the human neonate and fetus. *N. Engl. J. Med.* **317(21),** 1321–1329.
8. Anand, K. J. and Carr, D. B. (1989) The neuroanatomy, neurophysiology, and neurochemistry of pain, stress, and analgesia in newborns and children. *Pediatr. Clin. N. Am.* **36(4),** 795–822.
9. Stevens, B., Gibbins, S., and Franck, L. S. (2000) Treatment of pain in the neonatal intensive care unit. *Pediatr. Clin. N. Am.* **47(3),** 633–650.

10. Franck, L. S. (1987) A national survey of the assessment and treatment of pain and agitation in the neonatal intensive care unit. *J. Obstet. Gynecol. Neonatal. Nurs.* **16(6)**, 387–393.
11. Maxwell, L. G., Yaster, M., Wetzel, R. C., and Niebyl, J. R. (1987) Penile nerve block for newborn circumcision. *Obstet. Gynecol.* **70(3 Pt 1)**, 415–419.
12. Fitzgerald, M., Millard, C., and McIntosh, N. (1989) Cutaneous hypersensitivity following peripheral tissue damage in newborn infants and its reversal with topical anaesthesia. *Pain* **39(1)**, 31–36.
13. Fitzgerald, M. (1994) Neurobiology of fetal and neonatal pain, in *Textbook of Pain* (Wall, P. D. and Melzack, R., eds.), Churchill Livingstone, Edinburgh, pp. 153–164.
14. Coggeshall, R. E., Jennings, E. A., and Fitzgerald, M. (1996) Evidence that large myelinated primary afferent fibers make synaptic contacts in lamina II of neonatal rats. *Brain. Res. Dev. Brain Res.* **92(1)**, 81–90.
15. Fitzgerald, M., Shaw, A., and MacIntosh, N. (1988) Postnatal development of the cutaneous flexor reflex: comparative study of preterm infants and newborn rat pups. *Dev. Med. Child Neurol.* **30(4)**, 520–526.
16. Porter, F. L., Grunau, R. E., and Anand, K. J. (1999) Long-term effects of pain in infants. *J. Dev. Behav. Pediatr.* **20(4)**, 253–261.
17. Porter, F. L., Wolf, C. M., and Miller, J. P. (1999) Procedural pain in newborn infants: the influence of intensity and development. *Pediatrics* **104(1)**, e13.
18. Taddio, A., Katz, J., Ilersich, A. L., and Koren, G. (1997) Effect of neonatal circumcision on pain response during subsequent routine vaccination. *Lancet* **349(9052)**, 599–603.
19. Schechter, N. L., Allen, D. A., and Hanson, K. (1986) Status of pediatric pain control: a comparison of hospital analgesic usage in children and adults. *Pediatrics* **77(1)**, 11–15.
20. Pigeon, H. M., McGrath, P. J., Lawrence, J., and MacMurray, S. B. (1989) How neonatal nurses report infants' pain. *Am. J. Nurs.* **89(11)**, 1529–1530.
21. Reid, G. J., Hebb, J. P., McGrath, P. J., Finley, G. A., and Forward, S. P. (1995) Cues parents use to assess postoperative pain in their children. *Clin. J. Pain* **11(3)**, 229–235.
22. Zeltzer, L. K., Jay, S. M., and Fisher, D. M. (1989) The management of pain associated with pediatric procedures. *Pediatr. Clin. N. Am.* **36(4)**, 941–964.
23. Zeltzer, L. and LeBaron, S. (1982) Hypnosis and nonhypnotic techniques for reduction of pain and anxiety during painful procedures in children and adolescents with cancer. *J. Pediatr.* **101(6)**, 1032–1035.
24. Schechter, N. L., Weisman, S. J., Rosenblum, M., Bernstein, B., and Conard, P. L. (1995) The use of oral transmucosal fentanyl citrate for painful procedures in children. *Pediatrics* **95(3)**, 335–339.
25. Chen, E., Zeltzer, L. K., Craske, M. G., and Katz, E. R. (1999) Alteration of memory in the reduction of children's distress during repeated aversive medical procedures. *J. Consult. Clin. Psychol.* **67(4)**, 481–490.

26. Zeltzer, L. K., Altman, A., Cohen, D., LeBaron, S., Munuksela, E. L., and Schechter, N. L. (1990) American Academy of *Pediatrics* Report of the Subcommittee on the Management of Pain Associated with Procedures in Children with Cancer. *Pediatrics* **86(5 Pt 2),** 826–831.

27. Wilder, R. T. (2000) Local anesthetics for the pediatric patient. *Pediatr. Clin. N. Am.* **47(3),** 545–558.

28. Yaster, M., Tobin, J. R., Fisher, Q. A., and Maxwell, L. G. (1994) Local anesthetics in the management of acute pain in children. *J. Pediatr.* **124(2),** 165–176.

29. Blumer, J. L. (1999) The Therapeutic Orphan—30 Years Later. Proceedings of a joint conference of the Pediatric Pharmacology Research Unit Network, the European Society of Developmental Pharmacology, and the National Institute of Child Health and Human Development. Washington, D. C., May 2, 1997. *Pediatrics* **104(3 Pt 2),** 581–645.

30. Lietman, P. S. (1979) Chloramphenicol and the neonate—1979 view. *Clin. Perinatol.* **6(1),** 151–162.

31. Young, W. S. and Lietman, P. S. (1978) Chloramphenicol glucuronyl transferase: assay, ontogeny and inducibility. *J. Pharmacol. Exp. Ther.* **204(1),** 203–211.

32. Power, B. M., Forbes, A. M., van Heerden, P. V., and Ilett, K. F. (1998) Pharmacokinetics of drugs used in critically ill adults. *Clin. Pharmacokinet.* **34(1),** 25–56.

33. Wagner, B. K. and O'Hara, D. A. (1997) Pharmacokinetics and pharmacodynamics of sedatives and analgesics in the treatment of agitated critically ill patients. *Clin. Pharmacokinet.* **33(6),** 426–453.

34. Park, G. R. (1997) Sedation, analgesia and muscle relaxation and the critically ill patient. *Can. J. Anaesth.* **44(5 Pt 2),** R40–R51.

35. Volles, D. F. and McGory, R. (1999) Pharmacokinetic considerations. *Crit. Care Clin.* **15(1),** 55–75.

36. Cohen, S. N. (1999) The Pediatric Pharmacology Research Unit (PPRU) Network and its role in meeting pediatric labeling needs. *Pediatrics* **104(3 Pt 2),** 644–645.

37. Connor, J. D. (1999) A look at the future of pediatric therapeutics: an investigator's perspective of the new pediatric rule. *Pediatrics* **104(3 Pt 2),** 610–613.

38. Wilson, J. T., Kearns, G. L., Murphy, D., Yaffe, S. J. (1994) Paediatric labelling requirements. Implications for pharmacokinetic studies. *Clin. Pharmacokinet.* **26(4),** 308–325.

39. Yaksh, T. L., Al Rodhan, N. R., and Jensen, T. S. (1988) Sites of action of opiates in production of analgesia. *Prog. Brain Res.* **77,** 371–394.

40. Yaksh, T. L. (1993) New horizons in our understanding of the spinal physiology and pharmacology of pain processing. *Semin. Oncol.* **20(2 Suppl 1),** 6–18.

41. Sabbe, M. B. and Yaksh, T. L. (1990) Pharmacology of spinal opioids. *J. Pain. Symptom Manage.* **5(3),** 191–203.

42. Greene, R. F., Miser, A. W., Lester, C. M., Balis, F. M., and Poplack, D. G. (1987) Cerebrospinal fluid and plasma pharmacokinetics of morphine infusions in pediatric cancer patients and rhesus monkeys. *Pain* **30(3)**, 339–348.

43. Plummer, J. L., Cmielewski, P. L., Reynolds, G. D., Gourlay, G. K., and Cherry, D. A. (1990) Influence of polarity on dose-response relationships of intrathecal opioids in rats. *Pain* **40(3)**, 339–347.

44. Gourlay, G. K., Cherry, D. A., Plummer, J. L., Armstrong, P. J., and Cousins, M. J. (1987) The influence of drug polarity on the absorption of opioid drugs into CSF and subsequent cephalad migration following lumbar epidural administration: application to morphine and pethidine. *Pain* **31(3)**, 297–305.

45. Gourlay, G. K., Cherry, D. A., and Cousins, M. J. (1985) Cephalad migration of morphine in CSF following lumbar epidural administration in patients with cancer pain. *Pain* **23(4)**, 317–326.

46. Gourlay, G. K., Murphy, T. M., Plummer, J. L., Kowalski, S. R., Cherry, D. A., and Cousins, M. J. (1989) Pharmacokinetics of fentanyl in lumbar and cervical CSF following lumbar epidural and intravenous administration. *Pain* **38(3)**, 253–259.

47. Way, W. L., Costley, E. C., and Way, E. L. (1965) Respiratory senstivity of the newborn infant to meperidine and morphine. *Clin. Pharmacol. Ther.* **6,** 454–461.

48. Bragg, P., Zwass, M. S., Lau, M., and Fisher, D. M. (1995) Opioid pharmacodynamics in neonatal dogs: differences between morphine and fentanyl. *J. Appl. Physiol.* **79(5)**, 1519–1524.

49. Yaksh, T. L. (1997) Pharmacology and mechanisms of opioid analgesic activity. *Acta Anaesthesiol. Scand.* **41(1 Pt 2)**, 94–111.

50. Etches, R. C., Sandler, A. N., and Daley, M. D. (1989) Respiratory depression and spinal opioids. *Can. J. Anaesth.* **36(2)**, 165–185.

51. Cousins, M. J. and Mather, L. E. (1984) Intrathecal and epidural administration of opioids. *Anesthesiology* **61(3)**, 276–310.

52. Yaksh, T. L. (1992) The spinal pharmacology of acutely and chronically administered opioids. *J. Pain. Symptom Manage.* 7(6), 356–361.

53. Minto, C. F., Schnider, T. W., and Shafer, S. L. (1997) Pharmacokinetics and pharmacodynamics of remifentanil. II. Model application. *Anesthesiology* **86(1)**, 24–33.

54. Minto, C. F., Schnider, T. W., Egan, T. D., Youngs, E., Lemmens, H. J., Gambus, P. L., et al. (1997) Influence of age and gender on the pharmacokinetics and pharmacodynamics of remifentanil. I. Model development. *Anesthesiology* **86(1)**, 10–23.

55. Burkle, H., Dunbar, S., and Van Aken, H. (1996) Remifentanil: a novel, short-acting, mu-opioid. *Anesth. Analg.* **83(3)**, 646–651.

56. Tateishi, T., Nakura, H., Asoh, M., Watanabe, M., Tanaka, M., Kumai, T., et al. (1997) A comparison of hepatic cytochrome P450 protein expression between infancy and postinfancy. *Life Sci.* **61(26)**, 2567–2574.

57. Hakkola, J., Tanaka, E., and Pelkonen, O. (1998) Developmental expression of cytochrome P450 enzymes in human liver. *Pharmacol. Toxicol.* **82(5)**, 209–217.

58. Greeley, W. J. and de Bruijn, N. P. (1988) Changes in sufentanil pharmacokinetics within the neonatal period. *Anesth. Analg.* **67(1)**, 86–90.

59. Plummer, J. L., Gourlay, G. K., Cmielewski, P. L., Odontiadis, J., and Harvey, I. (1995) Behavioural effects of norpethidine, a metabolite of pethidine, in rats. *Toxicology* **95(1–3)**, 37–44.

60. Szeto, H. H., Inturrisi, C. E., Houde, R., Saal, S., Cheigh, J., and Reidenberg, M. M. (1977) Accumulation of normeperidine, an active metabolite of meperidine, in patients with renal failure of cancer. *Ann. Intern. Med.* **86(6)**, 738–741.

61. Tegeder, I., Lotsch, J., and Geisslinger, G. (1999) Pharmacokinetics of opioids in liver disease. *Clin. Pharmacokinet.* **37(1)**, 17–40.

62. McRorie, T. I., Lynn, A. M., Nespeca, M. K., Opheim, K. E., and Slattery, J. T. (1992) The maturation of morphine clearance and metabolism. *Am. J. Dis. Child* **146(8)**, 972–976.

63. Lynn, A. M. and Slattery, J. T. (1987) Morphine pharmacokinetics in early infancy. *Anesthesiology* **66(2)**, 136–139.

64. Haberkern, C. M., Lynn, A. M., Geiduschek, J. M., Nespeca, M. K., Jacobson, L. E., Bratton, S. L., et al. (1996) Epidural and intravenous bolus morphine for postoperative analgesia in infants. *Can. J. Anaesth.* **43(12)**, 1203–1210.

65. Dahlstrom, B., Tamsen, A., Paalzow, L., and Hartvig, P. (1982) Patient-controlled analgesic therapy, Part IV: pharmacokinetics and analgesic plasma concentrations of morphine. *Clin. Pharmacokinet.* **7(3)**, 266–279.

66. Koren, G., Butt, W., Chinyanga, H., Soldin, S., Tan, Y. K., and Pape, K. (1985) Postoperative morphine infusion in newborn infants: assessment of disposition characteristics and safety. *J. Pediatr.* **107(6)**, 963–967.

67. Koren, G., Butt, W., Pape, K., and Chinyanga, H. (1985) Morphine-induced seizures in newborn infants. *Vet. Hum. Toxicol.* **27(6)**, 519–520.

68. Bhat, R., Chari, G., Gulati, A., Aldana, O., Velamati, R., and Bhargava, H. (1990) Pharmacokinetics of a single dose of morphine in preterm infants during the first week of life. *J. Pediatr.* **117(3)**, 477–481.

69. Kupferberg, H. J. and Way, E. L. (1963) Pharmacologic basis for the increased sensitivity of the newborn rat to morphine. *J. Pharmacol. Exp. Ther.* **141**, 105–109.

70. Dagan, O., Klein, J., Bohn, D., Barker, G., and Koren, G. (1993) Morphine pharmacokinetics in children following cardiac surgery: effects of disease and inotropic support. *J. Cardiothorac. Vasc. Anesth.* **7(4)**, 396–398.

71. Geiduschek, J. M., Lynn, A. M., Bratton, S. L., Sanders, J. C., Levy, F. H., Haberkern, C. M., et al. (1997) Morphine pharmacokinetics during continuous infusion of morphine sulfate for infants receiving extracorporeal membrane oxygenation. *Crit. Care Med.* **25(2)**, 360–364.

72. Lynn, A. M., Opheim, K. E., and Tyler, D. C. (1984) Morphine infusion after pediatric cardiac surgery. *Crit. Care Med.* **12(10)**, 863–866.

73. Thornton, S. R., Compton, D. R., and Smith, F. L. (1998) Ontogeny of mu opioid agonist anti-nociception in postnatal rats. *Brain. Res. Dev. Brain Res.* **105(2)**, 269–276.

74. Martin, R. J., DiFiore, J. M., Jana, L., Davis, R. L., Miller, M. J., Coles, S. K., et al. (1998) Persistence of the biphasic ventilatory response to hypoxia in preterm infants. *J. Pediatr.* **132(6),** 960–964.

75. Martin, R. J., DiFiore, J. M., Korenke, C. B., Randal, H., Miller, M. J., and Brooks, L. J. (1995) Vulnerability of respiratory control in healthy preterm infants placed supine. *J. Pediatr.* **127(4),** 609–614.

76. Cohen, G., Malcolm, G., and Henderson-Smart, D. (1997) Ventilatory response of the newborn infant to mild hypoxia. *Pediatr. Pulmonol.* **24(3),** 163–172.

77. Moss, T. J., Jakubowska, A. E., McCrabb, G. J., Billings, K., and Harding, R. (1995) Ventilatory responses to progressive hypoxia and hypercapnia in developing sheep. *Respir. Physiol.* **100(1),** 33–44.

78. Hamilton, G. R. and Baskett, T. F. (2000) In the arms of Morpheus the development of morphine for postoperative pain relief. *Can. J. Anaesth.* **47(4),** 367–374.

79. Reisine, T. and Pasternak, G. (1996) Opioid analgesics and antagonists, in Goodman and Gilman's *The Pharmacologic Basis of Therapeutics* (Hardman, J. G. and Limbird, L. E., eds.), McGraw-Hill, New York, NY, pp. 521–555.

80. Yaster, M. and Deshpande, J. K. (1988) Management of pediatric pain with opioid analgesics. *J. Pediatr.* **113(3),** 421–429.

81. Berde, C. B. (1989) Pediatric postoperative pain management. *Pediatr. Clin. N. Am.* **36(4),** 921–940.

82. Mather, L. E. and Cousins, M. J. (1986) Pharmacology of opioids. Part 2. Clinical aspects. *Med. J. Aust.* **144(9),** 475–481.

83. Stoelting, R. K. (1999) Opioid Agonists and Antagonists, in *Pharmacology and Physiology in Anesthetic Practice* (Stoelting, R. K., ed.), Lippincott-Raven, Philadelphia, PA, pp. 77–112.

84. Pasternak, G. W. (1993) Pharmacological mechanisms of opioid analgesics. *Clin. Neuropharmacol.* **16(1),** 1–18.

85. Standifer, K. M. and Pasternak, G. W. (1997) G proteins and opioid receptor-mediated signalling. *Cell Signal* **9(3–4),** 237–248.

86. Nagasaka, H., Awad, H., and Yaksh, T. L. (1996) Peripheral and spinal actions of opioids in the blockade of the autonomic response evoked by compression of the inflamed knee joint. *Anesthesiology* **85(4),** 808–816.

87. Satoh, M. and Minami, M. (1995) Molecular pharmacology of the opioid receptors. *Pharmacol. Ther.* **68(3),** 343–364.

88. Harrison, L. M., Kastin, A. J., and Zadina, J. E. (1998) Opiate tolerance and dependence: receptors, G-proteins, and antiopiates. *Peptides* **19(9),** 1603–1630.

89. Mestek, A., Chen, Y., and Yu, L. (1996) Mu opioid receptors: cellular action and tolerance development. *NIDA Res. Monogr.* **161,** 104–126.

90. Chen, Y., Mestek, A., Liu, J., Hurley, J. A., and Yu, L. (1993) Molecular cloning and functional expression of a mu-opioid receptor from rat brain. *Mol. Pharmacol.* **44(1),** 8–12.

91. Raynor, K., Kong, H., Chen, Y., Yasuda, K., Yu, L., Bell, G. I., et al. (1994) Pharmacological characterization of the cloned kappa-, delta-, and mu-opioid receptors. *Mol. Pharmacol.* **45(2),** 330–334.

92. Yasuda, K., Raynor, K., Kong, H., Breder, C. D., Takeda, J., Reisine, T., et al. (1993) Cloning and functional comparison of kappa and delta opioid receptors from mouse brain. *Proc. Natl. Acad. Sci. USA* **90(14),** 6736–6740.

93. Callahan, P. and Pasternak, G. W. (1987) Opiate receptor multiplicity: evidence for multiple mu receptors. *Monogr. Neural. Sci.* **13,** 121–131.

94. Traynor, J. R. and Elliott, J. (1993) delta-Opioid receptor subtypes and crosstalk with mu-receptors. *Trends Pharmacol. Sci.* **14(3),** 84–86.

95. Knapp, R. J., Malatynska, E., Collins, N., Fang, L., Wang, J. Y., Hruby, V. J., et al. (1995) Molecular biology and pharmacology of cloned opioid receptors. *FASEB J.* **9(7),** 516–525.

96. Pasternak, G. W. (1988) Multiple morphine and enkephalin receptors and the relief of pain. *JAMA* **259(9),** 1362–1367.

97. Millan, M. J. (1986) Multiple opioid systems and pain. *Pain* **27(3),** 303–347.

98. Lord, J. A., Waterfield, A. A., Hughes, J., and Kosterlitz, H. W. (1977) Endogenous opioid peptides: multiple agonists and receptors. *Nature* **267(5611),** 495–499.

99. Wood, P. L. (1988) The significance of multiple CNS opioid receptor types: a review of critical considerations relating to technical details and anatomy in the study of central opioid actions. *Peptides* **9 Suppl 1,** 49–55.

100. Wood, P. L. (1982) Multiple opiate receptors: support for unique mu, delta and kappa sites. *Neuropharmacology* **21(6),** 487–497.

101. Snyder, S. H. (1984) Drug and neurotransmitter receptors in the brain. *Science* **224(4644),** 22–31.

102. Zhang, A. Z., and Pasternak, G. W. (1981) Ontogeny of opioid pharmacology and receptors: high and low affinity site differences. *Eur. J. Pharmacol.* **73(1),** 29–40.

103. Pasternak, G. W., Zhang, A., and Tecott, L. (1980) Developmental differences between high and low affinity opiate binding sites: their relationship to analgesia and respiratory depression. *Life Sci.* **27(13),** 1185–1190.

104. Pasternak, G. W. and Wood, P. J. (1986) Multiple mu opiate receptors. *Life Sci.* **38(21),** 1889–1898.

105. Fowler, C. J. and Fraser, G. L. (1994) Mu-, delta-, kappa-opioid receptors and their subtypes. A critical review with emphasis on radioligand binding experiments. *Neurochem. Int.* **24(5),** 401–426.

106. Esmail, Z., Montgomery, C., Courtrn, C., Hamilton, D., and Kestle, J. (1999) Efficacy and complications of morphine infusions in postoperative paediatric patients. *Paediatr. Anaesth.* **9(4),** 321–327.

107. Lynn, A. M., Nespeca, M. K., Opheim, K. E., and Slattery, J. T. (1993) Respiratory effects of intravenous morphine infusions in neonates, infants, and children after cardiac surgery. *Anesth. Analg.* **77(4),** 695–701.

108. Nichols, D. G., Yaster, M., Lynn, A. M., Helfaer, M. A., Deshpande, J. K., Manson, P. N., et al. (1993) Disposition and respiratory effects of intrathecal morphine in children. *Anesthesiology* **79(4),** 733–8; discussion 25A.

109. Yaster, M., Nichols, D. G., Deshpande, J. K., and Wetzel, R. C. (1990) Midazolam-fentanyl intravenous sedation in children: case report of respiratory arrest see comments]. *Pediatrics* **86(3)**, 463–467.

110. Yuan, C. S. and Foss, J. F. (2000) Antagonism of gastrointestinal opioid effects. *Reg. Anesth. Pain Med.* **25(6)**, 639–642.

111. Watcha, M. F. and White, P. F. (1992) Postoperative nausea and vomiting. Its etiology, treatment, and prevention. *Anesthesiology* **77(1)**, 162–184.

112. Jinks, S. L. and Carstens, E. (2000) Superficial dorsal horn neurons identified by intracutaneous histamine: chemonociceptive responses and modulation by morphine. *J. Neurophysiol.* **84(2)**, 616–627.

113. Kuraishi, Y., Yamaguchi, T., and Miyamoto, T. (2000) Itch-scratch responses induced by opioids through central mu opioid receptors in mice. *J. Biomed. Sci.* **7(3)**, 248–252.

114. Gunter, J. B., McAuliffe, J., Gregg, T., Weidner, N., Varughese, A. M., and Sweeney, D. M. (2000) Continuous epidural butorphanol relieves pruritus associated with epidural morphine infusions in children. *Paediatr. Anaesth.* **10(2)**, 167–172.

115. Joshi, G. P., Duffy, L., Chehade, J., Wesevich, J., Gajraj, N., and Johnson, E. R. (1999) Effects of prophylactic nalmefene on the incidence of morphine-related side effects in patients receiving intravenous patient-controlled analgesia. *Anesthesiology* **90(4)**, 1007–1011.

116. Gan, T. J., Ginsberg, B., Glass, P. S., Fortney, J., Jhaveri, R., and Perno, R. (1997) Opioid-sparing effects of a low-dose infusion of naloxone in patient-administered morphine sulfate. *Anesthesiology* **87(5)**, 1075–1081.

117. Bergasa, N. V., Alling, D. W., Talbot, T. L., Swain, M. G., Yurdaydin, C., Turner, M. L., et al. (1995) Effects of naloxone infusions in patients with the pruritus of cholestasis. A double-blind, randomized, controlled trial. *Ann. Intern. Med.* **123(3)**, 161–167.

118. Golianu, B., Krane, E. J., Galloway, K. S., and Yaster, M. (2000) Pediatric acute pain management. *Pediatr. Clin. N. Am.* **47(3)**, 559–587.

119. Berde, C. B., Lehn, B. M., Yee, J. D., Sethna, N. F., and Russo, D. (1991) Patient-controlled analgesia in children and adolescents: a randomized, prospective comparison with intramuscular administration of morphine for postoperative analgesia. *J. Pediatr.* **118(3)**, 460–466.

120. Collins, J. J., Geake, J., Grier, H. E., Houck, C. S., Thaler, H. T., Weinstein, H. J., et al. (1996) Patient-controlled analgesia for mucositis pain in children: a three- period crossover study comparing morphine and hydromorphone. *J. Pediatr.* **129(5)**, 722–728.

121. Mackie, A. M., Coda, B. C., and Hill, H. F. (1991) Adolescents use patient-controlled analgesia effectively for relief from prolonged oropharyngeal mucositis pain. *Pain* **46(3)**, 265–269.

122. McNeely, J. K. and Trentadue, N. C. (1997) Comparison of patient-controlled analgesia with and without nighttime morphine infusion following lower extremity surgery in children. *J. Pain. Symptom Manage.* **13(5)**, 268–273.

123. Yaster, M., Billett, C., and Monitto, C. (1997) Intravenous Patient Controlled Analgesia, in *Pediatric pain management and sedation handbook* (Yaster,

M., Krane, E. J., Kaplan, R. F., Cote, C. J., Lappe, D. G., eds.), Mosby Year Book, Inc., St. Louis, MO, pp. 89–112.

124. Monitto, C. L., Greenberg, R. S., Kost-Byerly, S., Wetzel, R., Billett, C., Lebet, R. M., et al. (2000) The safety and efficacy of parent-/nurse-controlled analgesia in patients less than six years of age. *Anesth. Analg.* **91(3)**, 573–579.

125. Gourlay, G. K., Wilson, P. R., and Glynn, C. J. (1982) Methadone produces prolonged postoperative analgesia. *Br. Med. J. (Clin. Res. Ed.)* **284(6316)**, 630–631.

126. Gourlay, G. K., Wilson, P. R., and Glynn, C. J. (1982) Pharmacodynamics and pharmacokinetics of methadone during the perioperative period. *Anesthesiology* **57(6)**, 458–467.

127. Gourlay, G. K., Willis, R. J., and Wilson, P. R. (1984) Postoperative pain control with methadone: influence of supplementary methadone doses and blood concentration—response relationships. *Anesthesiology* **61(1)**, 19–26.

128. Gourlay, G. K., Willis, R. J., and Lamberty, J. (1986) A double-blind comparison of the efficacy of methadone and morphine in postoperative pain control. *Anesthesiology* **64(3)**, 322–327.

129. Berde, C. B., Beyer, J. E., Bournaki, M. C., Levin, C. R., and Sethna, N. F. (1991) Comparison of morphine and methadone for prevention of postoperative pain in 3- to 7-year-old children. *J. Pediatr.* **119(1 (Pt 1)**, 136–141.

130. Gourlay, G. K., Cherry, D. A., and Cousins, M. J. (1986) A comparative study of the efficacy and pharmacokinetics of oral methadone and morphine in the treatment of severe pain in patients with cancer. *Pain* **25(3)**, 297–312.

131. Gourlay, G. K., Plummer, J. L., Cherry, D. A., Foate, J. A., and Cousins, M. J. (1989) Influence of a high-fat meal on the absorption of morphine from oral solutions. *Clin. Pharmacol. Ther.* **46(4)**, 463–468.

132. Gourlay, G. K. (1998) Sustained relief of chronic pain. Pharmacokinetics of sustained release morphine. *Clin. Pharmacokinet.* **35(3)**, 173–190.

133. Lundeberg, S., Beck, O., Olsson, G. L., and Boreus, L. O. (1996) Rectal administration of morphine in children. Pharmacokinetic evaluation after a single-dose. *Acta Anaesthesiol. Scand.* **40(4)**, 445–451.

134. Henderson, J. M., Brodsky, D. A., Fisher, D. M., Brett, C. M., and Hertzka, R. E. (1988) Pre-induction of anesthesia in pediatric patients with nasally administered sufentanil. *Anesthesiology* **68(5)**, 671–675.

135. Bates, B. A., Schutzman, S. A., and Fleisher, G. R. (1994) A comparison of intranasal sufentanil and midazolam to intramuscular meperidine, promethazine, and chlorpromazine for conscious sedation in children. *Ann. Emerg. Med.* **24(4)**, 646–651.

136. Glass, P. S. (1995) Remifentanil: a new opioid. *J. Clin. Anesth.* **7(7)**, 558–563.

137. Glass, P. S., Gan, T. J., and Howell, S. (1999) A review of the pharmacokinetics and pharmacodynamics of remifentanil. *Anesth. Analg.* **89(4 Suppl)**, S7–14.

138. Hughes, M. A., Glass, P. S., and Jacobs, J. R. (1992) Context-sensitive half-time in multicompartment pharmacokinetic models for intravenous anesthetic drugs. *Anesthesiology* **76(3)**, 334–341.

139. Scholz, J., Steinfath, M., and Schulz, M. (1996) Clinical pharmacokinetics of alfentanil, fentanyl and sufentanil. An update. *Clin. Pharmacokinet.* **31(4),** 275–292.

140. Santeiro, M. L., Christie, J., Stromquist, C., Torres, B. A., and Markowsky, S. J. (1997) Pharmacokinetics of continuous infusion fentanyl in newborns. *J. Perinatol.* **17(2),** 135–139.

141. Koehntop, D. E., Rodman, J. H., Brundage, D. M., Hegland, M. G., and Buckley, J. J. (1986) Pharmacokinetics of fentanyl in neonates. *Anesth. Analg.* **65(3),** 227–232.

142. Hertzka, R. E., Gauntlett, I. S., Fisher, D. M., and Spellman, M. J. (1989) Fentanyl-induced ventilatory depression: effects of age. *Anesthesiology* **70(2),** 213–218.

143. Gauntlett, I. S., Fisher, D. M., Hertzka, R. E., Kuhls, E., Spellman, M. J., and Rudolph, C. (1988) Pharmacokinetics of fentanyl in neonatal humans and lambs: effects of age. *Anesthesiology* **69(5),** 683–687.

144. Kuhls, E., Gauntlett, I. S., Lau, M., Brown, R., Rudolph, C. D., Teitel, D. F., et al. (1995) Effect of increased intra-abdominal pressure on hepatic extraction and clearance of fentanyl in neonatal lambs. *J. Pharmacol. Exp. Ther.* **274(1),** 115–119.

145. Yaster, M., Scherer, T. L., Stone, M. M., Maxwell, L. G., Schleien, C. L., Wetzel, R. C., et al. (1989) Prediction of successful primary closure of congenital abdominal wall defects using intraoperative measurements. *J. Pediatr. Surg* **24(12),** 1217–1220.

146. Masey, S. A., Koehler, R. C., Buck, J. R., Pepple, J. M., Rogers, M. C., and Traystman, R. J. (1985) Effect of abdominal distension on central and regional hemodynamics in neonatal lambs. *Pediatr. Res.* **19,** 1244–1249.

147. Yaster, M., Buck, J. R., Dudgeon, D. L., Manolio, T. A., Simmons, R. S., Zeller, P., et al. (1988) Hemodynamic effects of primary closure of omphalocele/ gastroschisis in human newborns. *Anesthesiology* **69(1),** 84–88.

148. Wilson, A. S., Stiller, R. L., Davis, P. J., Fedel, G., Chakravorti, S., Israel, B. A., et al. (1997) Fentanyl and alfentanil plasma protein binding in preterm and term neonates. *Anesth. Analg.* **84(2),** 315–318.

149. Wood, M. (1986) Plasma drug binding: implications for anesthesiologists. *Anesth. Analg.* **65(7),** 786–804.

150. Singleton, M. A., Rosen, J. I., and Fisher, D. M. (1987) Plasma concentrations of fentanyl in infants, children and adults. *Can. J. Anaesth.* **34(2),** 152–155.

151. Koehntop, D. E., Rodman, J. H., Brundage, D. M., Hegland, M. G., and Buckley, J. J. (1986) Pharmacokinetics of fentanyl in neonates. *Anesth. Analg.* **65(3),** 227–232.

152. Murphy, M. R. and Hug, C. C., Jr. (1983), McClain DA. Dose-independent pharmacokinetics of fentanyl. *Anesthesiology* **59(6),** 537–540.

153. McClain, D. A. and Hug, C. C., Jr. (1980) Intravenous fentanyl kinetics. *Clin. Pharmacol. Ther.* **28(1),** 106–114.

154. Gourlay, G. K., Kowalski, S. R., Plummer, J. L., Cousins, M. J., and Armstrong, P. J. (1988) Fentanyl blood concentration-analgesic response relationship in the treatment of postoperative pain. *Anesth. Analg.* **67(4)**, 329–337.

155. Glass, P. S., Estok, P., Ginsberg, B., Goldberg, J. S., and Sladen, R. N. (1992) Use of patient-controlled analgesia to compare the efficacy of epidural to intravenous fentanyl administration. *Anesth. Analg.* **74(3)**, 345–351.

156. Gronert, B. J., Davis, P. J., and Cook, D. R. (1992) Continuous infusions of alfentanil in infants undergoing inguinal herniorrhaphy. *Paediatr. Anaesth.* **2**, 105–109.

157. Davis, P. J., Killian, A., Stiller, R. L., Cook, D. R., Guthrie, R. D., and Scierka, A. M. (1989) Pharmacokinetics of alfentanil in newborn premature infants and older children. *Dev. Pharmacol. Ther.* **13(1)**, 21–27.

158. Kapila, A., Glass, P. S., Jacobs, J. R., Muir, K. T., Hermann, D. J., Shiraishi, M., et al. (1995) Measured context-sensitive half-times of remifentanil and alfentanil. *Anesthesiology* **83(5)**, 968–975.

159. Robinson, S. and Gregory, G. A. (1981) Fentanyl-air-oxygen anesthesia for ligation of patent ductus arteriosus in preterm infants. *Anesth. Analg.* **60(5)**, 331–334.

160. Yaster, M. (1987) The dose response of fentanyl in neonatal anesthesia. *Anesthesiology* **66(3)**, 433–435.

161. Stanley, T. H., Leiman, B. C., Rawal, N., Marcus, M. A., van den Nieuwenhuyzen, M., Walford, A., et al. (1989) The effects of oral transmucosal fentanyl citrate premedication on preoperative behavioral responses and gastric volume and acidity in children. *Anesth. Analg.* **69(3)**, 328–335.

162. Streisand, J. B., Stanley, T. H., Hague, B., van Vreeswijk, H., Ho, G. H., and Pace, N. L. (1989) Oral transmucosal fentanyl citrate premedication in children. *Anesth. Analg.* **69(1)**, 28–34.

163. Feld, L. H., Champeau, M. W., van Steennis, C. A., and Scott, J. C. (1989) Preanesthetic medication in children: a comparison of oral transmucosal fentanyl citrate versus placebo. *Anesthesiology* **71(3)**, 374–377.

164. Nelson, P. S., Streisand, J. B., Mulder, S. M., Pace, N. L., and Stanley, T. H. (1989) Comparison of oral transmucosal fentanyl citrate and an oral solution of meperidine, diazepam, and atropine for premedication in children. *Anesthesiology* **70(4)**, 616–621.

165. Bruera, E., Pereira, J., Watanabe, S., Belzile, M., Kuehn, N., and Hanson, J. (1996) Opioid rotation in patients with cancer pain. A retrospective comparison of dose ratios between methadone, hydromorphone, and morphine. *Cancer* **78(4)**, 852–857.

166. Goodarzi, M. (1999) Comparison of epidural morphine, hydromorphone and fentanyl for postoperative pain control in children undergoing orthopaedic surgery. *Paediatr. Anaesth.* **9(5)**, 419–422.

167. Caraco, Y., Sheller, J., and Wood, A. J. (1999) Impact of ethnic origin and quinidine coadministration on codeine's disposition and pharmacodynamic effects. *J. Pharmacol. Exp. Ther.* **290(1)**, 413–422.

168. Caraco, Y., Sheller, J., and Wood, A. J. (1996) Pharmacogenetic determination of the effects of codeine and prediction of drug interactions. *J. Pharmacol. Exp. Ther.* **278(3),** 1165–1174.
169. Krane, E. J. and Yaster, M. (1997) Transition to less invasive therapy, in *Pediatric pain management and sedation handbook* (Yaster, M., Krane, E. J., Kaplan, R. F., Cote, C. J., and Lappe, D. G., eds.), Mosby Year Book, Inc., St. Louis, MO, pp. 147–162.
170. Heubi, J. E., Barbacci, M. B., and Zimmerman, H. J. (1998) Therapeutic misadventures with acetaminophen: hepatoxicity after multiple doses in children. *J. Pediatr.* **132(1),** 22–27.
171. Kearns, G. L., Leeder, J. S., and Wasserman, G. S. (1998) Acetaminophen overdose with therapeutic intent. *J. Pediatr.* **132(1),** 5–8.
172. Rivera-Penera, T., Gugig, R., Davis, J., McDiarmid, S., Vargas, J., Rosenthal, P., et al. (1997) Outcome of acetaminophen overdose in pediatric patients and factors contributing to hepatotoxicity. *J. Pediatr.* **130(2),** 300–304.
173. Kirvela, M., Lindgren, L., Seppala, T., and Olkkola, K. T. (1996) The pharmacokinetics of oxycodone in uremic patients undergoing renal transplantation. *J. Clin. Anesth.* **8(1),** 13–18.
174. Leow, K. P., Cramond, T., and Smith, M. T. (1995) Pharmacokinetics and pharmacodynamics of oxycodone when given intravenously and rectally to adult patients with cancer pain. *Anesth. Analg.* **80(2),** 296–302.
175. Grond, S., Radbruch, L., and Lehmann, K. A. (2000) Clinical pharmacokinetics of transdermal opioids: focus on transdermal fentanyl. *Clin. Pharmacokinet.* **38(1),** 59–89.
176. Goldstein-Dresner, M. C., Davis, P. J., Kretchman, E., Siewers, R. D., Certo, N., and Cook, D. R. (1991) Double-blind comparison of oral transmucosal fentanyl citrate with oral meperidine, diazepam, and atropine as preanesthetic medication in children with congenital heart disease. *Anesthesiology* **74(1),** 28–33.
177. Stanley, T. H., Hague, B., Mock, D. L., Streisand, J. B., Bubbers, S., Dzelzkalns, R. R., et al. (1989) Oral transmucosal fentanyl citrate (lollipop) premedication in human volunteers. *Anesth. Analg.* **69(1),** 21–27.
178. Ashburn, M. A., Lind, G. H., Gillie, M. H., de Boer, A. J., Pace, N. L., and Stanley, T. H. (1993) Oral transmucosal fentanyl citrate (OTFC) for the treatment of postoperative pain. *Anesth. Analg.* **76(2),** 377–381.
179. Streisand, J. B., Varvel, J. R., Stanski, D. R., Le Maire, L., Ashburn, M. A., Hague, B. I., et al. (1991) Absorption and bioavailability of oral transmucosal fentanyl citrate. *Anesthesiology* **75(2),** 223–229.
180. Dsida, R. M., Wheeler, M., Birmingham, P. K., Henthorn, T. K., Avram, M. J., Enders-Klein, C., et al. (1998) Premedication of pediatric tonsillectomy patients with oral transmucosal fentanyl citrate. *Anesth. Analg.* **86(1),** 66–70.
181. Portenoy, R. K., Payne, R., Coluzzi, P., Raschko, J. W., Lyss, A., Busch, M. A., et al. (1999) Oral transmucosal fentanyl citrate (OTFC) for the treatment of breakthrough pain in cancer patients: a controlled dose titration study. *Pain* **79(2–3),** 303–312.

182. Epstein, R. H., Mendel, H. G., Witkowski, T. A., Waters, R., Guarniari, K. M., Marr, A. T., et al. (1996) The safety and efficacy of oral transmucosal fentanyl citrate for preoperative sedation in young children. *Anesth. Analg.* **83(6)**, 1200–1205.

183. Elenbaas, R. M., Iacono, C. U., Koellner, K. J., Pribble, J. P., Gratton, M., Racz, G., et al. (1991) Dose effectiveness and safety of butorphanol in acute migraine headache. *Pharmacotherapy* **11(1)**, 56–63.

184. Scott, J. L., Smith, M. S., Sanford, S. M., Shesser, R. F., Rosenthal, R. E., Smith, J. P., et al. (1994) Effectiveness of transnasal butorphanol for the treatment of musculoskeletal pain. *Am. J. Emerg. Med.* **12(4)**, 469–471.

185. Bennie, R. E., Boehringer, L. A., Dierdorf, S. F., Hanna, M. P., and Means, L. J. (1998) Transnasal butorphanol is effective for postoperative pain relief in children undergoing myringotomy. *Anesthesiology* **89(2)**, 385–390.

186. Zedie, N., Amory, D. W., Wagner, B. K., and O'Hara, D. A. (1996) Comparison of intranasal midazolam and sufentanil premedication in pediatric outpatients. *Clin. Pharmacol. Ther.* **59(3)**, 341–348.

187. Karl, H. W., Keifer, A. T., Rosenberger, J. L., Larach, M. G., and Ruffle, J. M. (1992) Comparison of the safety and efficacy of intranasal midazolam or sufentanil for preinduction of anesthesia in pediatric patients. *Anesthesiology* **76(2)**, 209–215.

188. Chandler, S. (1999) Nebulized opioids to treat dyspnea. *Am. J. Hosp. Palliat. Care* **16(1)**, 418–422.

189. Bostwick, D. G., Null, W. E., Holmes, D., Weber, E., Barchas, J. D., and Bensch, K. G. (1987) Expression of opioid peptides in tumors. *N. Engl. J. Med.* **317(23)**, 1439–1443.

190. Booth, S., Kelly, M. J., Cox, N. P., Adams, L., and Guz, A. (1996) Does oxygen help dyspnea in patients with cancer? *Am. J. Respir. Crit. Care Med.* **153(5)**, 1515–1518.

191. Zempsky, W. T., and Ashburn, M. A. (1998) Iontophoresis: noninvasive drug delivery. *Am. J. Anesthesiol.* **25(4)**, 158–162.

192. Ashburn, M. A., Gauthier, M., Love, G., Basta, S., Gaylord, B., and Kessler, K. (1997) Iontophoretic administration of 2% lidocaine HCl and epinephrine in humans. *Clin. J. Pain* **13(1)**, 22–26.

193. Ashburn, M. A., Streisand, J., Zhang, J., Love, G., Rowin, M., Niu, S., et al. (1995) The iontophoresis of fentanyl citrate in humans. *Anesthesiology* **82(5)**, 1146–1153.

194. Ashburn, M. A., Stephen, R. L., Ackerman, E., Petelenz, T. J., Hare, B., Pace, N. L., et al. (1992) Iontophoretic delivery of morphine for postoperative analgesia. *J. Pain. Symptom Manage.* **7(1)**, 27–33.

195. Arnold, J. H., Truog, R. D., Scavone, J. M., and Fenton, T. (1991) Changes in the pharmacodynamic response to fentanyl in neonates during continuous infusion. *J. Pediatr.* **119(4)**, 639–643.

196. Dagan, O., Klein, J., Bohn, D., and Koren, G. (1994) Effects of extracorporeal membrane oxygenation on morphine pharmacokinetics in infants. *Crit. Care Med.* **22(7)**, 1099–1101.

197. Franck, L. S., Vilardi, J., Durand, D., and Powers, R. (1998) Opioid withdrawal in neonates after continuous infusions of morphine or fentanyl during extracorporeal membrane oxygenation. *Am. J. Crit. Care* **7(5),** 364–369.
198. Paronis, C. A. and Holtzman, S. G. (1992) Development of tolerance to the analgesic activity of mu agonists after continuous infusion of morphine, meperidine or fentanyl in rats. *J. Pharmacol. Exp. Ther.* **262(1),** 1–9.
199. Sosnowski, M. and Yaksh, T. L. (1990) Differential cross-tolerance between intrathecal morphine and sufentanil in the rat. *Anesthesiology* **73(6),** 1141–1147.
200. Duttaroy, A. and Yoburn, B. C. (1995) The effect of intrinsic efficacy on opioid tolerance. *Anesthesiology* **82(5),** 1226–1236.
201. Suresh, S. and Anand, K. J. (1998) Opioid tolerance in neonates: mechanisms, diagnosis, assessment, and management. *Semin. Perinatol.* **22(5),** 425–433.

8

Patient Monitoring During Sedation

Kevin K. Tremper, MD, PhD

1. INTRODUCTION

Sedation of patients can only be accomplished safely if the physiologic effects of the sedative agents are continuously evaluated by a trained individual who is assisted by data provided by devices, that monitor the cardiopulmonary system *(1)*. Since sedation is on a continuum from the awake and alert state to general anesthesia, the monitors employed during sedation should be similar to those used during the provision of anesthesia. More than 15 years ago, the American Society of Anesthesiologists (ASA) published standards for monitoring during anesthesia *(2)*. These guidelines have been extended into the post-anesthesia care unit, and have more recently been applied to sedation *(1,3)*. It is important that the safety standards for monitoring be maintained regardless of the individuals providing sedation or the specific environment. This chapter reviews the current guidelines for monitoring during sedation and the specific devices used to monitor patients, including a brief description of how they work, and concludes with special recommendations for monitoring during magnetic resonance imaging (MRI).

2. MONITORING STANDARDS

In 1986, the ASA published standards for basic anesthetic monitoring *(2)*. At the time, it was considered somewhat revolutionary for a professional society to publish specific standards for the provision of medical care. This was done in the interest of patient safety. It had been well-documented that patients had been harmed by the inability of clinicians to evaluate oxygenation and ventilation by observation alone *(4)*. At the same time, two devices became available that allowed continuous monitoring of both oxygenation and ventilation: the pulse oximeter and the capnometer. The ASA took the position that all patients should be monitored objectively for oxygenation, ventilation, circulation, and temperature *(2)*. The devices recommended

From: *Contemporary Clinical Neuroscience: Sedation and Analgesia for Diagnostic and Therapeutic Procedures*
Edited by: S. Malviya, N. N. Naughton, and K. K. Tremper © Humana Press Inc., Totowa, NJ

Table 1
Monitoring Standards

I. Qualified personnel
II. Oxygenation, ventilation, circulation and temperature
   A. Oxygenation: pulse xximetry, SpO_2
   B. Ventilation: respiratory rate, capnography if intubated
   C. Circulation: blood pressure every 5 min, NIBP, pulse monitoring
      (pulse oximetry)
   D. Temperature

Basics of Anesthesia 4th ed., (Stoelting, R. K., and Miller, R. D., eds.), Churchill Livingston, NY, Appendix 2, p. 475.

to accomplish these monitoring standards were the pulse oximeter for oxygenation, the capnometer for ventilation, and a pulse plethysmograph, which is incorporated into a pulse oximeter for circulation. In addition, the ASA recommended that blood pressure should be monitored every 5 min and that temperature monitoring should be available whenever changes are anticipated in the patient's temperature. Although there is some controversy relating to the cause-and-effect relationship, there is no controversy regarding the improvement of patient safety that was documented over the subsequent 15 yr *(5)*. The standard application of a pulse oximeter to all patients who are receiving sedative anesthetic agents has been credited by many to be the primary reason for improved patient safety. In 1988, similar guidelines were adapted for the care of patients in the post-anesthesia care unit *(3)*. In this setting, patients recover from sedative agents and receive analgesics, and are therefore at high risk for cardiopulmonary depression. It should be noted that these are standards and not guidelines or recommendations—they are expressed as the minimum acceptable degree of monitoring, except in emergency situations, when lapses in the standard are unavoidable (Table 1).

Although these standards were developed for anesthesia care, that care encompasses both general anesthesia and intravenous (iv) sedation for operative procedures. Once anxiolytics or analgesics are given by any route, the physiologic result is on a continuum from mild sedation to general anesthesia, depending on the dose/response of the individual patient. In 1999, the ASA published an information bulletin describing the continuum of the depth of sedation *(6)* (Table 2). This table describes the continuum of sedation from minimal to general anesthesia by its effects on four physiologic processes: responsiveness of the patient, airway, spontaneous ventilation, and cardiovascular function. The method of evaluating each of these levels of sedation relies on a clinical evaluation of the physiologic effects of the

Table 2
Continuum of Depth of Sedation
Definition of General Anesthesia and Levels of Sedation/Analgesia

	Minimal sedation (anxiolysis)	Moderate Sedation/ Analgesia ("Conscious Sedation")	Deep Sedation/ Analgesia	General anesthesia
Responsiveness	Normal response to verbal stimuli	Purposeful response to verbal or tactile stimulation	Purposeful response following repeated or painful stimulation	Unarousable even with painful stimulus
Airway	Unaffected	No intervention required	Intervention may be required	Intervention often required
Spontaneous ventilation	Unaffected	Adequate	May be inadequate	Frequently inadequate
Cardiovascular function	Unaffected	Usually maintained	Usually maintained	May be impaired

Table 3
Monitoring Guidelines

Level of Consciousness	Spoken response and response to painful stimulus
Pulmonary ventilation	Observation of respiration. If patient is physically not in view, then an apnea monitor should be used
Oxygenation	Pulse oximetry
Hemodynamics	Vital signs: blood pressure, heart rate and pulse, electrocardiography monitoring in patients with cardiac disease

agents. As noted in Table 2, the difference between moderate sedation analgesia and deep sedation analgesia may be difficult to assess and may change very quickly, even when small doses of medications are administered. It therefore requires continuous observation by a trained individual who is not specifically involved in the procedure being performed. The ASA published practice guidelines for sedation and analgesia by non-anesthesiologists in 1996 *(4)*. A practice guideline is not as rigorous a statement as a standard. It would be difficult for one professional society to invoke standards on all other health care professionals. Nevertheless, since anesthesiologists are the specialists most trained and capable of providing sedation analgesia and managing the complications, it is reasonable that their society should make judicious recommendations *(4)*. These guidelines are divided into 14 sections starting with a patient pre-operative evaluation and continuing through procedure preparation, monitoring, staffing, training required, use of the medications, recovery, and special situations. These guidelines can be quickly found on the ASA website under the section entitled "Professional Information," which includes a variety of practice guidelines *(4)*. The section on monitoring covers the monitored variables as well as the recommended documentation of those parameters. The specifics of the monitoring are outlined in Table 3, and include level of consciousness, pulmonary ventilation, oxygenation, and hemodynamics. It is recommended that level of consciousness be monitored by an individual whose primary purpose is to monitor the patient and not be involved in the procedure, except for minor tasks that require only brief moments away from direct observation of the patient. The method of monitoring level of consciousness is by verbal response, and tactile response as described in Table 3. Although this level of consciousness monitoring is not objectified in a scale by the ASA, at the University of Michigan a numerical score has been developed to quantitate

Table 4
University of Michigan Sedation Scale

0	*Awake and alert*
1	*Lightly sedated:* Tired/sleepy, appropriate response to verbal conversation and/or sound
2	*Sedated:* Somnolent/sleeping, easily aroused with light tactile stimulation or a simple verbal command
3	*Deeply sedated:* Deep sleep, arousable only with significant physical stimulation
4	*Unarousable*

the levels of sedation that have been defined in a very similar way (Table 4). This scale has been very useful at the University of Michigan for both pediatric and adult patients *(7)*.

Ventilatory depression is the most common serious adverse consequence of providing sedation by any route. The ASA Task Force recommended that respiratory rate be monitored by visual observation at all times. When it is difficult or impossible to observe respiration because of physical limitations of the location (such as in MRI) the Task Force recommends the use of apnea monitoring using exhaled carbon dioxide. This technique is described in Subheading 6., page 210.

The most serious consequence of over-sedation and apnea is hypoxemia. For this reason, the pulse oximeter has become a ubiquitous device in all clinical situations in which apnea or hypoxemia is a potential concern. It is only logical that the Task Force recommends continuous monitoring by pulse oximeter, to provide continuous assessment of oxygenation as well as continuous monitoring of the patient's pulse. This Task Force emphasized that pulse oximetry does not substitute for monitoring ventilation—i.e., patients may have adequate hemoglobin saturation—especially when given supplemental oxygen—and at the same time become progressively hypercarbic because of respiratory depression.

The final monitoring recommendation involved methods of assessing hemodynamic stability. This group recommends that blood pressure be measured before the procedure, after the analgesics are provided, at "frequent intervals" during the procedure, at the end of the procedure, and prior to discharge. There is no specific definition of "frequent intervals"—it is therefore left to the judgement of the practitioner. The most recent pediatric sedation guidelines from the American Academy of Pediatrics (AAP) recommends that blood pressure be monitored before the procedure and during recovery. Blood pressure measurement during the procedure is left to the discretion of the monitoring individual because this procedure may rouse a sedated child, thus interfering with completion of the procedure. The task force also recommends that electrocardiogram (ECG) monitoring be used in patients with cardiovascular disease, but this is not required in patients with no cardiovascular disease.

Finally, there are recommendations regarding the recording of these monitored parameters. The specific frequency of recording these parameters is again left to the judgement of the practitioner, but the report recommends that at a minimum all cardio-respiratory parameters be recorded before the beginning of the procedure, after the administration of the sedative agents, upon completion of the procedure, during recovery, and at the time of discharge. If this recording is being accomplished by an automatic device, it should have alarms set to alert the team of critical changes in the measured parameters.

Even with the availability of a capnometer, pulse oximeter, ECG and a blood pressure device, safe monitoring of a sedated patient requires an individual who is dedicated to that purpose. It is specifically stated that the practitioner who performs the procedure should not be that individual. The individual dedicated to monitoring the patients may have interruptable tasks in assisting the practitioner who is performing the procedure, but these interruptions should be of very short duration. Clearly, the individual monitoring the patient and recording the physiologic parameters must understand the consequences of the sedative agents and know how to respond to an adverse event such as apnea or desaturation. This individual must therefore be trained in the pharmacology of the agents provided as well as their antagonists, and must be knowledgeable about the monitoring devices being used and how to recognize the common physiologic consequences of apnea, desaturation, and hypotension. At least one of the individuals involved must be capable of establishing a patent airway and providing positive pressure ventilation if apnea occurs. There must be an individual immediately available who has advanced life-support skills.

If the clinician could choose only one monitoring device to be used during sedation, it would clearly be pulse oximetry. Since this device continuously provides a measurement of oxygenation and pulse rate, it continuously evaluates the two essential aspects of cardiopulmonary physiology—oxygenation and peripheral perfusion. For this reason, the following section provides great detail, in the clinical as well as the technical aspects of the device.

3. OXYGENATION MONITORING: PULSE OXIMETRY

Since its development in the early 1980s, pulse oximetry has been widely adopted in clinical medicine *(8)*. It is currently the standard of care for monitoring all patients during surgical procedures, in recovery rooms, and critical care units, and in any situation in which oxygenation may be in question or at risk. It has been selected as the primary monitor to assess patients' physiologic well-being during sedation, and is an ideal technique for monitoring these patients because it continuously and noninvasively assesses oxygenation and pulse. Pulse oximetry does this without requiring calibration or technical skill by the user. However, it is important that caregivers using the technique to assess patient status are knowledgeable of the meaning of the data provided and the limitations of that data as well as the limitations of the device. To best understand the limitations of the device, it is useful to understand the fundamental principles that the device employs to determine saturation and pulse. Subheading 3.1. therefore reviews the definition and meaning of the term "hemoglobin saturation," the methods of measuring saturation, how pulse oximeters estimate saturation noninvasively, and finally situations in which the device may be unable to provide data or provide misleading data *(9)*.

3.1. Hemoglobin Saturation

Because oxygen is not effectively stored in the human body, aerobic metabolism depends on a constant supply. The amount of oxygen contained within blood-perfusing tissue is known as the oxygen content, which is defined as the number of ccs of oxygen contained within 100 ccs of blood.

$$CaO_2 = 1.34 \times Hb \times SaO_2 + 0.003 \times PaO_2 \tag{1}$$

CaO_2 = Oxygen content mL/dL
1.34 = The number of mL of oxygen contained on one saturated gram of hemoglobin per 1 dL of blood
Hb = The grams of hemoglobin per dL of blood
SaO_2 = Hemoglobin saturation, %
0.003 = The solubility constant of oxygen in water
PaO_2 = The arterial oxygen partial pressure in mmHg

Since oxygen has a very low solubility in water, the carrying capacity of blood is dramatically increased with the addition of hemoglobin. One gram of hemoglobin carries approximately $1^1/3$ cc of oxygen per dL, so that a patient with a normal hemoglobin of 15 g could carry approximately 20 cc of oxygen if the hemoglobin were completely filled (saturated) with oxygen. A hemoglobin molecule can carry four oxygen molecules. These sites are filled in a cooperative binding method as the oxygen tension surrounding the hemoglobin increases. Hemoglobin saturation is defined as the amount of hemoglobin with oxygen attached divided by the total amount of hemoglobin present per dL of blood. Hemoglobin with oxygen on it is termed oxyhemoglobin (HbO_2) and hemoglobin without oxygen on it is termed reduced hemoglobin (Hb).

$$\text{Hemoglobin Saturation} = [HbO_2/(HbO_2 + Hb)] \times 100\% \qquad (2)$$

This definition of hemoglobin saturation has been termed as functional hemoglobin saturation because it incorporates the two hemoglobin forms that function in oxygen transport—i.e., HbO_2 and Hb. Other forms of hemoglobin are present in small concentrations in healthy individuals, which may be in larger concentrations in pathologic conditions. Carbon monoxide has 800 times the affinity for hemoglobin than oxygen. Thus, if hemoglobin is exposed to carbon monoxide, it will form carboxyhemoglobin (COHb) and displace HbO_2. This form of hemoglobin does not contribute to oxygen transport. The iron in the heme of the hemoglobin is usually in the ferric form (Fe^{+++}). When it is reduced to the ferrous (Fe^{++}), it is called methemoglobin (metHb), and it will also not transport oxygen. When these hemoglobin species are present, they are part of the total measured hemoglobin and therefore must be considered when saturation is calculated. The term "fractional hemoglobin saturation" is defined as HbO_2 divided by total hemoglobin.

$$\text{Fractional Saturation} = [HbO_2/(HbO_2 + Hb + COHb + MetHb)] \times 100\% \quad (3)$$

Looking at Eq. 2 and Eq. 3, it is clear that even if all the reduced hemoglobin is oxygenated and functional saturation is 100%, the presence of significant amounts of metHb and COHb will produce a lower fractional saturation. It is important to understand the differences between functional and fractional saturation because the pulse oximeter provides different information when either metHb or COHb are present. This information may not correspond to that provided by saturation measured in the clinical chemistry lab.

Assuming that no metHb or COHb are present, the relationship between oxygen tension and hemoglobin saturation is represented by the sigmoidal hemoglobin dissociation curve shown in Fig. 1. When the oxygen tension increases above 90 mmHg, the hemoglobin is nearly 100% saturated. Normal healthy patients will have a saturation between 95% and 100% while breathing room air. A saturation of 95% corresponds to approximate PaO_2 of 75 mmHg, and a saturation of 90% corresponds to a PaO_2 of 60 mmHg. Once the PaO_2 drops below 60, the saturation drops more rapidly. A simplistic algorithm to remember the relationship between PaO_2 and saturation as the oxygen tension drops below 90 is given below.

$$PaO_2 \approx \text{saturation} - 30 \text{ (For a } PaO_2 \text{ from 60 to 45)} \qquad (4)$$

Normal mixed venous saturation is approx 75%, corresponding to a mixed venous oxygen tension ($P\bar{v}O_2$) of 40 mmHg. Note that the body usually ex-

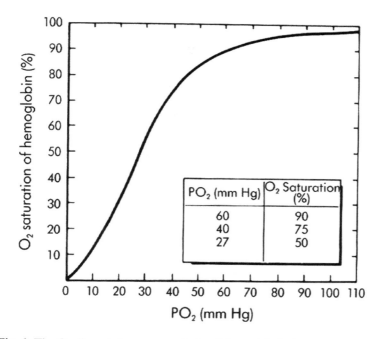

Fig. 1. The O_2 dissociation curve relation PO_2 and SaO_2 in man at 37° C, pH = 7.4. From ref. *(36)*.

tracts about 25% of the oxygen attached to the hemoglobin as it passes through the tissue—i.e., arterial saturation 98%, mixed venous saturation 73%. This allows for some margin of safety. If the arterial saturation declines, additional oxygen may be extracted from the hemoglobin. Unfortunately, this occurs at the expense of lower and lower PO_2 values at the tissue level.

Another important point on the HbO_2 association curve is the P50. This is defined as the oxygen tension at which 50% of the hemoglobin is saturated. The P50 is 26.7 mmHg at 37°C and 7.4 pH. The curve can shift to the right with increasing temperature, acidosis, and increasing 2–3 DPG (a protein that affects the affinity of hemoglobin for oxygen). Bank blood loses its 2–3 DPG very quickly and therefore can theoretically decrease the P50 of hemoglobin after a transfusion. This effect is not usually clinically significant, because the 2–3 DPG is quickly reestablished once the blood is in circulation. Fetal hemoglobin has a much lower P50 (a higher affinity for oxygen), thus shifting the curve to the left (P50 ≈ 19 mmHg). This is necessary so that the fetal blood can extract oxygen at a lower oxygen tension than the maternal blood perfusing the uterus.

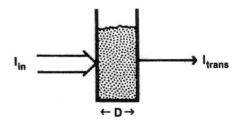

$$I_{trans} = I_{in}e^{-(D \times C \times a_\lambda)}$$

I_{trans} = intensity of light transmitted
I_{in} = intensity of incident light
D = distance light is transmitted through the liquid
C = concentration of solute (oxyhemoglobin)
a_λ = extinction coefficient of the solute (a constant)

Fig. 2. The concentration of a solute dissolved in a solvent can be calculated from the logarithmic relationship between the incident and transmitted light intensity and the solute concentration. From ref. *(36).*

3.2. Measurement of Hemoglobin Saturation

Equation 2 defines functional hemoglobin saturation. To measure this, it is necessary to measure the concentration of HbO_2 and Hb and then form the ratio of $HbO_2/(HbO_2 + Hb)$. Measuring the concentration of any of the hemoglobin species in solution can be accomplished by using the principle of optical absorption or Beer's Law. This law states that the concentration of a substance dissolved in a solution can be determined if a light of known wavelength and intensity is transmitted through a known distance through the solution. Fig. 2 illustrates this principle. If hemoglobin is placed in a cuvet of known dimensions and light is shined through the container, the concentration of hemoglobin can be calculated if the incident light intensity and the transmitted light intensity are both measured.

$$I_t = I_ie^{-dc\alpha} \qquad (5)$$
$$c = 1/dx \ln I_i/I_t \qquad (5a)$$

The above equation is known as Beer's Law, where:

I_i = the incident light intensity
I_t = the transmitted light intensity
d = the path length of light
α = the absorption coefficient for hemoglobin
c = the concentration of hemoglobin that is being determined

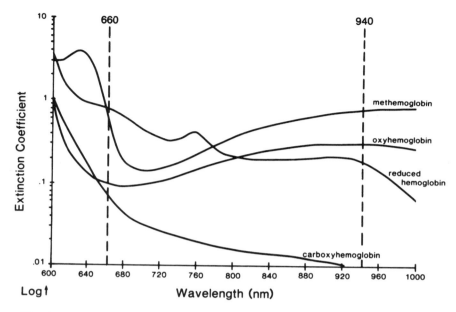

Fig. 3. Transmitted light absorbance spectra of four hemoglobin species; oxyhemoglobin, reduced hemoglobin, carboxyhemoglobin, and methemoglobin. From ref. *(37)*.

Therefore, if the incident and transmitted light intensity are known and the path length of light is known, then the concentration of hemoglobin can be measured if the absorption coefficient α is known. The absorption coefficient for Hb, HbO_2 and metHb and COHb are presented in Fig. 3. All of these absorption coefficients vary as a function of the wavelength of light used. If the light is of a known wavelength, then one hemoglobin concentration can be measured for each wavelength of light used—i.e., one equation and one unknown. If we need to measure both HbO_2 and Hb, then it would require at least two wavelengths of light to form two Beer's Law equations and solve for the two unknown concentrations—i.e., Hb and HbO_2. If met Hb and COHb are also present we would want to measure fractional saturation (Eq. 3) and require at least four wavelengths of light to produce four equations to solve for the four concentrations of the hemoglobin species present. The device that uses this method of measuring hemoglobin concentration and hemoglobin saturation is called a co-oximeter. This optical absorption technique is used to measure the concentration of many substances in science and in medicine—for example, the capnometer that will be described in a later section and bilirubin concentration in the plasma. When an arterial blood sample is sent to a blood gas laboratory, the PaO_2, PCO_2 (carbon dioxide tension) and pH are measured and the saturation is often presented with the blood gas results. This saturation is usually not measured but determined from the HbO_2 dissociation curve, Fig. 1. If the clinician wants to know the measured saturation—including metHb and COHb concentration, then a blood saturation measurement must be requested and the results will be presented in the form of percent saturation for all the constituents—i.e., HbO_2, metHb, COHb. These results usually do not present a reduced hemoglobin—it is what is left over after the other hemoglobin saturations are added, because they all must sum to 100%.

3.3. Pulse Oximeters

Some of the first clinical measurements in hemoglobin saturation were done noninvasively through human tissue. During World War II, aviation research needed a device that could determine at what altitude supplemental oxygen was required. To accomplish this, an oximeter was developed which transilluminated the human ear. The device effectively used the ear as the test tube containing hemoglobin. A light source was placed on one side of the earlobe and a light detector on the opposite side. Since the light was absorbed not only by hemoglobin in the blood but also by skin and other tissues, the device needed to be zeroed to the light absorbance of the non-blood tissue. This was accomplished by compressing the ear to eliminate all the blood and then measuring the absorbance resulting from the bloodless tissue. This absorbance was considered the zero point and when the pressure was relieved, the additional absorbance was caused by the blood returning to the ear. This blood was not only arterial blood, but also venous and capillary blood. To obtain a signal that was related to arterial hemoglobin saturation, the device was heated to 40° centigrade, thereby making the ear hyperemic and producing a signal that was predominately related to arterial blood. This ear oximeter was used after World War II in clinical physiologic studies and in early studies monitoring patients in the operating room *(8)*. Unfortunately, this early ear oximeter was difficult to use as a clinical monitor because it required calibration on each patient, and heating of the ear which often caused burns if it is left in one place too long.

In the mid 1970s, an engineer working in Japan was using an ear oximeter as a noninvasive method to measure cardiac output. The proposed technique involved injecting a dye in a vein and then using the ear oximeter to detect the light absorption caused by that dye as it circulated and perfused the ear. This noninvasive ear dye dilution cardiac output technique was not successful, but the engineer noted an interesting phenomena during his stud-

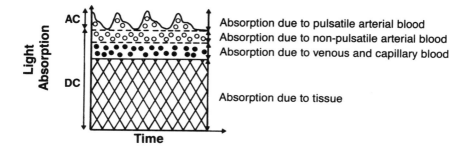

Fig. 4. Light absorption through living tissue. The alternating current signal is caused by the pulsatile component of the arterial blood; the direct current signal comprises all the non-pulsatile absorbers in the tissue, non-pulsatile arterial blood, non-pulsatile venous and capillary blood and all other tissues (Modified from *Ohmeda Pulse Oximeter Model 3700 Service Manual,* 1986, pp. 22.)

ies. There was a pulsatile absorbance signal from the oximeter that fluctuated with the heart rate. He then postulated that if this pulsatile component were analyzed, it would be related to arterial blood, thereby negating the necessity to compress the ear or to heat the probe when trying to determine an arterial signal from the oximeter. By the early 1980s, this technique of analyzing the pulsatile absorbance signal became known as pulse oximetry, and was being developed as a routine clinical monitor for intra-operative and postoperative use. Therefore, the basic premise of a pulse oximeter is that the pulsatile component of the absorption signal must be produced by arterial blood (Fig. 4). Although the pulsatile signal is related to arterial blood, determining actual arterial saturation from this signal is not easily accomplished. Pulse oximeters use two frequencies of light in the red and infrared range, 660 nm red light and 940 nm infrared light. It was clear that the amplitude of the signal in the red range of light and the infrared range of light changed as the amount of HbO_2 and Hb changed. The pulse-added absorbance in these two frequency changes with the change in arterial saturation, but the specific relationship must be determined empirically from data derived from human volunteer studies. Pulse oximeters were placed on subjects as they breathed low inspired oxygen and arterial blood samples were drawn. Samples were analyzed by laboratory co-oximeters to determine the actual arterial saturation relative to the pulse oximeter reading. Fig. 5 illustrates a calibration curve between the ratio of pulse-added red and infrared absorbance signal (R) from the pulse oximeter and measured arterial blood saturation.

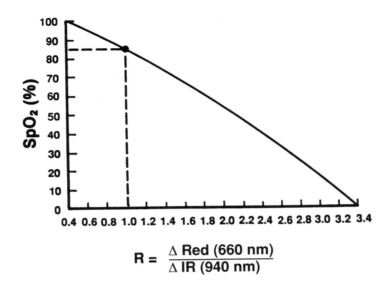

$$R = \frac{\Delta \text{ Red (660 nm)}}{\Delta \text{ IR (940 nm)}}$$

Fig. 5. This is a typical pulse oximeter calibration curve. Note that the SaO_2 estimate is determined from the ratio (R) of the pulse-added red absorbance at 660 nm to pulse-added infrared absorbance at 940 nm. The ratios of red to infrared absorbances vary from approx 0.4 at 100% to 3.4 at 0% saturation. Note that the ratio of red to infrared absorbance is one at a saturation of approx 85%. This curve can be approximated on a theoretical basis, but for accurate predications of SpO_2, experimental data are required. Adapted from ref. *(38)*.

$$R = \Delta \text{Red}/\Delta \text{IR} \qquad\qquad (6)$$

Note that when the ratio of pulse added red to pulse added infrared light is one, the saturation is approx 85%. This fact has interesting clinical consequences, which will be noted on page 205 when methemoglobin is discussed.

The principles of pulse oximeters can be summarized with the following three simple statements. First, the device measures the pulsatile component of light absorbance in two frequencies. Second, it assumes that that pulsatile absorbance is produced by the arterial blood pulsations in that tissue. Third, this ratio of absorbances is empirically calibrated to arterial hemoglobin saturation (SaO_2) so that the device can present saturation values, SpO_2.

3.4. Problems with Pulse Oximetry

Pulse oximeters have become so valuable clinically because they are easy to use and easy to interpret, and are fairly reliable in providing valuable information regarding oxygenation and pulse. There are several circumstances in which the device may have difficulty providing an accurate SpO_2 value or may even provide a misleading saturation value. Problem areas can be divided into three types: the presence of dyes or abnormal hemoglobins within the blood; low perfusion signals; and artifacts resulting from motion or light. These last two problems both involve signal-to-noise ratio—i.e., either low signal or high noise.

When dye is injected intravenously, it may very likely provide a transient error in pulse oximetry if that dye absorbs light in the red or infrared range. The most common dye to produce this problem is methylene blue, which will cause a transient (few minute) drop in saturation to as low as 50% saturation. Since this is only a transient effect, it is not a significant clinical issue. Carboxy or methemoglobin poisoning may cause a more significant and complex problem with pulse oximeters *(10,11)*. COHb is bright red and is interpreted by the pulse oximeter as HbO_2. Therefore, in a patient who is suffering from carbon monoxide poisoning, the pulse oximeter will not be able to detect the presence of COHb and will give the false impression that the patient has a normal hemoglobin saturation. The SpO_2 value will present a value which is the sum of HbO_2 and COHb. Methemoglobin has a more interesting effect on pulse oximeters. Methemoglobin produces a dark brownish color of blood, which strongly absorbs light in both the red and infrared range. Thus, it causes a very large pulsatile absorbance that is equally distributed in both light ranges and overwhelms the HbO_2 and Hb signal usually detected by the pulse oximeter. Because this large absorbance is equal in both the numerator and the denominator (Eq. 6) it forces the ratio to one, which is interpreted by the pulse oximeter as a saturation of approx 85% (Fig. 5). Therefore, if a patient is suffering from metHb toxicity, the pulse oximeter usually reads in the mid 80s, regardless of the patient's actual saturation *(11)*. This problem has a significant clinical potential because metHb toxicity can be easily caused by an overdose of the local anesthetic benzocaine. Benzocaine is the main constituent of the topical spray known as Hurricane Spray®. This anesthetic spray is frequently used to topicalize the airway during endoscopic procedures. Unfortunately, this spray contains 20% benzocaine—i.e., 200 mg/mL per cc, and can quickly produce high levels of metHb when systemically absorbed *(12)*.

A low perfusion or low-pulse amplitude signals will make it difficult for a pulse oximeter to determine an accurate saturation value. The device will go into a pulse-search mode and ultimately produce no saturation value. Modern devices have low signal cutoffs that will not allow the device to "guess" at a saturation if the signal strength is too weak. This can occur when patients have severe peripheral vascular disease or shock syndrome, or are cold. If pulse oximeters cannot produce a signal when placed on a finger, they may derive a signal on the ear or may work when placed on the bridge of the nose.

Large artifacts resulting from motion are probably the most troublesome problem for pulse oximetry. When patients move their extremities, they cause pulsations of the venous blood that are superimposed on the pulsations of the arterial blood. The pulse oximeter has significant difficulty in discriminating between the two pulsatile signals, one at a low saturation at the motion rate and the other at the arterial saturation at the pulse rate. Because there is more venous blood in tissue than arterial blood, the device may frequently choose to present a value that is more like the venous saturation than the arterial saturation. Therefore when patients move their extremities, it is not uncommon to see the saturation drop to the low 90s and into the 80s very quickly, but when the extremity stops moving the saturation will quickly jump back to the 90s. This is most likely a result of the motion artifact causing venous pulsations. Newer-generation devices are specifically designed to identify venous pulsations during motion and eliminate them from the signal *(13–15)*. As these second-generation pulse oximeters become more readily available, the problems with motion artifact should be significantly reduced.

Finally, pulse oximeters will have difficulty in detecting the fluctuating absorbance signal of the red and infrared light if they have a large ambient background light producing a noise signal. Therefore, whenever the pulse oximeter probe is in the presence of a bright light that may be fluctuating at a high frequency, it is best to cover the probe with an opaque material to eliminate that light "noise" and allow the device to calculate its ratios of pulsatile absorbances and present a more accurate saturation.

4. BLOOD PRESSURE MONITORING: NONINVASIVE BLOOD PRESSURE MONITORING (NIBP)

Blood pressure and heart rate are the primary physiologic parameters used to document hemodynamic stability. A blood pressure reading in the normal range documents adequate perfusion pressure and implies adequate cardiac output (assuming a normal systemic vascular resistance). Arterial blood pressure can be measured in a variety of ways, but unfortunately the results differ slightly with each technique, whether it is invasive or noninvasive *(16,17)*. The gold standard is still the manual measurement, using a Riva-Rocci cuff and listening for Korotkoff sounds. The width of the blood pressure cuff should be 20–30% of the circumference of the limb, and the pneumatic bladder should span at least half the circumference while it is centered over the artery *(17)*. If the cuff is too narrow, the blood pressure values will be too high and vice versa. The deflation rate can affect accuracy. If the pressure in the cuff is deflated too quickly, the estimated blood pressure is usually too low. The recommended deflation rate is approx 3 mmHg per s *(18,19)*.

Korotkoff sounds consist of a complex series of audible frequencies that are produced by turbulent blood flow on the arterial wall and a shock wave created as the external occluding pressure is reduced on the major artery being compressed. The Phase I sound (the first sound) is heard as the cuff is deflated, and is defined as a systolic blood pressure. As the cuff is fully deflated, the character of the sound changes, becomes muffled, and finally is absent. The diastolic pressure is recorded as the sound becomes muffled or becomes absent. Clearly there is significant subjectivity in the measurement as well as patient-to-patient variation and tester-to-tester variation. In spite of these limitations the manual measurement of blood pressure by auscultating Korotkoff sounds is still considered the gold standard.

4.1. NIBP

In the late 1970s, continuous noninvasive automatic blood pressure devices became available. The first devices were developed using two different technologies. One relied upon a small microphone placed within a blood pressure cuff, which attempted to identify Korotkoff sounds. This method was known as auscultatory NIBP. Unfortunately, because of a variety of technical problems and errors associated with multiple artifacts, this technique was not widely accepted. The second technique, known as oscillometric blood pressure, has become the standard of NIBP measurement. In this method a cuff is automatically inflated and the pressure oscillations within the cuff are measured as the pressure is reduced. The onset of oscillation occurs just before the systolic pressure. As the cuff is deflated further, there is an increase in cuff oscillation pressure as noted in Fig. 6 *(17)*. These cuff pressure oscillations increase to a maximum which occurs at the mean arterial pressure (MAP). Further reduction in cuff pressure reduces the oscillations until they are back to a baseline amplitude at the point near the diastolic pressure. These devices most accurately measure the MAP and use sophisticated algorithms programmed into the microprocessors to predict systolic and diastolic pressure with a high level of consistency. Although these blood pressure data are not equal to those obtained with a manual method, they are consistent. Movement of the arm during blood pressure measurement causes significant error, which will usually result in a non-reported value. The devices can be programmed for repeating blood pressure measurements at any time interval down to 1 min. There are concerns that repeated blood pressure measurements at high frequencies can result in ulnar nerve palsies, superficial thrombophlebitis, and even compartment syndrome. Fortunately, these are very rare problems. In general, blood pressure is checked every 5 min during sedation

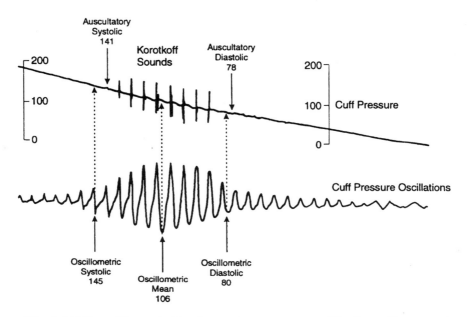

Fig. 6. NIBP, oscillometric blood pressure measurement. The figure illustrates the method for oscillometric blood pressure measurement. The upper graph measures the total pressure in the blood pressure cuff, and the lower graph represents the oscillating pressure within the cuff. Starting on the right depicts the point at which the blood pressure cuff is fully inflated to a point higher than the systolic blood pressure. As the pressure in the cuff is progressively lowered at the point, *Oscillometric Systolic (145)*, systolic pressure oscillations are felt within the cuff. Those oscillations increase as the total pressure in the cuff decreases to peak oscillations, which occurs at the MAP. With further cuff deflation the oscillations decrease until they are back to baseline, the point known as the diastolic blood pressure. The most accurate pressure measurement is the mean pressure; the systolic and diastolic are estimates. The upper portion of the figure also depicts the point at which Korotkoff sounds are heard, initiating at the systolic pressure and decreasing at the diastolic pressure. (Reproduced with permisison from ref. *[39]*, Churchill Livingston, 2000).

or anesthesia and only more frequently when there is hemodynamic instability. The primary advantages of NIBP devices are their uniformity in data presentation and their ability to produce a blood pressure measurement while practitioners are free to do other tasks such as treating the patient.

5. ECG MONITORING

It is important to document heart rate in all patients who are receiving sedation. Generally, this is accomplished continuously by the pulse oximeter and intermittently by the measurement of NIBP. Both of these devices generate a pulse rate that is a byproduct of their primary determinations of saturation and blood pressure, respectively. In patients with a history of cardiac disease, it is recommended that an ECG also be used to monitor the patient *(4)*. An in-depth discussion of the ECG and electrocardiographic monitoring is beyond the scope of this chapter. There are several excellent texts on this subject *(20–22)*. In the setting of sedation for minor surgical and medical procedures ECG monitoring should be used for the gross detection of dysrhythmias and potentially myocardial ischemia. If the patient becomes symptomatic with chest pain or shortness of breath, the procedure should be discontinued for a more in-depth evaluation of the patient's cardiac status and a 12-lead ECG. A three-electrode system is generally sufficient to monitor patients for these short procedures even if they have a history of significant cardiac disease. The leads are placed on the right arm (white), left arm (black), and the left leg (red). Lead two is generally monitored for it provides a good view of the P-wave and the ability to detect dysrhythmias. Unfortunately, this three-lead system is not sensitive for detecting myocardial ischemia frequently occurring in the left ventricle. For this reason, there have been several modifications of lead placement recommended to improve the ability to detect ischemia *(22)*. Most of these modifications attempt to represent a standard V5-lead view of the heart (Fig. 7). The most popular placement is known as the CS_5 modification. In this situation, the right arm lead (white lead) is kept at its standard location, while the left arm lead (the black lead) electrode is placed in the V5 position—i.e., the anterior axillary line at the fifth intercostal space (Fig. 8). The left leg electrode is left in its standard position. This CS_5 modification has been demonstrated to be as accurate as a V5 lead for detecting left ventricular ischemia *(23)*.

In patients with a more significant potential of ischemia, it is best to use a five-lead ECG system illustrated in Fig. 7. With a five-lead configuration, it is recommended that both leads II and V be monitored continuously to detect ischemia. It has been reported that 75% of the 12-lead ECG detectable ischemia is detected by a single V5 lead. This can be increased to 80% if both lead II and lead V5 are continuously monitored *(23,24)*.

It is important to realize that ECG monitoring only monitors the electrical activity of the heart and does not ensure oxygenation, ventilation, or hemodynamic stability. It is for this reason that the other monitors—i.e., blood pressure and pulse oximetry and observation of ventilation—are essential monitors during sedation, and ECG monitoring is only added when a patient has a significant history of cardiac disease.

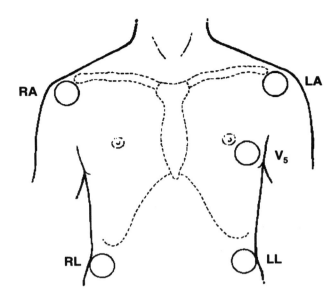

Fig. 7. Standard five-lead ECG system consisting of four extremity electrodes and the V5 lead. The V5 lead detects left ventricular ischemia. RA = right arm, LA = left arm, RL = right leg, LL = left leg. (Reproduced with permisison from ref. *[40]*, Mosby Year Book, 1992).

6. VENTILATION MONITORING—CAPNOGRAPHY

Continuously sampling the carbon dioxide from the airway is known as capnography, although referred to clinically as end-tidal CO_2 monitoring. Capnometry is derived the Greek word "kapnos," meaning smoke, carbon dioxide (CO_2) being the "smoke" of cellular metabolism. After it is produced in the mitochondria, CO_2 is removed from the tissue by diffusion down a partial pressure gradient to the capillary blood. The venous circulation then transports carbon dioxide to the right heart, where it is then pumped through the pulmonary circulation equilibrating with the alveolar gas. It is then ventilated to the atmosphere with each expiration. The shape and physiologic significance of the capnogram had to await the development of rapidly responding CO_2 analyzers. Today these devices are readily available using infrared absorption to measure CO_2. To obtain an accurate capnogram and avoid contamination with room air, patients must be intubated. Since this is usually not the case for patients undergoing sedation, the discussion of the interpretation of the capnogram is beyond the scope of this chapter. The reader is referred to excellent texts on this topic *(25,26)*. When capnography is applied to non-intubated patients it is used as a method of measuring res-

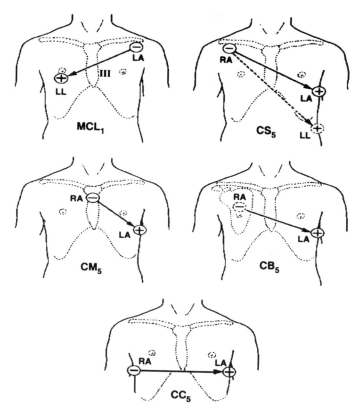

Fig. 8. Modified bipolar standard limb lead system: MCL_1, CS_5, CM_5, CB_5, CC_5. (Reproduced with permisison from ref. *[41]*, Churchill Livingston, 1987).

piratory rate by counting the peaks in the CO_2 wave with each expiration. It is important to remember that the presence of a capnogram also ensures pulmonary perfusion and thus cardiac output. A depression in the peak of the CO_2 tracing can be caused by either a contamination of the expired gas sample with room air (air has virtually no carbon dioxide) or more importantly, a depression in cardiac output.

6.1. Capnography in Non-Intubated Patients

When a capnometer is used to monitor ventilation in a non-intubated patient, there are technical problems in obtaining an accurate continuous sample of the respiratory gases. In intubated patients the system is "closed," and therefore the expired gas sample at the endotracheal tube is a very accurate measurement of the respiratory gases. In non-intubated patients a sampling

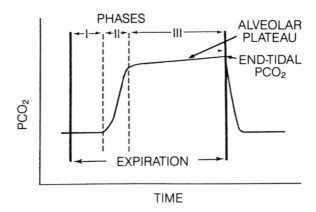

Fig. 9. Above is a plot of carbon dioxide partial pressure versus time during one respiratory cycle. This tracing is known as a capnogram. The capnogram tracing starts at zero during the beginning of the expiratory cycle, then rapidly rises to a plateau as alveolar gas is sampled. The capnogram quickly drops down to zero during inspiration. The three types of pulmonary dead space in the tidal volume are known as apparatus dead space (V_{appDS}), anatomical dead (V_{anaDS}) and alveolar dead space (V_{alvDS}). The first two types of dead space are caused by the respiratory equipment that the patient breathes through and the conducting airways. Alveolar dead space is produced by the alveoli that are ventilated but not perfused and therefore do not participate in CO_2 exchange. If there were no alveolar dead space, the end-tidal plateau value of CO_2 would be nearly identical to the arterial CO_2. As the patient develops more alveolar dead space, the end-tidal CO_2 drops and the difference between the arterial and end-tidal CO_2 widens. Adapted from ref. *(26)*.

device must be inserted in the airway—either the mouth or nose—which aspirates respiratory gases without aspirating additional room air or the supplemental oxygen. Aspirating these additional gases will dilute the sample and cause a lower capnogram or a capnogram that is rounded as opposed to the appropriate square wave as depicted in Fig. 9. Despite of these limitations seeing a repeated CO_2 wave form of any shape ensures that there is ventilation occurring, and can document the frequency of the respiratory rate. For this reason, despite of the less than optimal capnographic wave forms produced in non-intubated patients, capnography is still very useful in confirming ventilation.

A variety of methods of securing sampling tubes have been recommended. Fig. 10 illustrates how a sampling tube can be made using a standard nasal canula, which provides supplemental oxygen to the patient and an iv catheter and sampling tube inserted through one of the nasal prongs *(27)*. Fig. 11 shows a specialized nasal canula, which is available, which

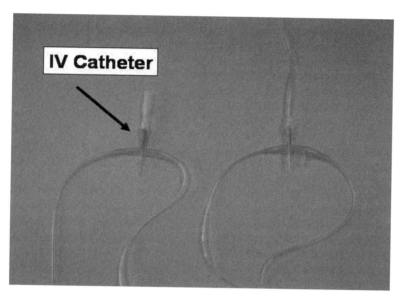

Fig. 10. A standard oxygen nasal cannula can be adapted to monitor end-tidal carbon dioxide in a spontaneously breathing patient. An iv catheter is inserted into one of the nasal prongs. The metal needle is then removed, the catheter is trimmed, and the gas aspirating tubing is attached to the iv catheter. It should be noted that this system works only with the aspirating or sidestream type of gas analyzers. (Reproduced with permission from ref. *[27]*, Mosby Year Book, 1993).

uses one of the nasal prongs to supply oxygen and the other one to sample carbon dioxide. This type of device is especially useful when managing patients who require deeper sedation, who are also in a difficult to observe location (as in MRI). This topic is discussed in the following section.

7. MONITORING PATIENTS IN MRI

Providing sedation for patients undergoing radiologic studies with MRI is challenging for a variety of reasons *(28)*. First, the enclosed space obscures the patient from the individual who is trying to provide and monitor the sedation. That same enclosed space also requires a deeper level of sedation in many patients because of the severe claustrophobic environment. Since most MRIs will take at least 30 min, most children will be unable to remain still for the duration of the procedure, also necessitating a deeper level of sedation. The environment is not only logistically hostile but also electro-magnetically hostile to most standard monitors. Thus, the high magnetic field may not only cause erroneous readings because of its interaction with ferrous metals, but in some cases may be dangerous if large ferrous objects are attracted to the magnet. The radiofrequency (RF) field, which is imposed on the magnetic field to produce the image, can interfere with and be subject to interference from monitoring devices. Finally, this RF field may also induce currents if monitoring wires are in the field and looped. These currents have caused patient burns *(29)*. This section systematically reviews the problems with monitoring patients during MRI and provide recommendations for specific equipment.

It is likely that there will be an even greater demand for sedation for MRI in the future because there are a growing number of applications, such as functional MRI and procedures being conducted under MRI guidance. To be able to provide safe patient care, practitioners must understand some of the basic physics involved in the MRI and the problems associated with the technique.

7.1. Magnetic Fields

The magnetic field strength is measured in teslet (T). One teslet equals 10,000 gauss (G). The earth's magnetic field at the surface is 0.5 to 2G. Clinical magnetic resonance imaging systems operate between 0.5T and 2T. At 5G, pacemakers may become dysfunctional, electrical equipment may start to malfunction, and magnetic tape will be erased. When the magnetic field strength approaches 50G, the attractive force on ferrous metal becomes significant. Clearly, a 1T MRI unit will cause significant problems. In addition, since the devices produce a magnetic field by cooled superconducting coils, the magnetic field is always on.

7.2. Implants

Patients with electrical and ferrous device implants are at high risk for problems and should be excluded from MRI exams. These include patients with pacemakers, AICDs, implanted pumps, or stimulators. Many implanted prosthetic devices are non-ferrous, Shellock recently published a review evaluating the ferromagnetic qualities of metal implants *(30)*. When there is a question, the patient should not be taken into MRI.

7.3. Induced Currents

The change in magnetic field gradient is used for image location and the RF currents used to excite the proton nuclei also cause significant problems when trying to monitor patients during MRI. Currents can be induced in monitoring wires, which can be heated to the extent of causing burns. For this reason, all probes and wire leads should be placed as far away from the exam area as possible, and cables should not be formed in loops within the

Table 5
Classification of Monitoring Problems
in the Magnetic Resonance Imaging Environment

Interaction of monitoring equipment with the MRI system
    Radio-frequency interference—monitoring produces RF or leads act as an
        aerial for stray RF
    Magnetic Field effects—distortion of the magnetic field by ferro magnetic
        equipment
Interaction of MRI system with monitoring equipment
    Static field—effects on some electronic circuitry, and cathode ray tube displays
    RF effects—artifact and interference particularly ECG and pulse oximetry
    Gradient field effects
Potential patient safety hazards
    Leakage currents
    Heating and burns
    Magnetic components "missile effect"—secure ferro magnetic or battery-
        operated equipment

magnet. All wires should also be kept away from the patient's skin. It is useful for ECG leads to be braided together to minimize this potential of forming a loop *(31–33)*.

The currents in the monitoring equipment can also generate RF signals that can deteriorate the MRI image. Batteries are strongly ferromagnetic; therefore, battery-powered equipment must be firmly secured if it is near the MRI unit. Problems involved in monitoring patients in MRI can be classified into three basic types: Interaction of monitoring equipment with the MRI system; interaction of the MRI system with the monitoring equipment; and potential safety hazards (Table 5). To minimize the possibility of any of these problems, MRI-compatible equipment should be used. MRI compatible is defined as equipment which is able to be used in a MRI unit without causing any risk to the patient and without causing any problems to the MRI scan. MRI-safe equipment is equipment that is safe for the patient but may cause problems with scanning. Canale has published a magnetic resonance safety website, which can provide updated information regarding monitor compatibility and safety issues as well as references to available equipment *(34)*.

7.4. ICU Patients in MRI Units

The most difficult patients to sedate for procedures are probably those who are already critically ill and require monitoring devices for their care. Invasive monitoring catheters may make it easier to evaluate the effect sedative agents have on patients undergoing procedures; however, for patients in MRI units these monitoring catheters may cause additional concern. Pulmonary artery catheters have wires embedded in the catheter, which are connected to the thermistor tip to measure blood temperature. There is significant concern that these wires could cause harm by producing microshock to the heart, or even being heated to the point of melting as they coil through the heart *(35)*. It is therefore recommended that pulmonary artery catheters be withdrawn from patients who are undergoing MRI.

REFERENCES

1. Practice guidelines for sedation and analgesia by non-anesthesiologists. A report by the American Society of Anesthesiologists Task Force on Sedation and Analgesia by Non-Anesthesiologists. (1996) *Anesthesiology* **84(2)**, 459–471.
2. Website: American Society of Anesthesiologists standards for intraoperative monitoring. http://www.asahq.org/standards/homepage.
3. Website: American Society of Anesthesiologists standards for post anesthesia care unit monitoring. http://www.asahq.org/standards/homepage.
4. Website: American Society of Anesthesiologists guidelines for non-operating room anesthetizing locations. http://www.asahq.org/standards/homepage.
5. Eichorn, J. H., Cooper, J. B., Colen, D. J., Maier, W. R., Phillip, J. H., and Seman, R. G. (1986) Standards for patient monitoring during anesthesia at Harvard Medical School. *JAMA* **256**, 1017–1020.
6. Website: American Society of Anesthesiologists Continuum of Depth of Sedation. http://www.asahq.org/standards/homepage.
7. Malviya, S., Voepel-Lewis, T., Tait, A. R., Merkel, S., Tremper, K. K., and Naughton, N. (2002) Validity and Reliability of the University of Michigan Sedation Scale (UMSS) in children undergoing sedation for computerized tomography. *Br. J. Anaesth.* **88(2)**, 241–245.
8. Tremper, K. K., and Barker, S. J. (1989) Pulse Oximetry. *Anesthesiology* **70**, 98–108.
9. Tremper, K. K., and Barker, S. J. (1994) Monitoring of oxygen, in *Clinical Monitoring for Anesthesia and Critical Care*, 2nd ed. (Lake, C., ed.), W. B. Saunders Co., Philadelphia, PA, pp. 196–212.
10. Barker, S. J., and Tremper, K. K. (1987) The effect of carbon monoxide inhalation on pulse oximeter signal depiction. *Anesthesiology* **67**, 559–603.
11. Barker, S. J., Tremper, K. K., and Hyatt, J. (1989) Effects of methemoglobin anemia on pulse oximetry and mixed venous oximetry. *Anesthesiology* **70**, 112–117.
12. Anderson, S. T., Hajduczek, J., and Barker, S. J. (1988) Benzocaine-induced methemoglobinemia in an adult: accuracy of pulse oximetry with methemoglobinemia. *Anesth. Analg.* **67(11)**, 1099–1101.
13. Barker, S. J., and Shah, N. K. (1997) The effects of motion on the performance of pulse oximeters in volunteers (revised publication). *Anesthesiology* **86(1)**, 101–108.

14. Dumas, C., and Wahr, J. A. Tremper, K.K. (1996) Clinical evaluation of a prototype motion artifact resistant pulse oximeter in the recovery room. *Anesth. Analg.* **83(2),** 269–272.
15. Malviya, S., Reynolds, P. I., Voepel-Lewis, T., Siewert, M., Watson, D., Tait, A. R., et al. (2000) False alarms and sensitivity of conventional pulse oximetry versus the Masimo SET technology in the pediatric postanesthesia care unit. *Anesth. Analg.* **90(6),** 1336–40.
16. Davis, R. F. (1985) Clinical comparison of automated auscultatory and oscillometric and catheter transducer measurements of arterial pressure. *J. Clin. Monitoring* **1,** 114–120.
17. Breuner, J. M. R., Kernis, L. J., and Kusman, J. M. (1981) Comparison of direct and indirect methods of measuring arterial pressure, Part III. *Med. Instruments.* **15,** 183–190.
18. Stanley, T. E., and Reves, J. G. (1994) Cardiovascular monitoring, in *Anesthesia* 4th ed. (Miller, R, ed.), Churchill Livingston, New York, NY, pp. 1164–1165.
19. Young, P. G., and Gedes, L. A. (1987) The effect of cuff pressure deflation rate on accuracy in indirect measurement of blood pressure with auscultatory effort. *J. Clin. Monitoring.* **3,** 155–160.
20. Rapid interpretation of EKG. (1981) Dale Dubin, Cover Publishing Company, Tampa, FL.
21. Practical Electrocardiography, 7th ed. (1983) (Marriott, Henry, J. L., ed.), Williams & Wilkins, Baltimore/London.
22. Hillel, Z., and Thys, D. M. (2000) Electrocardiography, in *Anesthesia* 5th ed., Volume 1 (Miller, R. D., ed.), Churchill Livingston, Philadelphia, PA, pp. 1231–1254.
23. Griffin, R. N., and Kaplan, J. A. (1986) Comparison of ECG V_5, CS_5, CV_5 and II by computerized ST segment analysis (abstract). *Anesth. Analg.* 65S1.
24. London, N. J., Hollenberg, M., and Wong, N. G., et al. (1988) Intraoperative myocardial ischemia: localization by continuous 12 lead electrocardiography. *Anesthesiology* **69,** 232–238.
25. Gravenstein, J. S., Panlus, D. A., and Hayes, J. J. (1989) Capnography, in *Clinical Practice.* Butterworks.
26. Good, M. L., Gravenstein, N. (1993) Capnography, in *Anesthesia Equipment—Principles and Applications* (Ehrenwerth, J., and Eisenkraft, J. B., eds.), CV Mosby-Year Book, St. Louis, MO, pp. 237–248.
27. Hughes, C. W., and Bell, C. (1993) Anesthesia equipment in remote hospitals, in *Anesthesia Equipment—Principles and Applications* (Ehrenwerth, J., and Eisenkraft, J. B., eds.), CV Mosby Year Book, St. Louis, MO, pp. 565–587.
28. Peden, C. J. (1999) Monitoring patients during anesthesia for radiological procedures. *Curr. Opin. Anes.* **12,** 405–410.
29. Basheim, G., and Syrovy, G. (1991) Burns associated with pulse oximetry during magnetic resonance imaging. Anesthesiology (75), 382–383.
30. Shellock, F. G. (1998) MR imaging of metallic implants and materials: a compilation of the literature. *Am. J. Roentgenol.* **151,** 811–814.
31. Menon, D. K., Peden, C. J., Halls as, Sargentoni, J., et al. (1992) Magnetic resonance for anesthetists, Part I: physical principles, applications, safety aspects. *Anaesthesiology* **47,** 240–255.

32. Canal, E., and Shellock, F. G. (1992) Patient monitoring during clinical MR imaging. *Radiology* **85,** 623–629.

33. Keller, E. K., Casey, F. X., Engels, H., Lauder, E., et al. (1998) Accessory equipment considerations with respect to MRI compatibility. *J. Magn. Resonance Imaging* **8,** 12–18.

34. Website: Canale magnetic resonance safety web site. http://www.canal.arad. upmc.edu/mr-safety/.

35. Shellock, F. G., and Shellock, V. J. (1998) Cardiovascular catheters and accessories: ex vivo testing of ferromagnetism, heating, and artifacts associated with MRI. *J. Magn. Resonance Imaging* **8(6),** 1338–1342.

36. Tremper, K. K., and Barker, S. J. (1986) Pulse Oximetry and oxygen transport, in *Pulse Oximetry.* (Payne, J. P., Severinghaus, J. W., eds.), Springer-Verlag, Berlin, pp. 19–27.

37. Barker, S. J., and Tremper, K. K. (1987) Pulse oximetry: applications and limitations, in *Advances in Oxygen Monitoring,* (Barker, S. J., Tremper, K. K., eds.), *Int. Anesthesiology Clin.* **25,** 155–175.

38. Pologe, J. A. (1987) Pulse *Oximetry: Technical Aspects of Machine Design, International Anesthesiology Clinics, Advances in Oxygen Monitoring.* (Tremper, K. K., and Barker, S. J., eds.), Little, Brown and Company, pp. 142).

39. Mark, J. B., Slaughter, T. F., and Reves, J. G. (2000) Cardiovascular Monitoring, in *Anesthesia,* Fifth Edition, Volume 1, (Miller, R. D., ed.), Churchill Livingston, Philadelphia, PA, p. 1122, Figure 30–3.

40. Narang, J., and Thys, D. M. (1992) Electrocardiographic monitoring, in *Anesthesia Equipment: Principles and Applications.* (Ehrenwerth, J., and Eisenkraft, J. B., eds.), CV Mosby Year Book, St. Louis, pp. 284.

41. Thys, D. M., and Kaplan, J. A. (1987) *The ECG in Anesthesia and Critical Care,* Churchill Livingston, New York, NY.

9
Assessment of Sedation Depth

Lia H. Lowrie, MD and Jeffrey L. Blumer, MD, PhD

1. INTRODUCTION

Dosing of medications for sedation and analgesia has always been based on a clinical assessment of patient response. The proliferation of medications with specific hypnotic or analgesic effects and the continued development of diagnostic and therapeutic procedures requiring some degree of patient sedation and pain control have resulted in wide variations in management. Although toxicity and safety are easily monitored by trained clinicians using standard cardiopulmonary equipment, efficacy is more difficult to standardize. The desired "level" of sedation and analgesia depends on the psychological and physiological state of the patient and the procedure being performed, and varies during the procedure itself.

Ideally, to monitor sedation efficacy, the desired "level" of sedation and analgesia should be quantified in a manner that is easily reproduced from patient to patient, procedure to procedure, and clinician to clinician. A number of clinical scales exist that describe the apparent level of consciousness, degrees of patient responsiveness, and effectiveness of pain control. These scales depend on the hypothesis that sedation and anesthesia represent a linear continuum that can be conceptualized in graduated terms of "level" and "depth." More modern hypotheses separate anesthesia into a simultaneous and interconnected triad of i) level of consciousness and volitional response, ii) pain or stimulus response that may be in large part reflexic, and iii) muscle relaxation (1). Terms may then be interpreted as follows: "sedation" to imply alteration of the level of consciousness and volitional response, "analgesia" to indicate alteration of pain and stimulus response, and "anesthesia," a more global alteration of all three parts of the triad. For the purposes of this chapter, however, where applicable, the terms "sedation" or "anesthesia" will be used as described in the referenced citation. It is generally assumed that the "deeper levels" of sedation are associated with an increased risk of respiratory depression, loss of airway control, and hemodynamic

From: *Contemporary Clinical Neuroscience: Sedation and Analgesia for Diagnostic and Therapeutic Procedures*
Edited by: S. Malviya, N. N. Naughton, and K. K. Tremper © Humana Press Inc., Totowa, NJ

instability *(2,3)*. The ability to monitor the "level" of sedation may allow change in medication administration or increased vigilance for cardiopulmonary events during the procedure. Current clinical scales are imprecise and poorly sensitive or specific. Neurophysiologic monitoring using electroencephalographic variables or evoked potential responses may provide a rigorous and reproducible quantification of the state of anesthesia that may more clearly delineate the parts of the anesthesia triad and increase the sensitivity of sedation efficacy and safety monitoring.

2. CLINICAL EVALUATIVE TOOLS

Many approaches to measuring the pharmacodynamic response to sedatives and analgesics have been published. These rating systems have been variably applied to patients who are undergoing anesthesia for specific procedures, to evaluate speed and completeness of recovery after anesthesia, and during relatively long-term sedation in the intensive care unit (ICU). Although some have been carefully validated for a specific purpose, many have simply been applied in a given situation for which the system may or may not have been appropriately validated. Table 1 lists several published sedation scoring systems divided into categories that depend on the degree of patient participation and objectiveness of observer ratings. Scoring systems that depend on patient participation may not be convenient for clinical use during a procedure, and are affected by patient effort and learning the response over time. Observer ratings of sedation, particularly if not tested for interobserver variability, are affected by interobserver interpretation and bias. In attempts to overcome these inherent problems with clinical testing, some clinical tools combine observer-based ratings with physiologic variables that change during sedation and are presumably not open to observer interpretation *(4)*.

2.1. Patient Tasks

The digit symbol substitution test (DSST), which is frequently used in drug evaluation studies, particularly of benzodiazepines, requires the patient to match a number with a symbol from a code involving the numbers 1 through 9 matched to single symbols. The patient must also draw the symbol on the test paper. Scoring involves both the number of attempts and correct answers. Psychomotor impairment is effectively measured with DSST *(5)*. Choice reaction time (CRT), another common psychometric test, has been used to differentiate among hypnotic agents and reflects the sedating potential of a drug. A tight dose-effect curve may be obtained using CRT and several benzodiazepine dose levels *(6)*. These types of psychomet-

Table 1
Some Published Sedation Scoring Systems

Subjective observer rating

Visual analog scales
Steward
Ramsay
Harris
Modified Glasgow Coma Scale
Observer's Assessment of Alertness/Sedation Scale (OAA/S)
Cambridge
Bloomsbury
Cook/Newcastle
Neurobehavioral Assessment Scale (NAS)
Sedation-Agitation Scale (SAS)

Patient task performance

Digital symbol substitution test (DSST)
Choice reaction time (CRT)
Memory tests
Visual analog scales

Physiologic measures included

COMFORT
Nisbet and Norris
Heart rate variability
Esophageal sphincter contractility
PRST (Pressure, rate, sweat, tearing)

ric tests, although well-validated, have not been applied frequently in clinical situations involving anesthesia or sedation for procedures. During periods of heavy sedation, the patient cannot participate enough to produce results, and patient activity at other times may interfere with the completion of the procedure or study.

Many studies have used visual analog scales (VAS) completed by the patient at various points during anesthetic administration and the procedure *(7)*. These scales are usually 10-cm lines capped at each end by a statement intended to reflect the extremes of the effect measured. The distance measured from the negative end of the scale to the point marked by the patient is the "score" recorded. For instance, Smith used VAS labeled "wide awake" and "almost asleep" during a study of the sedative effects of propofol *(8)*.

The patient is asked to indicate the point on the line that correlates with his or her current state. VAS have shown remarkable consistency in the comparison of scores simultaneously assessed by the patient and an independent observer *(9)*. Simple recall of several objects or words over time, or the ability to acquire memory, is another psychometric technique that has been used as a measure of anesthesia during procedures *(10)*. However, eliciting implicit or explicit memory following a sedation or anesthetic event after the fact does little to monitor the depth of sedation or anesthesia during the procedure.

Problems with these types of psychometric tests include the effects of patient learning and effort, group comparison effects, and probably even the time of day performed *(11)*. Psychomotor function will improve over time as the patient repeatedly performs the same task (practice). This effect can be lessened in drug evaluation studies by designing the placebo score as the maximum possible score, but clinical sedation studies rarely utilize placebo. The degree of effort the patient uses to complete the task will affect the results. It is difficult to separate effort from drug effects during sedation. Finally, particular task performance will vary by patient type. Both the elderly and children will have different psychomotor performance than healthy adults. The effects of chronic illness are poorly understood. It is possible to use psychometric scoring to compare group data if the individual's score is expressed as a change from baseline ability.

2.2. Observer Ratings

VAS are also used by clinicians to rate the level of sedation and have been used to assess inter-rater validity for new anesthetic techniques *(12)*. The end caps of the scale can be more inclusive when someone other than the patient is rating sedation, as degrees of unresponsiveness can be included. When VAS are used to evalutate a single patient over time by many clinicians, the raters must be careful to ensure that they are rating the same variable. Pain, agitation, and degree of sedation may be confused.

When reporting the use of a particular sedative regimen during mechanical ventilation in an ICU in 1974, Ramsay used the sedation ratings shown in Table 2 *(13)*. This scoring system has been used extensively in ICUs and in the recovery room during anesthesia emergence. As the need for precise monitoring of the efficacy of sedatives and anesthetics has grown, scrutiny of the Ramsay scale as an assessment tool has escalated *(14)*. The Ramsay scale will provide a numerical label for a subjective assessment of a level of sedation. As such, it may be useful as a tool for inter-personnel discussions of patient status. However, even for this use the scale is not precise, particularly for critically ill patients. It is frequently criticized for having only one

Table 2
The Ramsay Score[a]

1. Patient anxious and agitated or restless or both
2. Patient cooperative, oriented, and tranquil
3. Patient responds to commands only
4. Brisk response to light glabellar tap or loud auditory stimulus
5. Sluggish response to light glabellar tap or loud auditory stimulus
6. No response to light glabellar tap or loud auditory stimulus

[a]Adapted from ref. *(13)*.

level of agitation assessment *(15)*. The six levels of sedation are not mutually exclusive. Patients may be agitated and restless (Level 1), but not awake at the same time they are responsive to light glabellar tap (Level 5). The rater using the scale may not provide an identical stimulus in the "light" glabellar tap or "loud" auditory stimulus as previously applied or applied by another rater. Interpretation of "brisk" or "sluggish" adds bias to the scale. Table 3 lists several other published scores similar to the Ramsay score in the use of a numerical value attached to a semisubjective rater assessment of the patient at that moment. Varying degrees of rater/patient interaction are required. Scores reported by Cohen, Cambridge, and Newcastle are all specific to patients supported with mechanical ventilation *(16)*.

The Sedation-Agitation Scale (SAS) (Table 4) was developed to describe the patient's state of agitation and sedation during a study of haloperidol use in an adult ICU *(17)*. A later paper reported the reliability and validity of a revised SAS for patients in ICUs *(18)*. It showed acceptable interrater reliability and for ICU use, it has the advantage of including several degrees of agitation. Despite the perceived benefit in critically ill patients of multiple levels of agitation assessment (Levels 5–7), it is interesting to note that in actual usage, patients were only scored using Levels 1–5 *(19)*. It was validated against the two unvalidated but commonly used Ramsay and Harris Scales *(20)* (Table 5) and has since been correlated with bispectral index (BIS) monitoring in ICU patients *(19)*.

The Observer's Assessment of Alertness/Sedation Scale (OAA/S Scale) (Table 6) was developed to assess the ability of a benzodiazepine antagonist to reverse sedation. It was tested for reliability and validity against VAS, DSST, and Serial Sevens Subtraction Test *(21)*. It has been used to assess the level of sedation achieved with propofol in adult patients *(22)*, and to assess sedation efficacy in a double-blind, placebo-controlled protocol using an opioid and a benzodiazepine during elective biopsy procedures *(23)*. As

Table 3
Sedation Scales

Cohen sedation score[a]

0 Asleep, no response to tracheal
   suction
1 Arousable, coughs with tracheal
   suction
2 Awake, spontaneously coughs or
   triggers ventilator
3 Actively breathes against ventilator
4 Unmanageable

Bloomsbury sedation score[a]

3 Agitated and restless
2 Awake and uncomfortable
1 Aware but calm
0 Roused by voice, remains calm
−1 Roused by movement or suction
−2 Roused by painful stimuli
−3 Unarousable
A Natural sleep

Cambridge sedation score[a]

1 Agitated
2 Awake
3 Roused by voice
4 Roused by tracheal suction
5 Unarousable
6 Paralyzed
7 Asleep

*Simplified post-anesthesia recovery
score[a]*

Consciousness
2 Awake
1 Responding to stimuli
0 Not responding

Airway
2 Coughing on command or crying
1 Maintaining good airway
0 Airway requires maintenance

Movement
2 Moving limbs purposefully
1 Non-purposeful movements
0 Not moving

[a]Adapted from refs. *(16,69).*

with the Ramsay Scale, inadequately sedated or agitated, uncooperative patients are not well-assessed with the OAA/S Scale.

Chernik then developed the Neurobehavioral Assessment Scale (NAS) specifically to evaluate patients across the full range of behavioral functioning. The NAS was tested for interrater reliability and evaluated against two scores believed to be most effective at the extreme ends of the range of neurobehavior, the Glascow Coma Score (GCS) and DSST *(24).* The NAS was tested during induction of anesthesia before a surgical procedure. The GCS is believed to rate more unresponsive or comatose patients well. However, it correlated poorly with NAS in lightly sedated patients. On the other hand, the DSST that requires a fair degree of alertness showed good correlation with NAS. Therefore, Chernik concluded that NAS is an effective scale,

Table 4
The Sedation-Agitation Scale[a]

7 Dangerous agitation	Pulling an ET tube, trying to remove catheters, climbing over bed rail, striking at staff, thrashing side-to-side
6 Very agitated	Does not calm despite frequent verbal reminding of limits; requires physical restraints, biting ET tube
5 Agitated	Anxious or mildly agitated, attempting to sit up, calms down to verbal instructions
4 Calm and cooperative	Calm, awakens easily, follows commands
3 Sedated	Difficult to arouse, awakens to verbal stimuli or gentle shaking but drifts off again, follows simple commands
2 Very sedated	Arouses to physical stimuli but does not communicate or follow commands, may move spontaneously
1 Unarousable	Minimal or no response to noxious stimuli, does not communicate or follow commands

[a]Adapted from ref. *(17)*.

Table 5
Harris Scale[a]

A. General condition

1. Confused and uncontrollable
2. Anxious and agitated
3. Conscious, oriented, and calm
4. Asleep but arousable to speech, obeys commands
5. Asleep but responds to loud auditory stimulus or sternal pressure
6. Unarousable

B. Compliance with mechanical ventilation

1. Unable to control ventilation
2. Distressed, fighting ventilator
3. Coughing when moved but tolerating ventilation for most of the time
4. Tolerating movement

C. Response to endotracheal suctioning

1. Agitation, distress, prolonged coughing
2. Coughs, distressed, rapid recovery
3. Coughs, not distressed
4. No cough

[a]Adapted from ref. *(20)*.

Table 6
The Observer's Assessment of Alertness/Sedation Scale[a]

Responsiveness	Speech	Facial expression	Eyes	Composite score level
Responds readily to name spoken in normal tone	Normal	Normal	Clear No ptosis	5 (Alert)
Lethargic response to name spoken in normal tone	Mild slowing or thickening	Mild relaxation	Glazed or mild ptosis (<half the eye)	4
Responds only after name is called loudly and/or repeatedly	Slurring or prominent slowing	Marked relaxation (Slack jaw)	Glazed and marked ptosis (>half the eye)	3
Responds only after mild prodding or shaking	Few recognizable words	—	—	2
Does not respond	—	—	—	1 (Deep sleep)

[a]Adapted from ref. (21).

226

Table 7
Glasgow Coma Score[a]

Activity	Best response	Score
Eye opening	Spontaneous	4
	To verbal stimuli	3
	To pain	2
	None	1
Verbal	Oriented	5
	Confused	4
	Inappropriate words	3
	Nonspecific sounds	2
	None	1
Motor	Follows commands	6
	Localizes pain	5
	Withdraws in response to pain	4
	Flexion in response to pain	3
	Extension in response to pain	2
	None	1

[a]Adapted from ref. *(26)*.

particularly at more alert ranges of sedation. The scale scores an interview process with specific questions on the orientation to person, place, and time, and includes asking the patient to repeat a sentence to enable the rater to judge the quality of speech. The rater must also judge 4–5 levels of alertness, disorientation, speech articulation, and psychomotor retardation.

The GCS has been used to assess sedation efficacy *(25)* and as a validation tool for new sedation scales as noted previously. The original GCS was a nonvalidated scale intended to allow interrater reliability in the assessment of coma without extensive staff training *(26)*. Subsequently, predictions of severity of outcome after head trauma have been linked to GCS scores on presentation *(27)*. It is a scale of three parts: motor response, verbal response and eye opening (Table 7). Various scales have been denoted the "modified" Glasgow Coma Scale and have been used in different settings to rate the efficacy of a particular drug combination for sedation in mechanically ventilated patients in the ICU by omitting the verbal section *(28)*. It is doubtful that "levels" of coma and sedation are synonymous enough to make this a valid technique.

Techniques that require an observer to rate a patient characteristic or degree of response to an applied stimulus are all subject to variability in observer skill, experience, and judgment. Although training and interobserver validity testing make these types of scoring systems more accurate, precise application of these scores to the clinical situation for which they were intended is even more necessary. Sedation and analgesia in the intubated patient over time in the ICU is a very different process than short-term sedation and analgesia or anesthesia of the same patient undergoing a procedure. Sedation in the ICU is necessary not only to allow patient tolerance of prolonged immobilization and invasive monitoring devices, but also to possibly prevent and certainly alleviate "ICU stress delirium" believed by many to be an indication of cerebral failure *(15)*. Regulation of sleep cycles and a "semi-alert" but calm state of being are now believed to be most beneficial in ICU patients as opposed to the coma deemed desirable in earlier years of ICU medicine *(29)*. Sedation and analgesia for short procedures encompass only the goals of patient comfort, ability to complete the procedure, and possibly amnesia. With expectant cardiopulmonary management, during short nonoperative procedures, it is unclear that there is a meaningful difference between deeper levels of sedation rated by an observer rating score developed for ICU patients (SAS, for instance) when patients arouse to physical stimuli and move spontaneously (SAS Level 2) or are calm and awaken easily, following commands (SAS Level 4) but allow the procedure to occur. It is generally believed that deeper levels of sedation predict longer recovery time but newer short-acting anesthetics have facilitated early recovery to a large extent *(30)*.

It is recommended that observer rating scales be used only in the population and clinical situation for which they are validated. Furthermore, pain vs anxious agitation, and sleepiness vs unconsciousness are not easily distinguished by assigning a score to one specific patient characteristic or response. Inappropriate medications may be used when the cause of the patient response is not understood. For instance, large doses of potent anxiolytics may be used inappropriately to "sedate" a somnolent or confused patient who is agitated because of pain. Separate quantitative scales of pain, somnolence, and anxiety more in keeping with the modern hypotheses of an anesthesia "triad" may be necessary to appropriately manage the variety of sedatives and analgesics available today *(7)*.

2.3. Physiologic Variables

Sedation assessment methods that use physiologic responses to stimulus or medication are usually viewed as more objective than the observer ratings described here. Anesthesiologists have long described the hemodynamic changes that occur during varying levels of general anesthesia *(4)*.

Table 8
PRST Scale[a]

Systolic blood pressure (mmHg)	< Control + 15	0
	> Control + 15	1
	> Control + 30	2
Heart rate (beats/min)	< Control + 15	0
	> Control + 15	1
	> Control + 30	2
Sweating	Nil	0
	Skin moist to touch	1
	Visible beads of sweat	2
Tears	No excess of tears in open eyes	0
	Excess of tears in open eyes	1
	Tear overflow from closed eyes	2

[a]Adapted from ref. *(4)*.

For instance, Table 8 shows a simple means of evaluating the level of anesthesia using change in blood pressure and heart rate from baseline, degree of sweating and tearing referred to as PRST. Utility may be limited in the presence of hemodynamically active medications or underlying disease that directly affects vital signs *(31)*. Nisbet developed a scoring system that incorporated physiologic changes for preoperative and intra-operative use *(32)* (Table 9). A score of 0–4 correlated with "poor" sedation, 5–6 "fair" and 7–10 "good" sedation. He attempted to validate this scoring system against an observer's subjective assessment of sedation (drowsy, wide awake, anxious). However, the statistical analysis used was incomplete.

The COMFORT score was developed and validated against observer VAS ratings for use in assessing sedation in mechanically ventilated children *(33,34)* (Table 10). A score between 17 and 26 was considered indicative of optimal sedation in ventilated patients in the unit in which it was developed. The 2-min observation period for accurate score reporting has contributed to the concern that the score is too complex for routine use, adding to the ICU nursing workload *(29)*. The COMFORT score has not been validated in adults or during procedures, where the level of stimulus may change quickly and frequently.

Another physiologic variable that has been studied in the context of depth of anesthesia is lower esophageal sphincter contractility, which is increased by physiologic stress *(35)*. Deepening levels of anesthesia lowers esophageal contractility. The correlation between sphincter contractility and clinical signs of deep anesthesia was at first believed to be quite strong *(36)*.

Table 9
A Scoring System for Objective Measurement of Sedation[a]

A.	Subjective state in operating room	
	Apprehensive	0
	Fully awake	1
	Drowsy	2
B.	Change in state after premedication	
	Apparent improvement, change in state 1–2 or 2–3	2
	No change	1
	Apparent deterioration change in state 2–1	0
C.	Change after premedication	
	Fall in blood pressure >10 mmHg	2
	No change	1
	Rise in blood pressure >10 mmHg	0
	Fall in heart rate >10/min	2
	No change	1
	Rise in heart rate >10/min	0
D.	After stimulation	
	Rise in blood pressure >10 mmHg	0
	No change	1
	Rise in heart rate >10/min	0

[a]Adapted from ref. (32).

Table 10
The COMFORT Scale[a]

ALERTNESS	
Deeply asleep	1
Lightly asleep	2
Drowsy	3
Fully awake and alert	4
Hyper-alert	5

CALMNESS/AGITATION	
Calm	1
Slightly anxious	2
Anxious	3
Very anxious	4
Panicky	5

(continued)

Table 10 (cont.)

RESPIRATORY RESPONSE	
No coughing and no spontaneous respiration	1
Spontaneous respiration with little or no response to ventilation	2
Occasional cough or resistance to ventilator	3
Actively breathes against ventilator or coughs regularly	4
Fights ventilator; coughing or choking	5

PHYSICAL MOVEMENT	
No movement	1
Occasional, slight movement	2
Frequent, slight movement	3
Vigorous movement limited to extremities	4
Vigorous movements including torso and head	5

BLOOD PRESSURE (MAP) BASELINE	
Blood pressure below baseline	1
Blood pressure consistently at baseline	2
Infrequent elevations (1–3) of ≥15%	3
Frequent elevations (>3) of ≥15%	4
Sustained elevation ≥ 15%	5

HEART RATE BASELINE	
Heart rate below baseline	1
Heart rate consistently at baseline	2
Infrequent elevations (1–3) of ≥15% above baseline during observation period	3
Frequent elevations (>3) of ≥15% above baseline	4
Sustained elevation of ≥ 15%	5

MUSCLE TONE	
Muscles totally relaxed, no muscle tone	1
Reduced muscle tone	2
Normal muscle tone	3
Increased muscle tone and flexion of fingers and toes	4
Extreme muscle rigidity and flexion of fingers and toes	5

FACIAL TENSION	
Facial muscles totally relaxed	1
Facial muscle tone normal, no facial muscle tension evident	2
Tension evident in some facial muscles	3
Tension evident throughout facial muscles	4
Facial muscles contorted and grimacing	5

[a]Adapted from ref. *(34).*

However, further study has shown wide interpatient and interagent variability *(37,38)*, and that atropine ablates the ability to monitor change in esophageal contractility *(39)*. The value of this modality as a measure of depth of anesthesia is therefore questionable.

Reduction of heart rate variation has been shown with induction of anesthesia and increased variation is seen with recovery *(40)*. Recent development of computer real time analysis of heart-rate variation may provide an objective physiologic index of depth of anesthesia. Stimulation with chest physiotherapy of sedated and paralyzed ICU patients produced marked increases in respiratory sinus arrhythmia without significant changes in electrocardiogram (ECG) R-R interval *(41)*. Commercially available analyzing equipment was used to correlate beat-to-beat variability of heart rate and Ramsay scores in 20 mechanically ventilated ICU patients during awakening from midazolam sedation *(42)*. Prediction of Ramsay score was poor. Perhaps the use of hemodynamically active medications or co-existing disease that may have altered heart rate variability confounded the ability to assess anesthesia effects alone with this tool. On the other hand, the Ramsay score may simply be too insensitive to correlate well with this type of index.

Although physiologic methods of assessment of sedation efficacy are desirable in terms of objectivity, these techniques have not been used to assess patients at "lighter" levels of sedation during short procedures, not involving muscle relaxation or neuromuscular blockade. Their ability to discriminate effectively between levels of sedation remains inconclusive.

3. NEUROPHYSIOLOGIC MONITORING

3.1. Modalities

Clinical monitoring tools are in general poor predictors of patient awareness of sensations, experiences, and pain in the operating room. Use of neuromuscular blockade in the ICU renders most nonphysiologic clinical tools useless. Once the patient exhibits a change in physiology (heart rate or blood pressure increase) or response to stimulus (movement or follows a command), awareness may have already occurred. The technique of isolating an arm from the effects of neuromuscular blockade with a tourniquet has demonstrated response to commands during a variety of anesthetic regimens and poor correlation with clinical assessments of the "depth" of anesthesia *(44)*. The incidence of awareness during anesthesia averages 0.25–1%, but may be as high as 43% in certain populations *(1)*. Particularly during the use of neuromuscular blockade, the electroencephalogram (EEG) as an indicator of brain function may offer more precise measurement of the individual's response to sedation and analgesia.

The EEG is a plot of voltage of the electrical activity of the cerebral cortex against time. The resulting waveforms are traditionally interpreted on the basis of amplitude, frequency, and location of origin and pattern recognition. All medications used for anesthesia alter the EEG and many, with increasing drug concentration, will eventually produce burst suppression. The burst suppression pattern is closely associated with unconsciousness, but is not usually considered a desirable level of even general anesthesia, as patients may become hemodynamically unstable and recover slowly. The changes exhibited in frequency, amplitude, and EEG pattern during dose escalation are both drug- and patient-specific *(44)*. The traditionally formatted EEG is a complex, cumbersome record that requires a high level of training and attention for accurate interpretation. Standardization, reproducibility, and electrical interference in the operating room or ICU are also problematic.

Computer analysis of EEG raw data has been developed to overcome some of the difficulties inherent to EEG interpretation. The cerebral function monitor (CFM) is an early simple example of processed EEG information, which used a single EEG channel and integrated EEG frequency and amplitude to produce a single tracing. This system was further modified to produce the cerebral function analyzing monitor (CFAM) that used two EEG channels and analyzed different frequency bands along with amplitude to produce a trend over time *(45)*. Although developed for use in the ICU, impairment of cerebral function by changes in perfusion or oxygenation blunts the CFAM tracing, and deep sedation cannot be differentiated from general anesthesia (unconsciousness) *(9,31)*. Other methods of EEG processing are considered superior techniques.

Fast Fourier transformation can be performed in real time for several EEG channels by microprocessors. Power spectrum analysis involves Fourier analysis of an epoch of EEG raw waveform defined by amplitude, frequency, and phase angle, and resolved into a set of sinusoids that when added together equal the original EEG complex. This information may be displayed as a compressed spectral array that is a histogram of power (amplitude^2) vs frequency or as a density spectral array, where a color change represents power for each frequency. Compressed spectral array and density spectral array are essentially very compact displays of an EEG, yet they require a good deal of training and judgment by the practitioner for correct interpretation.

Numerical parameters have been derived from statistical analysis of the power spectrum to simplify pattern recognition. The epoch of EEG signal is assumed to be stationary or linear, and its variables normally distributed. Commonly derived variables include the peak power frequency or the frequency with the highest power in the epoch, median power frequency or the frequency that divides the power spectrum in two halves, and spectral edge frequency defined by the frequency below which 95% of the power is located.

Power spectrum analysis also assumes that frequency bands of the EEG are independent variables. Because the EEG is not completely stationary and there are interrelationships between frequency components (phase coupling where the phase of one component depends on the phase angle of other components), power spectrum analysis may analyze two complex waveforms with different phase structures as identical. Bispectral analysis allows for the influence of these nonlinear interrelationships, and can produce a multivariate index single number called the bispectral index (BIS). A commercially available algorithm provides a BIS score. It is important to understand that this algorithm was derived from analyzing a large database of EEGs from patients receiving hypnotic agents that were intended to produce degrees of lack of awareness and recall (unconsciousness) *(46,47)*. The interaction of analgesia in BIS (reduction in pain perception manifested by decreased autonomic responses to noxious stimuli) is unclear *(48)*. Bispectral analysis is a classic form of EEG interpretation. A complete discussion of EEG signal processing including a detailed description of BIS specific to anesthesia has recently been published *(49)*.

The electrophysiologic response to external sensory stimuli—auditory, peripheral nerve stimulation, visual—is represented by evoked potentials. Anesthetics produce dose- and agent-specific changes in the amplitudes and latencies of evoked potential waveforms. Some authors believe that evoked responses may be able to differentiate the analgesic and hypnotic effects of a variety of medications *(50,51)*. Somatosensory-evoked potentials (SSEP) have been used most often as a monitor of neurologic function during procedures involving spinal cord manipulation, and the cortically generated SSEP amplitude is suppressed with analgesics but not some hypnotics *(52)*. Auditory-evoked potentials (AEP) have been best characterized in relationship to sedation *(53)*. The AEP tracing is produced by delivering specific clicks or tones through earphones. The resulting scalp signal is processed to cancel out background EEG signal, and a representative waveform is produced. Early AEP generated from the brainstem are not affected by anesthetics. The late AEP that arise from the frontal cortex vary from individual to individual and are quite dependent on the degree of attention and alertness. The midlatency AEP represent noncognitive cortical processing of the auditory signal, are highly reproducible from patient to patient, and correlate closely with consciousness and implicit memory during anesthesia. Some training is needed for interpretation of waveform changes unless the latencies and amplitudes are indexed. Evoked potential monitoring is also technically difficult in the electrically active environment of the operating room and ICU, making this technique in its currently available mode less attractive than processed EEG techniques for general use *(54)*.

3.2. Clinical Comparisons

Many systems have been designed to titrate anesthetic medications to target serum drug concentrations or mean alveolar concentrations of inhaled gases that have been shown to produce the desired level of anesthesia *(55)*. In a study designed to evaluate the relationship of BIS to measured drug concentration and clinically assigned levels of sedation, 72 volunteers were given isoflurane, propofol, midazolam, or alfentanil in a dose-ranging manner to achieve target concentrations *(56)*. Compared to an OAA/S score of 2 or less (defined as unconsciousness in this study), BIS correlated better than propofol concentration and equally well with midazolam and isoflurane concentrations. Ninety-five percent of participants were unconscious, with a BIS of 50. Target-controlled infusion of propofol was also used with and without the addition of narcotic in a volunteer study assessing BIS, OAA/S, and memory function *(57)*. BIS correlated better than drug concentration with OAA/S. These investigators noted that the increase in BIS induced with painful stimulus was blunted in the presence of alfentanil, lending support to use of BIS as a monitor of depth of consciousness and not of pain response. The use of BIS monitoring and target-controlled infusion technology may facilitate more closely controlled drug delivery and consistent sedation levels *(58,59)*.

Theoretically, because BIS considers phase coupling and the nonlinear nature of the EEG, it should describe anesthesia-induced changes in the EEG better than power spectrum analysis. Studies directly comparing the correlation of BIS, 95% spectral-edge frequency (SEF), and median frequency (MF) with OAA/S during sedation with midazolam or propofol show much better correlation between BIS and clinical scores during induction and recovery *(60,61)*. Similar comparisons of BIS, power spectrum indices, and AEP have shown very poor specificity and sensitivity of 95% spectral edge and median frequency in predicting unconsciousness, whereas AEP was somewhat better than BIS *(62–64)*.

Retrospective group correlation of one monitor with another monitor may indicate improved sensitivity and specificity. Monitors of anesthesia are potentially most helpful if they can predict patient response. In a study that compared BIS, AEP, 95% SEF and median frequency, Doi used target-controlled infusions of propofol and alfentanil and evaluated movement at laryngeal mask insertion *(65)*. Although all patients had loss of eyelash reflex confirming unconsciousness before attempted insertion, only the AEP index 30 s before insertion discriminated between movers and non-movers. However, Kochs could not demonstrate good prediction of movement response to skin incision during isoflurane anesthesia using AEP *(66)*. Similar findings were reported in 1998 during sevoflurane anesthesia *(67)*. BIS, SEF, MF, and OAA/S did not predict movement at skin incision.

BIS represents the most accurate neurophysiologic monitor currently available for monitoring of anesthesia level. Although it may not completely accurately predict response to painful stimulus (incision) or deep reflexic response (laryngeal stimulus), it may allow more tightly controlled anesthesia delivery, resulting in a shorter recovery time. Higher BIS scores at the end of clinically controlled anesthesia with propofol and desflurane predicted fast-track eligibility in outpatient tubal ligation patients *(30)*. In a randomized, multi-institutional study comparing standard practice during propofol-alfentanil-nitrous oxide anesthesia to standard practice plus BIS targeting of propofol infusions, anesthesiologists attempted to achieve the fastest possible recovery times *(68)*. The intra-operative course was similar between the two groups; however, the propofol infusion rate was reduced (134 and 116 ug/kg/min), extubation occurred sooner (11 and 7 min), more patients were oriented on arrival in the recovery room (43% and 23%) and eligibility for discharge was earlier (38 and 32 min) in the group that received BIS monitoring.

4. CONCLUSION

The ideal monitor of sedation and analgesia will need to differentiate level of consciousness and pain. It must be easily used across many patient types and during a variety of procedures, and be easily understood by a variety of clinical practitioners. It should be predictive of response to stimuli, not simply an alarm to indicate a threshold has been reached. It must be equally able to monitor patients who are in the process of becoming conscious and those who may be slowly reaching undesirable levels of unconsciousness. Current clinical scoring systems certainly do not provide this degree of accuracy or flexibility. The BIS and indexed AEP represent the currently available technology useful for patients receiving neuromuscular blockade who are most likely to experience undetected awareness during ICU sedation and anesthesia and for producing very tightly controlled levels of effective and uniform anesthesia. Whether BIS and AEP are useful for targeting sedation (implying a higher level of consciousness than anesthesia) remains to be demonstrated. Further work must be done to apply BIS and AEP to children, specific anesthetic regimens, and critically ill patients whose disease process may affect cerebral blood flow and function.

REFERENCES

1. Glass, P. S. A. (1999) Why and how we will monitor the state of anesthesia in 2010? *Acta Anaesthesiol. Belg.* **50,** 35–44.
2. American Academy of Pediatrics, Committee on Drugs. (1992) Guidelines for monitoring and management of pediatric patients during and after sedation for diagnostic and therapeutic procedures. *Pediatrics* **89,** 1110–1115.
3. American Society of Anesthesiologists Task Force on Sedation and Analgesia by Non-Anesthesiologists. (1996) Practice guidelines for sedation and analgesia by non-anesthesiologists. *Anesthesiology* **84,** 459–471.
4. Wang, D. Y. (1993) Assessment of sedation in the ICU. Intensive Care World **10,** 193–196.
5. Johnson, L. C. and Chernik, D. A. (1982) Sedative-hypnotics and human performance. *Psychopharmacology* **76,** 101–113.
6. Hindmarch, I. (1994) Instrumental assessment of psychomotor functions and the effects of psychotropic drugs. *Acta Psychiatr. Scand.* **(89 Suppl) 380,** 49–52.
7. Wansbrough, S. R. and White, P. F. (1993) Sedation scales: Measures of calmness or somnolence? *Anesth. Analg.* **76,** 219–221.
8. Smith, I., Monk, T. G., White, P. F., and Ding, Y. (1994) Propofol infusion during regional anesthesia: sedative, amnestic, and anxiolytic properties. *Anesth. Analg.* **79,** 313–319.
9. Avramov, M. N. and White, P. F. (1995) Methods for monitoring the level of sedation. *Crit. Care Clin.* **11,** 803–826.
10. Bailey, A. R. and Jones, J. G. (1997) Patients' memories of events during general anaesthesia. *Anaesthesia* **52,** 460–476.
11. Laurijssen, B. E. and Greenblatt, D. J. (1996) Pharmacokinetic-pharmacodynamic relationships for benzodiazepines. *Clin. Pharmacokinet.* **1,** 52–76.
12. Wehrmann, T., Kokabpick, S., Lembcke, B., Caspary, W. F., and Seifert, H. (1999) Efficacy and safety of intravenous propofol sedation during routine ERCP: a prospective, controlled study. *Gastrointest. Endosc.* **49,** 677–683.
13. Ramsay, M. A. E., Savege, T. M., Simpson, B. R. J., and Goodwin, R. (1974) Controlled sedation with alphaxalone-alphadolone. *Br. Med. J.* **2,** 656–659.
14. Hansen-Flaschen, J., Cowen, J., and Polomano, R. C. (1994) Beyond the Ramsay scale: need for a validated measure of sedating drug efficacy in the intensive care unit. *CCM* **22,** 732–733.
15. Crippen, D. W. (1994) Neurologic monitoring in the intensive care unit. *New Horizons* **2,** 107–120.
16. Schulte-Tamburen, A. M., Schier, J., Briegel, J., Schwender, D., and Peter, K. (1999) Comparison of five sedation scoring systems by means of auditory evoked potentials. *Intensive Care Med.* **25,** 377–382.
17. Riker, R. R., Fraser, G., and Cox, P. M. (1994) Continuous infusion haloperidol controls agitation in critically ill patients. *Crit. Care Med.* **22,** 433–440.
18. Riker, R. R., Picard, J. T., and Fraser, G. L. (1999) Prospective evaluation of the sedation-agitation scale for adult critically ill patients. *Crit. Care Med.* **27,** 1325–1329.

19. Simmons, L. E., Riker, R. R., Prato, S., and Fraser, G. L. (1999) Assessing sedation during intensive care unit mechanical ventilation with the bispectral index and the sedation-agitation scale. *Crit. Care Med.* **27,** 1499–1504.

20. Harris, C. E., O'Donnell, C., Macmillan, R., et al. (1991) Use of propofol by infusion for sedation of patients undergoing haemofiltration—Assessment of the effect of haemofiltration on the level of sedation and on blood propofol concentration. *J. Drug Dev.* **4(Suppl 3),** 37–39.

21. Chernik, D. A., Gillings, D., Laine, H., Hendler, J., Silver, J. M., Davidson, A. B., et al. (1990) Validity and reliability of the observer's assessment of alertness/sedation scale: Study with intravenous midazolam. *J. Clin. Psychopharmacol.* **10,** 244–251.

22. Casati, A., Fanelli, G., Casaletti, E., Colnaghi, E., Cedrati, V., and Torri, G. (1999) Clinical assessment of target-controlled infusion of propofol during monitored anesthesia care. *Can. J. Anesth.* **46,** 235–239.

23. Avramov, M. N., Smith, I., and White, P. F. (1996) Interactions between midazolam and remifentanil during monitored anesthesia care. *Anesthesiology* **85,** 1283–1289.

24. Chernik, D. A., Tucker, M., Gigli, B., Yoo, K., Paul, K., Laine, H., et al. (1992) Validity and reliability of the neurobehavioral assessment scale. *J. Clin. Psychopharmacol.* **12,** 43–48.

25. Lerman, B., Yoshida, D., and Levitt, M. A. (1996) A prospective evaluation of the safety and efficacy of methohexital in the emergency department. *Am. J. Emerg. Med.* **14,** 351–354.

26. Teasdale, G. and Jennett, B. (1974) Assessment of coma and impaired consciousness: a practical scale. *Lancet* July **13,** 81–84.

27. Alvarez, M., Nava, J. M., Rue, M., and Quintana, S. (1998) Mortality prediction in head trauma patients: Performance of Glasgow coma score and several severity systems. *Crit. Care Med.* **26,** 142–148.

28. Edbrooke, D. L., Newby, D. M., Mather, S. J., Dixon, A. M., and Hebron, B. S. (1982) Safer sedation for ventilated patients. A new application for etomidate. *Anaesthesia* **37,** 765–771.

29. Lowson, S. M. and Sawh, S. (1999) Adjuncts to analgesia. *Crit. Care Clin.* **15,** 119–141.

30. Song, D., van Vlymen, J., and White, P. F. (1998) Is the bispectral index useful in predicting fast-track eligibility after ambulatory anesthesia with propofol and desflurane? *Anesth. Analg.* **87,** 1245–1248.

31. Habibi, S. and Coursin, D. B. (1996) Assessment of sedation, analgesia, and neuromuscular blockade in the perioperative period. *Int. Anesth. Clinics* **34,** 215–241.

32. Nisbet, H. L. A. and Norris, W. (1963) Objective measurement of sedation II: A simple scoring system. *Br. J. Anaesth.* **35,** 618–623.

33. Ambuel, B., Hamlett, K. W., Marx, C. M., and Blumer, J. L. (1992) Assessing distress in pediatric intensive care environments: The COMFORT scale. *J. Pediatr. Psychol.* **17,** 95–109.

34. Marx, C. M., Smith, P. G., Lowrie, L. H., Hamlett, K. W., Ambuel, B., Yamashita, T. S., and Blumer, J. L. (1994) Optimal sedation of mechanically ventilated pediatric critical care patients. *CCM* **22**, 163–170.
35. Faulkner, W. B. (1940) Objective oesophageal changes due to psychic factors. *American Journal of Medical Science* **200**, 796–803.
36. Evans, J. M., Bithell, J. F., and Vlachonikolis, I. G. (1987) Relationship between lower oesophageal contractility, clinical signs and halothane concentration during general anesthesia and surgery in man. *Br. J. Anaesth.* **59**, 1346–1355.
37. Isaac, P. A. and Rosen, M. (1990) Lower oesophageal contractility and detection of awareness during anaesthesia. *Br. J. Anaesth.* **65**, 319–324.
38. Cox, P. N. and White, D. C. (1986) Do oesophageal contractions measure "depth" of anaesthesia? *Br. J. Anaesth.* **58**, 131P-132P.
39. Aitkenhead, A. R., Lin, E. S., and Thomas, D. (1987) Relationship between lower esophageal contractility and clinical signs of light anaesthesia. *Anesthesiology* **67**, A671.
40. Pomfrett CJD, Beech, M. J., and Healy, T. E. J. (1991) Variation in respiratory sinus arrhythmia may reflect levels of anaesthesia. *Br. J. Anaesth.* **67**, 646–647.
41. Wang, D. Y., Pomfrett, C. J. D., and Healy, T. E. J. (1993) Respiratory sinus arrhythmia: A new, objective sedation score. *Br. J. Anaesth.* **71**, 354–358.
42. Haberthur, C., Lehmann, F., and Riz, R. (1996) Assessment of depth of midazolam sedation using objective parameters. *Intensive Care Med.* **22**, 1385–1390.
43. Winchell, R. J. and Hoyt, D. B. (1996) Spectral analysis of heart rate variability in the ICU: a measure of autonomic function. *J. Surg. Res.* **63**, 11–16.
44. Heier, T. and Steen, P. A. (1996) Assessment of anaesthesia depth. *Acta Anaesthesiol. Scand.* **40**, 1087–1100.
45. Maynard, D., Prior, P. F., and Scott, D. F. (1969) A device for continuous monitoring of cerebral activity in resuscitated patients. *Br. Med. J.* **4**, 545–546.
46. Kearse, L. A., Rosow, C., Zaslavsky, A., Connors, P., Dershwitz, M., and Denman, W. (1998) Bispectral analysis of the electroencephalogram predicts conscious processing of information during propofol sedation and hypnosis. *Anesthesiology* **88**, 25–34.
47. Leslie, K., Sessler, D. I., Smith, W. D., Larson, M. D., Ozaki, M., Blanchard, D., et al. (1996) Prediction of movement during propofol/nitrous oxide anesthesia. *Anesthesiology* **84**, 52–63.
48. Shapiro, B. A. (1999) Bispectral index: better information for sedation in the intensive care unit? *Crit. Care Med.* **27**, 1663–1664.
49. Rampil, I. J. (1998) A primer for EEG signal processing in anesthesia. *Anesthesiology* **89**, 980–1002.
50. Crabb, I., Thornton, C., Konieczko, K. M., Chan, A., Aquilina, R., Frazer, N., et al. (1996) Remifentanil reduces auditory and somatosensory evoked responses during isoflurane anaesthesia in a dose-dependent manner. *Br. J. Anaesth.* **76**, 795–801.
51. Thornton, C. and Sharpe, R. M. (1998) Evoked responses in anaesthesia. *Br. J. Anaesth.* **81**, 771–781.

52. Thornton, C. and Jones, J. G. (1993) Evaluating depths of anesthesia: Review of methods. *Int. Anesthesiol. Clin.* **31,** 67–88.

53. Schwender, D., Weninger, E., Daunderer, M., Klasing, S., Poeppel, E., and Peter, K. (1995) Anesthesia with increasing doses of sufentanil and midlatency auditory evoked potentials in humans. *Anesth. Analg.* **80,** 499–505.

54. Stanski, D. R. (2000) Monitoring depth of anesthesia, in *Anesthesia* (Miller, R. D., ed.), Churchill Livingstone, Philadelphia, PA, pp. 1087–1116.

55. Newson, C., Joshi, G. P., Victory, R., and White, P. F. (1995) Comparison of propofol administration techniques for sedation during monitored anesthesia care. *Anesth. Analg.* **81,** 486–491.

56. Glass, P. S., Bloom, M., Kearse, L., Rosow, C., Sebel, P., and Manberg, P. (1997) Bispectral analysis measures sedation and memory effects of propofol, midazolam, isoflurane, and alfentanil in healthy volunteers. *Anesthesiology* **86,** 836–847.

57. Iselin-Chaves, I. A. (1998) Flaishon, R., Sebel, P. S., Howell, S., Gan, T. J., Sigl, J., et al. The effect of the interaction of propofol and alfentanil on recall, loss of consciousness, and the bispectral index. *Anesth. Analg.* **87,** 949–955.

58. Mortier, E., Struys, M., De Smet, T., Versichelen, L., and Roly, G. (1998) Closed-loop controlled administration of propofol using bispectral analysis. *Anaesthesia* **53,** 749–754.

59. Struys, M., Versichelen, L., Byttebier, G., Mortier, E., Moerman, A., and Rolly, G. (1998) Clinical usefulness of the bispectral index for titrating propofol target effect-site concentration. *Anaesthesia* **53,** 4–12.

60. Liu, J., Singh, H., and White, P. F. (1997) Electroencephalographic bispectral index correlates with intraoperative recall and depth of propofol-induced sedation. *Anesth. Analg.* **84,** 185–189.

61. Liu, J., Singh, H., and White, P. F. (1996) Electroencephalogram bispectral analysis predicts the depth of midazolam-induced sedation. *Anesthesiology* **84,** 64–69.

62. Schraag, S., Bothner, U., Gajraj, R., Kenny, G. N., and Georgieff, M. (1999) The performance of electroencephalogram bispectral index and auditory evoked potential index to predict loss of consciousness during propofol infusion. *Anesth. Analg.* **89,** 1311–1315.

63. Gajraj, R. J., Doi, M., Manzaridis, H., and Kenny, G. N. C. (1998) Analysis of the EEG bispectrum, auditory evoked potentials and the EEG power spectrum during repeated transitions from consciousness to unconsciousness. *Br. J. Anaesth.* **80,** 46–52.

64. Doi, M., Gajraj, R. J., Mantzaridis, H., and Kenny, G. N. C. (1997) Relationship between calculated blood concentration of propofol and electrophysiological variables during emergence from anaesthesia: comparison of bispectral index, spectral edge frequency, median frequency and auditory evoked potential index. *Br. J. Anaesth.* **78,** 180–184.

65. Doi, M., Gajraj, R. J., Mantzaridis, H., and Kenny, G. N. C. (1999) Prediction of movement at laryngeal mask airway insertion: comparison of auditory evoked potential index, bispectral index, spectral edge frequency and median frequency. *Br. J. Anaesth.* **82,** 203–207.

66. Kochs, E., Kalkman, C. J., Thornton, C., Newton, D., Bischoff, P., Kuppe, H., et al. (1999) Middle latency auditory evoked responses and electroencephalographic derived variable do not predict movement to noxious stimulation during 1 minimum alveolar anesthetic concentration isoflurane/nitrous oxide anesthesia. *Anesth. Analg.* **88,** 1412–1417.

67. Katoh, T., Suzuki, A., and Ikeda, K. (1998) Electroencephalographic derivatives as a tool for predicting the depth of sedation and anesthesia induced by sevoflurane. *Anesthesiology* **88,** 624–650.

68. Gan, T. J., Glass, P. S., Windsor, A., Payne, F., Rosow, C., Sebel, P., and Manberg, P. (1997) BIS Utility Study Group. Bispectral index monitoring allows faster emergence and improved recovery from propofol, alfentanil, and nitrous oxide anesthesia. *Anesthesiology* **87,** 808–815.

69. Steward, D. J. (1975) A simplified scoring system for the post-operative recovery room. *Can. Anaesth. Soc. J.* **22,** 111–113.

10

Nursing Perspectives
on the Care of Sedated Patients

Terri Voepel-Lewis, MSN, RN

1. INTRODUCTION

Recent changes in the health care environment have increased the demand for sedation to facilitate medical and diagnostic procedures. First, there has been an increased availability and utilization of various diagnostic and therapeutic procedures. Furthermore, it has become widely accepted that sedation and analgesia decrease the patient's anxiety, enhance the patient's comfort, and may thereby improve the success of any procedure *(1)*. Additionally, the costs associated with sedation are less than those associated with general anesthesia for similar procedures *(2)*, and the amount of disruption in daily life is also perceived to be less. Finally, several short-acting sedative agents have been introduced during the last few of decades that may offer safer alternatives for use during procedures.

This increased demand for sedation requires the involvement of knowledgeable and skilled teams of care providers to assure the provision of safe and high-quality care *(3)*. Typically, a primary care provider orders the procedure. However, an attending physician in the diagnostic procedures area is responsible for the procedure itself and for the overall management of the sedated patient. Additionally, it is the direct care provider, generally a nurse, who is responsible for pre-procedural preparation, administration of sedative agents, ongoing patient monitoring, discharge assessment, and patient education. Although several providers may be involved with sedation of a patient, in a practical sense it is the nurse who ensures appropriateness of care, and implementation and compliance with practice guidelines for every patient. Therefore, it is important that the nurse be fully aware of institutional sedation practice guidelines, and be knowledgeable about all aspects of sedation care. This chapter examines the role and responsibilities of the nurse who provides care for patients requiring sedation for a medical procedure,

From: *Contemporary Clinical Neuroscience: Sedation and Analgesia for Diagnostic and Therapeutic Procedures*
Edited by: S. Malviya, N. N. Naughton, and K. K. Tremper © Humana Press Inc., Totowa, NJ

and emphasizes the important risk factors and special considerations associated with sedation outside of the operating room.

2. PERSONNEL

Existing practice guidelines *(1,4–7)* recommend that one trained person is responsible for the provision of care and monitoring of the patient throughout a sedation episode; however, there is no consensus regarding the qualifications for sedation personnel *(8)*. Recent literature suggests that in most settings, this primary sedation care provider is a registered nurse *(3,9–12)*. Additionally, recent standards from the Joint Commission on the Accreditation of Health Care Organizations (JCAHO) state that sufficient numbers of qualified personnel, in addition to the licensed independent practitioner performing the procedure, must be present during procedures using moderate or deep sedation *(7)*.

Competency-based training programs should be established in settings providing sedation care, and nurses and other caregivers must demonstrate proficiency prior to caring for sedated patients *(12,13)*. Competency should include knowledge of the pharmacology of the medications used and of factors that increase the potential for risks associated with sedation. Furthermore, the sedation care provider must be trained in the use of monitoring and emergency equipment, and be able to recognize and respond to complications associated with sedation. National guidelines recommend minimal training in basic life support (BLS), but some organizations require advanced cardiac life support (ACLS) training for the sedation care provider. At the least, the care provider must be capable of establishing a patent airway and maintaining ventilation and oxygenation. Furthermore, an individual who is capable of establishing intravenous (iv) access and one who is trained in ACLS must be immediately available.

The nurse or sedation care provider should also be aware of state policies on administration of sedation *(12)*, as there are restrictions and policies regarding sedation practices in many states *(1)*. For instance, some states mandate that a physician must be present in the room throughout a procedure performed under sedation, and others simply require a physician to be in the vicinity. Some states have policy statements regarding the authorized involvement of unlicensed personnel in the care of sedated patients, and others do not address this issue. Recent guidelines of the JCAHO mandate that anesthesiology departments are responsible for ensuring the consistency of sedation care throughout the institution. Furthermore, the JCAHO stipulates that individuals who provide moderate to deep sedation must have the appropriate credentials to manage patients at whatever level of sedation or

Table 1
Qualifications of Individuals Providing Moderate or Deep Sedation (7)

Qualified individuals are trained in professional standards and techniques to:

1. Evaluate patients prior to performing moderate or deep sedation
2. Administer pharmacologic agents to predictably achieve desired levels of sedation
3. Monitor sedated patients carefully and maintain them at the desired level of sedation
4. Perform moderate or deep sedation to include methods and techniques required to rescue patients who unavoidably or unintentionally slip into a deeper level of sedation or analgesia than desired
   - Individuals who are permitted to administer moderate sedation must be able to rescue patients from deep sedation (i.e., must be competent to manage a compromised airway and provide adequate oxygenation and ventilation; basic life support)
   - Individuals who are permitted to administer deep sedation must be able to rescue patients from general anesthesia (i.e., must be competent to manage an unstable cardiovascular system as well as a compromised airway and inadequate oxygenation and ventilation; advanced life support)

anesthesia is achieved, either intentionally or unintentionally (*see* Table 1). In many settings, this has resulted in the formation of privileging systems for non-anesthesiology physicians who provide sedation care.

3. PRE-PROCEDURE ASSESSMENT

3.1. Patient Selection

When deciding whether to use sedation to facilitate a procedure, it is important to consider the nature of the procedure (i.e., whether it is painful, and its duration), the patient's traits (such as age and anxiety level), and the patient's risk factors *(14)*. Although certain procedures, such as electrophysiologic studies, may call for sedation or even general anesthesia in every case, others such as computerized tomography (CT) may require sedation only in select cases. It is imperative to include the patient—or in the case of children, the parent—in the decision to use sedation vs other alternatives for the procedure. Some patients may require little to no sedation for their procedure, particularly if it is painless. However, young children, cognitively impaired individuals, or very anxious adults may require deep sedation, or, in some cases, general anesthesia in order to complete brief diagnostic procedures. Some patients with co-existent painful conditions such as arthritis

Table 2
Considerations for Determining the
Need for Sedation and Choice of Sedative Agent(s)

Procedure characteristics

Duration
Invasiveness/Pain
Required cooperation
Immobility
Environment/noise

Sedative Properties

Available routes of administration
Onset/duration of action
Ability to titrate
Risks/side effects
Reversibility

Patient factors

Age
Anxiety
Temperament
Allergies
Previous sedation experience
Risk factors/co-existing disease

may require sedation or analgesics even for noninvasive procedures to permit them to lie still for the duration of the procedure. Table 2 presents a summary of some of the factors that should be considered when determining whether a given patient will need sedation for a procedure.

3.2. Risk Factors

Prior to the procedure, the patient's physical status should be carefully evaluated to determine whether the patient is an appropriate candidate for sedation. The health history and physical examination will highlight factors that increase the risks associated with sedation, and facilitate the appropriate classification of risk using the American Society of Anesthesiologists (ASA) physical status categorization (*see* Chapter 3, Appendix 3). An ASA classification of 3 or greater indicates a greater risk for adverse events from sedation than an ASA status of 1–2 *(15,16)*. Following is a brief summary of specific risk factors for sedation-related adverse events. Patients who present with these conditions require special consideration and individualized plans for sedation, and in some cases may warrant consultation with an anesthesiologist.

Certain patients present with conditions that place them at increased risk for respiratory adverse events during sedation. Tonsillar hypertrophy has been shown to predispose the patient to airway obstruction during sedation *(17)*. A history of sleep apnea, stridor, or snoring should therefore be obtained. It is important to assess for craniofacial abnormalities and musculoskeletal disease such as arthritis of the cervical spine, because these traits may make airway management difficult and thus place the patient at higher risk if airway management becomes necessary. Pulmonary disease, a history of asthma, or smoking may also predispose the patient to respiratory complications. Additionally, a history of alcohol or narcotic use within the past 24 h places the patient at risk for apnea *(18)*. Infants, particularly those who were pre-term, are at increased risk for apnea and hypoxemia.

Other populations may be at increased risk for cardiovascular complications associated with sedation. In patients with congenital heart disease, respiratory depression, hypoxemia, and hypercarbia associated with sedation may lead to increased pulmonary vascular resistance (PVR), increased right-to-left shunting, and worsening cyanosis. A history of cardiovascular disease, particularly left main coronary artery disease and/or unstable angina, places the patient at risk for complications during cardiovascular procedures *(19)*. The elderly or patients who are hypovolemic may be susceptible to sedation-induced hypotension.

Patients with morbid obesity or gastroesophageal reflux and those who have not fasted prior to emergent procedures may not be suitable candidates for sedation without a protected airway because of the increased risk of aspiration. Patients with neurological impairment such as a history of seizure disorders or conditions with a potential for increased intracranial pressure also require special attention. Hypoventilation and hypercarbia that may occur with sedation place these patients at risk for increased intracranial pressure and neurologic compromise. The young infant as well as the elderly adult require special consideration, because studies have found these age groups to be at greater risk for adverse events following administration of sedative agents *(16,19)*. Altered hepatic or renal function in these populations may cause variable drug metabolism and clearance, warranting close monitoring of drug response. These patients may be at risk for prolonged effects of sedatives.

Some patients may be at increased risk for difficult sedation or sedation failure. The patient's previous experience with sedation as well as their medication history may help to determine this risk. Young children who have had difficult sedation experiences or paradoxical reactions with certain agents warrant consideration of alternative agents or general anesthesia. Several populations, including children older than 3 yr of age, neurologi-

Table 3
Pre-Sedation Instruction to Patients

Procedure-specific information (including bowel preparation, etc.)

NPO times

Suggested:	Solids and non-clear liquids*	6–8 h
	Clear liquids	2–3 h
	Breast milk	4 h

Arrival time
Medications/alternatives for sedation
Complications or side effects during and following sedation
Recovery characteristics (duration, potential for delayed side effects)
Resuming regular activities (activities to avoid, when to resume work, school, etc.)

*Includes non-human milk and infant formula.

cally or cognitively impaired children, children with less adaptable temperaments, and patients with a higher ASA physical status have been shown to have a higher incidence of sedation difficulties and failure *(16,20–22)*. Although little is known about paradoxical reactions, there is some evidence to suggest that genetic predisposition may play a role in such responses to benzodiazepines *(23)*. Soliciting a family history of sedation-related problems may therefore help to establish a risk profile for potential adverse events.

3.3. Education

Detailed patient education that begins when the procedure is first scheduled is invaluable because it allays anxiety and allows both the patient and the sedation care provider to be prepared for the procedure. The information that is most helpful to the patient is presented in Table 3. Pre-procedure instruction should include a detailed discussion regarding the procedure, including its anticipated duration, the environment in which it is performed, the associated pain, and the need for immobility and cooperation. This will enable the patient and the provider to determine whether sedation will be required. The patient should be fully informed of the anticipated side effects of the sedatives commonly used for the procedure, the risks associated with sedation and the procedure itself, and the measures that will be taken to minimize these risks. Early teaching regarding the anticipated duration of action of sedative(s) and the potential for delayed recovery *(24)* will enable the patient to arrange for appropriate time away from work or school, and for a support person to be present following the procedure if necessary. Pre-procedure directions should also include preparation for the test itself, such as bowel preparation or oral contrast agents, and specific directions regarding when to discontinue oral solids and liquids prior to the procedure. Additionally, patient preparation should include information about the recovery period, which is reviewed in detail in Chapter 11.

Children who are undergoing sedation should be provided with developmentally appropriate information about what will happen during the procedure, so that they will be less anxious and therefore more likely to cooperate *(25)*. The young child may benefit most from concrete information that is given close to the time of the procedure or during the procedure. However, older children may need more detailed information ahead of time so that any questions or concerns can be addressed prior to the procedure. In either case, children should be informed about what may cause pain or discomfort and how that pain will be treated. Although sleep deprivation in children has been advocated to increase the success of sedation during procedures, one descriptive study has refuted this notion *(26)*. The role of sleep deprivation prior to the procedure, therefore, remains unclear.

3.4. Informed Consent

Except in emergency situations, individual states often mandate that written consent be obtained from the patient prior to administering a sedative agent for a procedure *(4,5,10)*. In many cases, the nurse is responsible for obtaining consent for sedation, and should therefore be knowledgeable regarding the elements of consent. First, it is important to establish that the patient or parent has the capacity to understand the given information. In cases involving children or cognitively impaired adults, a parent, guardian, or surrogate must be available to provide consent *(27)*. Information regarding the risks and benefits of sedation and alternatives for treatment should be disclosed in a manner that the patient/parent can understand. When a written consent document is used, the reading level of the material should be no higher than the 8th-grade level. When the patient is a child, the procedure should be explained to the child and assent should be obtained from those who are able to understand the risks and benefits of sedation *(27)*. Parents can generally help the care provider decide whether or not the child will be able to understand enough of the information in order to provide assent.

3.5. Choice of Sedative

Although a wide variety of sedative agents are available for use, there is a tendency for practitioners to select among only a few *(28)*. This tendency may be the result of the success rate and/or relative safety record associated with certain agents, or perhaps to practitioner comfort related to experience with the agent selected. The choice of sedative should be individualized to the patient and based on the requirements for the specific procedure (Table 2). Factors such as the anticipated duration of and potential pain associated with the procedure, the degree of cooperation required from the patient, and/or whether complete immobility is necessary, should be considered when choosing the appropriate sedative agent. Although the use of a topical anesthetic agent, such as Eutectic Mixture of Local Anesthetics (EMLA(tm)) can facilitate placement of an iv catheter in young children, initial oral or intranasal administration of a sedative may be necessary in cases where iv access is anticipated to be difficult. During certain procedures, such as electrophysiological studies, titration of a short-acting agent such as midazolam, fentanyl, or perhaps propofol may be desirable so that depth of sedation can be better titrated *(29)*. For procedures that require a deeply sedated patient for a longer duration, pentobarbital or chloral hydrate may be appropriate choices *(21,30,31)*. In any case, the patient's health status, risk factors, and age, as well as previous experience with sedation, should be considered prior to prescribing any sedative medication.

The success and safety of the sedation experience is probably less dependent on the specific agent used, but more importantly related to selecting the appropriate drug for the patient, monitoring its effectiveness, and augmenting sedation carefully *(9)*. It is imperative that the nurse responsible for sedative administration and care of the patient be knowledgeable about the pharmacology of the agent(s) used. Chapters 7 and 8 provide in-depth descriptions of sedative and analgesic agents used to facilitate procedures. It is important to note that most institutions require the involvement of an anesthesiologist when agents with a narrower margin of safety, such as propofol or ketamine, are used.

3.6. Environment

The sedation care provider must ensure that all of the facilities, equipment, and supplies necessary to manage sedation as well as potential emergencies are available prior to sedating the patient. A list of suggested equipment and supplies is presented in Table 4. The nurse must document that emergency equipment is maintained and is functioning on a scheduled basis. Emergency medications and supplies, including agents used to reverse sedative effects, must also be routinely checked and maintained.

In addition to assuring a well-equipped diagnostic suite for the promotion of safety, other environmental considerations can facilitate a successful sedation experience for children and adults alike. Once a sedative medication is

Table 4
Suggested Emergency Equipment

Appropriately sized stretcher or crib
Standard monitoring equipment (i.e., pulse oximeter, noninvasive blood pressure
  monitor, stethoscope)
Electrocardiograph
Positive pressure oxygen delivery system
Bag valve mask device and face masks*
Artificial airways* (nasopharyngeal, oropharyngeal, endotracheal tubes)
Intubation equipment*
Suction equipment and supplies*
Defibrillator
Supplies necessary to establish/maintain iv access
Emergency medications including reversal agents

*All sizes.

Table 5
Non-Pharmacologic Techniques to Facilitate Conscious Sedation

Infants	Rocking, patting, swaddling, sucking on a pacifier, music
Toddler	Rocking, stuffed toy or favorite blanket, music or singing, storytelling, parental presence
Preschool and school-aged children	Touch/stroking, distraction, guided imagery, music, video, stories, parental presence, relaxation (older children)
Adolescents and adults	Touch, massage, distraction (music, video), imagery, relaxation, hypnosis

administered, a quiet, non-threatening setting should be maintained to the extent possible. Music, storytelling, and, during some procedures, video movies, may provide effective distraction techniques for the sedated patient. Some children may feel more comfortable if they are allowed to bring a small toy or blanket with them for the procedure, and when possible, allowing a parent to stay with the child may facilitate the child's ability to cope with the procedure *(32–34)*. Incorporation of behavioral techniques such as progressive relaxation or guided imagery may enhance the comfort of selected patients who are undergoing conscious sedation. Table 5 suggests some of

Table 6
The University of Michigan Sedation Scale *(39)*

0 *Awake/alert*
1 *Lightly sedated*: Tired/sleepy, appropriate response to verbal conversation and/
   or sounds
2 *Sedated*: Somnolent/sleeping, easily aroused with light tactile stimulation
3 *Deeply sedated*: Deep sleep, arousable only with significant physical stimulation
4 *Unarousable*

the behavioral-cognitive techniques that may help to reduce the stress and pain imposed by the medical procedure.

4. DURING THE PROCEDURE

The requirements for monitoring the patient during sedation have been described previously in Chapters 2, 3, and 8. However, it must be emphasized that monitoring should not be considered a substitute for the constant vigilance of a care provider or nurse who is responsible solely for the patient's well-being and who may be only peripherally involved with tasks associated with the procedure itself.

4.1. Monitoring and Maintaining Sedation

Deep sedation places the patient at risk for loss of protective reflexes, and has been associated with higher risk for adverse events such as respiratory depression *(35)*. For most adults and many children, it is thus desirable that the patient remain responsive to verbal stimulation throughout the procedure. Throughout the procedure, and until discharge criteria are met, the nurse must evaluate the patient's depth of sedation at regular intervals. Chapter 9 presents an overview of the assessment of sedation depth. Sedation assessment tools must be sensitive enough to detect the patient's progression from light sedation, during which the patient remains responsive to verbal stimulation, to deeper sedation, in which there is response only to physical stimulation or no response. Furthermore, the tool must be easy to score and document because frequent assessment is imperative, yet should also facilitate a reliable, objective assessment of sedation depth. Although several sedation assessment tools have been developed for use in clinical and research settings, some have not been validated *(36)*, while others may be cumbersome for use in a busy clinical setting *(37,38)*. The University of Michigan Sedation Scale has recently been developed for assessing the depth of sedation throughout diagnostic and therapeutic procedures, and was recently tested for validity and reliability (Table 6) *(39)*.

Maintaining a depth of sedation that promotes the patient's comfort while maintaining responsiveness can be challenging. Titration of short-acting iv agents throughout the procedure may be the best method to produce this level of sedation. The advantage of this method is that the desired effect can be achieved while avoiding unwanted side effects associated with higher bolus doses of medication *(40)*. It is important that such titration be done carefully and with patience. Small doses of medication should be administered at intervals that allow the peak effect of the previous bolus to be assessed *(5)*. Bolus doses that are administered too closely together may produce a deeper than intended level of sedation with associated increased risks. When non-parenteral routes are used to administer medications, the time required for drug absorption should be considered prior to supplementation with additional medications.

When deep sedation is required to complete the procedure, a larger bolus of medication prior to the procedure is generally warranted. However, maintaining deep sedation during long procedures or for those that are painful or stimulating frequently requires augmentation of sedation with additional doses of sedatives or analgesics. For painful procedures adding a short-acting opioid such as fentanyl provides analgesia as well as adjunctive sedation. For nonpainful procedures, a short-acting benzodiazepine or barbiturate can effectively supplement sedation in many patients. With any combination of medications used, it is important to consider the potential for increased risks for prolonged sedation or synergistic respiratory depression *(41)*. Augmenting sedation with a drug that can be reversed may therefore be in the best interest of the patient.

Occasionally, the sedative agent(s) fail to produce a depth of sedation that is necessary to complete the procedure. The incidence of failed sedation in children has been reported to be between 5% and 15% of cases *(16,21,42–44)*, and failed sedation in adults is not well-documented. Paradoxical reactions to the sedative agent may cause the patient to become agitated, restless, and/ or hyperactive, which may pose a risk of injury to the patient since motor imbalance may be also be present. Such reactions can be very challenging to manage, and frequently result in sedation failure. The etiology of paradoxical reactions is poorly understood, but is believed to be related to the interference with neurotransmitters or neuromodulators in various regions of the brain, predisposing susceptible individuals to unusual reactions to the agent *(23,45)*. Medical management of paradoxical reactions is not well-documented, and consists primarily of case reports *(45–47)*. Flumazenil has been successfully used to reverse such reactions to midazolam in adult patients *(47,48)*. Haloperidol reversed midazolam-induced agitation in another case *(45)*, and morphine sulphate was effective in another *(49)*. Physostigmine has been successfully used to treat scopolamine-induced delirium in postoperative patients; however, reports of its use for benzodiazepine reactions have been conflicting *(46,50)*. Paradoxical reactions can be anxiety-producing for the patient, or when children are involved, for the parents. Indeed, a previous report has suggested that postsedation agitation contributes to parental dissatisfaction with the sedation experience *(24)*. In cases of sedation-induced agitation, the nurse should provide emotional support and maintain a quiet, soothing environment until the reaction subsides *(51)*. It is important to note that patients who experience paradoxical reactions may still be at risk for other adverse effects of sedatives and must therefore be monitored according to guidelines until the effects of the medication wear off, and the patient meets discharge criteria. Furthermore, if a reversal agent is used to reverse a paradoxical reaction, it is important to continue monitoring the patient for the duration of action of the sedative(s) administered, because resedation may occur once the effects of the reversal agent have worn off.

Cases of failed sedation and aborted procedures are particularly frustrating for the patient and family, as well as the care provider. The cost of sedation failure to the family in terms of repeated trips to the hospital, time away from work, or other family responsibilities and, more importantly, the impact of delayed diagnoses are immeasurable. The nurse must be aware of these concerns when dealing with cases of failed sedation. Decisions for follow-up may necessitate consultation with an anesthesiologist. In some instances, the patient's procedure may need to be rescheduled for completion with an alternative sedative agent. In the pediatric setting, a greater number may need to be rescheduled for a general anesthetic *(24)*.

4.2. Physiologic Assessment and Management of Complications

The widespread implementation of continuous pulse oximetry has markedly improved the safety of sedation by facilitating the early detection of respiratory depression and hypoxemia, and in turn, allowing early intervention and prevention of clinically significant sequelae *(16)*. Even with such monitoring, the nurse must frequently assess the ventilatory status of the patient *(5)*. Hypoxemia is a late symptom of apnea, particularly in patients receiving supplemental oxygen *(52–54)*. In the absence of capnography that can readily detect apnea and airway obstruction, the nurse must evaluate the patient's respiratory rate and depth, and observe for suprasternal or intercostal retractions, or paradoxical abdominal movement, which may indicate obstruction. Restlessness may also indicate hypoxemia or hypercarbia. Both respiratory depression and airway obstruction place the patient at risk for cardiac dysrhythmias and neurologic sequelae, and therefore warrant immediate intervention. Initial supportive interventions for respiratory depression or airway obstruction include administration of supplemental oxygen, stimulating the patient, and measures to ensure a patent airway such as the head-tilt, chin lift maneuver, or in the case of young children, use of the sniffing position with the jaw forward. If initial measures fail, placement of an oral or nasopharyngeal airway and ventilation with bag-valve-mask may become necessary.

Some practitioners recommend routinely supplementing sedated patients with oxygen, because this practice has been shown to reduce the incidence of hypoxemia *(54)*. However, current guidelines do not address supplemental oxygen for all sedated patients, and this intervention is generally reserved for higher-risk patients or for patients who experience hypoxemia during the procedure *(5)*. It is important to remember that administration of oxygen to patients with chronic obstructive pulmonary disease (COPD) should be done with caution, since high flow rates may diminish the patient's respiratory drive.

The patient's blood pressure should generally be monitored at routine intervals throughout the sedation episode, since hypotension is a potential side effect of many sedative agents. However, in young children who may be easily awakened, it may be necessary to postpone blood pressure monitoring until the procedure is completed. Patients with pre-existing hypovolemia, the elderly, and patients who receive propofol are at greatest risk for hypotension. In these high-risk patients, volume replacement prior to sedative administration may help to prevent hemodynamic instability. In some cases, acute hypotension may warrant intervention with vasoactive medications, and possibly reversal of the sedative agent.

A deeper level of sedation increases the risk for pulmonary aspiration, which can lead to life-threatening complications. Obese patients, obstetric patients, and those with a history of reflux, are at higher risk for aspiration. Additionally, patients who have not fasted prior to the procedure and those who are given oral contrast for abdominal scans are also at increased risk, and may require special consideration or consultation with an anesthesiologist. Interventions to reduce the risk of aspiration include elevation of the head, when not contraindicated, administration of medications that lower gastric pH, or administration of metoclopramide to facilitate gastric emptying *(55)*. If the sedated patient vomits, immediate suctioning is warranted, and airway protection may be indicated if sedation is deep enough to cause loss of protective airway reflexes. Suspected aspiration should be aggressively treated with antibiotic therapy, pulmonary toilet, and oxygen supplementation if needed.

Reversal of the sedative agent may be warranted in certain cases of excessive sedation. The occurrence of respiratory depression or a life-threatening adverse event calls for sedative reversal when feasible. However, it must be emphasized that administration of reversal agents should not delay or be considered a substitute for aggressive supportive interventions such as bag-and-mask ventilation. Paradoxical reactions may also be treated with administration of a reversal agent. Previous investigators have reported shortened recovery following sedation for short procedures when flumazenil was used to reverse sedation (56), suggesting a potential role for reversal in facilitating recovery and discharge. However, the half-life of the reversal agent may be shorter than that of the sedative drug thereby predisposing the patient to re-sedation after discharge to an unmonitored setting. Reversal agents must therefore be used with caution, and carefully titrated to achieve the desired effect. Slow titration of naloxone will facilitate reversal of side effects such as excessive sedation and respiratory depression, while preserving the analgesic effects of the opioid. Conversely, rapid administration of this reversal agent can trigger adverse reactions including hypotension, hypertension, ventricular tachycardia, fibrillation, and seizures. The benzodiazepine reversal agent, flumazenil, can be titrated to diminish sedation without completely reversing all sedative and anxiolytic effects of the benzodiazepine. Administration of this reversal agent in small doses is warranted to minimize the possibility of adverse effects. Flumazenil must be used with caution in patients with underlying seizure disorders, since it has been reported to precipitate seizures in this population.

4.3. Documentation

National guidelines stipulate aspects of the procedure that must be documented (4,5). Careful documentation throughout the procedure is necessary in order to ensure continuity of care in cases in which multiple caregivers may be involved, to facilitate subsequent procedures that may require sedation by permitting review of the patient's response to the sedative agents used, and for medico-legal reasons. Table 7 presents the important aspects of the sedation experience that must be documented. National guidelines and institutional policy should be referred to for further information regarding documentation.

5. SUMMARY

The care of sedated patients presents a unique set of challenges and responsibilities to the professional nurse. Given appropriate training and experience, the nurse who is committed to safe care of the patient can effec-

Table 7
Documenting the Sedation Procedure

I. History/risk assessment	Underlying conditions ASA status Allergies Current medications Consultations as indicated History of sedation/anesthesia
II. Physical status	Review of systems Airway assessment NPO status Baseline vital signs Weight
III. During sedation	Medications dose/time/route Vital signs Oxygen saturation Other monitoring as indicated Adverse events and interventions Paradoxical reactions
IV. Discharge status	Patient's level of alertness Vital signs Patient's general condition Discharge criteria Where patient is going (i.e., home/inpatient bed)
V. Patient Instructions	Pre-procedure and at discharge Verbal and written Responsible person Emergency contacts

tively meet these challenges, and perhaps, reduce the risk associated with sedation. Although institutional guidelines provide a framework for safe practice, and monitoring devices improve the ability to detect unsafe conditions, it is the nurse's observations and judgment that remain the most important factors in facilitating safe and effective sedation of each patient.

REFERENCES

1. Bubien, R. S., Fisher, J. D., Gentzel, J. A., Murphy, E. K., Irwin M. E., Shea, J. B., et al. (1998) NASPE expert consensus document: use of iv (conscious) sedation/analgesia by nonanesthesia personnel in patients undergoing arrhythmia

specific diagnostic, therapeutic, and surgical procedures. *Pacing Clin. Electrophysiol.* **21(2)**, 375–385.

2. Smith, P. R. (1997) The cost of administering intravenous conscious sedation. *Crit. Care Nurs. Clin. N. Am.* **9(3)**, 423–427.

3. Sury, M. R., Hatch, D. J., Deeley, T., Dicks-Mireaux, C., and Chong, W. K. (1999) Development of a nurse-led sedation service for paediatric magnetic resonance imaging. *Lancet* **353(9165)**, 1667–1671.

4. American Academy of Pediatrics Committee on Drugs: Guidelines for monitoring and management of pediatric patients during and after sedation for diagnostic and therapeutic procedures. (1992) *Pediatrics* **89(6 Pt 1)**, 1110–1115.

5. Practice guidelines for sedation and analgesia by non-anesthesiologists. (1996) A report by the American Society of Anesthesiologists Task Force on Sedation and Analgesia by Non-Anesthesiologists. *Anesthesiology* **84(2)**, 459–471.

6. Clinical policy for procedural sedation and analgesia in the emergency department. (1998) American College of Emergency Physicians. *Ann. Emerg. Med.* **31(5)**, 663–677.

7. Joint Commission on Accreditation of Healthcare Organizations. (2001) Comprehensive Accreditation Manual for Hospitals, in *The Official Handbook,* Oakbrook Terrace, IL, JCAHO, http://www.jcaho.org/standards_frm.html.

8. Litman, R. S. (1999) Sedation and anesthesia outside the operating room: answers to common questions. *Semin. Pediatr. Surg.* **8(1)**, 34–39.

9. Hollman, G. A., Elderbrook, M. K., and VanDenLangenberg, B. (1995) Results of a pediatric sedation program on head MRI scan success rates and procedure duration times. *Clin. Pediatr. (Phila.)* **34(6)**, 300–305.

10. Dlugose, D. (1997) Risk management considerations in conscious sedation. *Crit. Care Nurs. Clin. N. Am.* **9(3)**, 429–440.

11. Odom, J. (1997) Conscious sedation in the ambulatory setting. *Crit. Care Nurs. Clin. N. Am.* **9(3)**, 361–370.

12. Shaw, C., Weaver, C. S., and Schneider, L. (1996) Conscious sedation: a multidisciplinary team approach. *J. Post. Anesth. Nurs.* **11(1)**, 13–19.

13. Algren, C. L. and Algren, J. T. (1997) Pediatric sedation. Essentials for the perioperative nurse. *Nurs. Clin. N. Am.* **32(1)**, 17–30.

14. Coté, C. J. (1994) Sedation for the pediatric patient. A review. *Pediatr. Clin. N. Am.* **41(1)**, 31–58.

15. Gilger, M. A., Jeiven, S. D., Barrish, J. O., and McCarroll, L. R. (1993) Oxygen desaturation and cardiac arrhythmias in children during esophagogastroduodenoscopy using conscious sedation. *Gastrointest. Endosc.* **39(3)**, 392–395.

16. Malviya, S., Voepel-Lewis, T., and Tait, A. R. (1998) Adverse events and risk factors associated with the sedation of children by nonanesthesiologists [published erratum appears in *Anesth. Analg.* Feb;**86(2)**, 227. *Anesth. Analg.* **85(6)**, 1207–1213.

17. Fishbaugh, D. F., Wilson, S., Preisch, J. W., and Weaver, J. M., 2nd. (1997) Relationship of tonsil size on an airway blockage maneuver in children during sedation. *Pediatr. Dent.* **19(4)**, 277–281.

18. Lerman, B., Yoshida, D., and Levitt, M. A. (1996) A prospective evaluation of the safety and efficacy of methohexital in the emergency department. *Am. J. Emerg. Med.* **14(4)**, 351–354.

19. Kixmiller, J. M. and Schick, L. (1997) Conscious sedation in cardiovascular procedures. *Crit. Care Nurs. Clin. N. Am.* **9(3),** 301–312.
20. Greenberg, S. B., Faerber, E. N., Radke, J. L., Aspinall, C. L., Adams, R. C., and Mercer-Wilson, D. D. (1994) Sedation of difficult-to-sedate children undergoing MR imaging: value of thioridazine as an adjunct to chloral hydrate. *AJR Am. J. Roentgenol.* **163(1),** 165–168.
21. Rumm, P. D., Takao, R. T., Fox, D. J., and Atkinson, S. W. (1990) Efficacy of sedation of children with chloral hydrate. *South. Med. J.* **83(9),** 1040–1043.
22. Voepel-Lewis, T., Malviya, S., Prochaska, G., and Tait, A. R. (2000) Sedation failures in children undergoing MRI and CT: is temperament a factor? *Paediatr. Anaesth.* **10(3),** 319–323.
23. van der Bijl, P. and Roelofse, J. A. (1991) Disinhibitory reactions to benzodiazepines: a review. *J. Oral Maxillofac. Surg.* **49(5),** 519–523.
24. Malviya, S. (2000) Prolonged recovery and delayed side effects of sedation for diagnostic imaging studies in children. *Pediatrics* **105(3),** http://www.pediatrics.org/cgi/content/full/105/3/e42.
25. Deady, A. and Gorman, D. (1997) Intravenous conscious sedation in children. *J. Intraven. Nurs.* **20(5),** 245–252.
26. Sanders, B. J., Potter, R. H., and Avery, D. R. (1994) The effect of sleep on conscious sedation. *J. Clin. Pediatr. Dent.* **18(3),** 211–214.
27. Informed consent, parental permission, and assent in pediatric practice. (1995) Committee on Bioethics, American Academy of Pediatrics. *Pediatrics* **95(2),** 314–317.
28. Keeter, S., Benator, R. M., Weinberg, S. M., and Hartenberg, M. A. (1990) Sedation in pediatric CT: national survey of current practice. *Radiology* **175(3),** 745–752.
29. Tung, R. T. and Bajaj, A. K. (1995) Safety of implantation of a cardioverter-defibrillator without general anesthesia in an electrophysiology laboratory. *Am. J. Cardiol.* **75(14),** 908–912.
30. Hollman, G. A., Elderbrook, M. K., and VanDenLangenberg, B. (1995) Results of a pediatric sedation program on head MRI scan success rates and procedure duration times. *Clin. Pediatr. (Phila.)* **34(6),** 300–305.
31. Strain, J. D., Harvey, L. A., Foley, L. C., and Campbell, J. B. (1986) Intravenously administered pentobarbital sodium for sedation in pediatric CT. *Radiology* **161(1),** 105–108.
32. Bauchner, H., Vinci, R., Bak, S., Pearson, C., and Corwin, M. J. (1996) Parents and procedures: a randomized controlled trial. *Pediatrics* **98(5),** 861–867.
33. Kuttner, L. (1989) Management of young children's acute pain and anxiety during invasive medical procedures. *Pediatrician* **16(1–2),** 39–44.
34. Zeltzer, L. K., Jay, S. M., and Fisher, D. M. (1989) The management of pain associated with pediatric procedures. *Pediatr. Clin. N. Am.* **36(4),** 941–964.
35. Graff, K. J., Kennedy, R. M., and Jaffe, D. M. (1996) Conscious sedation for pediatric orthopaedic emergencies. *Pediatr. Emerg. Care* **12(1),** 31–35.
36. Ramsay, M. A., Savege, T. M., Simpson, B. R., and Goodwin, R. (1974) Controlled sedation with alphaxalone-alphadolone. *Br. Med. J.* **2(920),** 656–659.

37. Chernik, D. A., Tucker, M., Gigli, B., Yoo, K., Paul, K., Laine, H., et al. (1992) Validity and reliability of the Neurobehavioral Assessment Scale. *J. Clin. Psychopharmacol.* **12(1),** 43–48.

38. Macnab, A. J., Levine, M., Glick, N., Phillips, N., Susak, L., and Elliott, M. (1994) The Vancouver sedative recovery scale for children: validation and reliability of scoring based on videotaped instruction. *Can. J. Anaesth.* **41(10),** 913–918.

39. Malviya, S., Voepel-Lewis, T., Tait, A., Merkel, S., Tremper, K., and Naughton N. Depth of Sedation in Children Undergoing Computerized Tomography: Validity and Reliability of the University of Michigan Sedation Scale (UMSS). *Br. J. Anaesth.* in press;in press:in press.

40. Higgins, T. L., Hearn, C. J., and Maurer, W. G. (1996) Conscious sedation: What an internist needs to know. *Clevel. Clin. J. Med.* **63(6),** 355–361.

41. Yaster, M., Nichols, D. G., Deshpande, J. K., and Wetzel, R. C. (1990) Midazolam-fentanyl intravenous sedation in children: case report of respiratory arrest. *Pediatrics* **86(3),** 463–467.

42. Greenberg, S. B., Faerber, E. N., and Aspinall, C. L. (1991) High dose chloral hydrate sedation for children undergoing CT. *J. Comput. Assisted Tomogr.* **15(3),** 467–469.

43. Greenberg, S. B., Faerber, E. N., Aspinall, C. L., and Adams, R. C. (1993) High-dose chloral hydrate sedation for children undergoing MR imaging: safety and efficacy in relation to age. *AJR Am. J. Roentgenol.* **161(3),** 639–641.

44. Hubbard, A. M., Markowitz, R. I., Kimmel, B., Kroger, M., and Bartko, M. B. (1992) Sedation for pediatric patients undergoing CT and MRI. *J. Comput. Assisted Tomogr.* **16(1),** 3–6.

45. Khan, L. C. and Lustik, S. J. (1997) Treatment of a paradoxical reaction to midazolam with haloperidol. *Anesth. Analg.* **85(1),** 213–215.

46. Knaack-Steinegger, R. and Schou, J. (1987) [Therapy of paradoxical reactions to midazolam in regional anesthesia]. *Anaesthesist* **36(3),** 143–146.

47. Thurston, T. A., Williams, C. G., and Foshee, S. L. (1996) Reversal of a paradoxical reaction to midazolam with flumazenil. *Anesth. Analg.* **83(1),** 192.

48. Honan, V. J. (1994) Paradoxical reaction to midazolam and control with flumazenil. *Gastrointest. Endosc.* **40(1),** 86–88.

49. Doyle, W. L., and Perrin, L. (1994) Emergence delirium in a child given oral midazolam for conscious sedation. *Ann. Emerg. Med.* **24(6),** 1173–1175.

50. Pandit, U. A., Kothary, S. P., Samra, S. K., Domino, E. F., and Pandit, S. K. (1983) Physostigmine fails to reverse clinical, psychomotor, or EEG effects of lorazepam. *Anesth. Analg.* **62(7),** 679–685.

51. Zeigler, V. L. and Brown, L. E. (1997) Conscious sedation in the pediatric population. Special considerations. *Crit. Care Nurs. Clin. N. Am.* **9(3),** 381–394.

52. Anderson, J. A. and Vann, W. F., Jr. (1988) Respiratory monitoring during pediatric sedation: pulse oximetry and capnography. *Pediatr. Dent.* **10(2),** 94–101.

53. Hart, L. S., Berns, S. D., Houck, C. S., and Boenning, D. A. (1997) The value of end-tidal CO_2 monitoring when comparing three methods of conscious sedation for children undergoing painful procedures in the emergency department. *Pediatr. Emerg. Care* **13(3),** 189–193.

54. Rohlfing, G. K., Dilley, D. C., Lucas, W. J., and Vann, W. F., Jr. (1998) The effect of supplemental oxygen on apnea and oxygen saturation during pediatric conscious sedation. *Pediatr. Dent.* **20(1),** 8–16.
55. Page, B. and Dallara, J. (1996) Metoclopramide in trauma CT scanning: preventing emesis of oral radiographic contrast. *Am. J. Emerg. Med.* **14(4),** 373–376.
56. Reversal of central nervous system effects by flumazenil after intravenous conscious sedation with midazolam: report of a multicenter clinical study. (1992) The Flumazenil in Intravenous Conscious Sedation with Midazolam Multicenter Study Group I. *Clin. Ther.* **14(6),** 861–877.

11

Recovery and Transport of Sedated Patients

Loree A. Collett, BSN, RN, Sheila A. Trouten, BSN, RN, and Terri Voepel-Lewis, MSN, RN

1. INTRODUCTION

Patients who receive sedation or analgesia for diagnostic and medical procedures remain at significant risk for associated adverse events until the pharmacologic effects of the sedative or analgesic agent(s) subside *(1)*. In some circumstances, patients may be at greater risk for problems after the procedure is completed, when painful or other stimuli are removed *(2,3)*. Vigilant physiologic monitoring and care of the sedated patient must therefore continue during transportation to recovery areas, and throughout the postprocedure period until the patient can be safely discharged to an unmonitored setting. Recent sedation guidelines and standards of care stipulate that such care be provided by qualified individuals throughout the sedation episode until discharge criteria are met *(1,4–7)*. The current emphasis on cost containment and efficiency in most health care settings may result in increased risk to the patient *(8)*. Transportation of sedated patients by nonqualified personnel or premature discharge of the patient may occur in busy diagnostic settings that prioritize rapid patient turnover. Such "production pressure" should never circumvent the caregiver's ability to provide adequate monitoring to sedated patients. This chapter examines important considerations for the monitoring and care of sedated patients during transportation and recovery.

2. TRANSPORTATION OF SEDATED PATIENTS

In some settings, patients remain in the procedure area for the duration of sedation including recovery. In others, patients must be moved from the diagnostic or treatment area to a centralized recovery area, a short stay unit, or an inpatient unit following completion of the procedure. Regardless of where the patient recovers, the patient's safety during transport must be assured *(9)*. Furthermore, unstable or medically compromised patients

From: *Contemporary Clinical Neuroscience: Sedation and Analgesia for Diagnostic and Therapeutic Procedures*
Edited by: S. Malviya, N. N. Naughton, and K. K. Tremper © Humana Press Inc., Totowa, NJ

Table 1
Information to Include in a Verbal Report
Upon Transferring the Care of the Sedated Patient

General information
Patient's age
Weight
Medication allergies
Pertinent medical history and risk factors for sedation
Total fasting time

Procedure
Sedative and analgesic agents; total dose and last time of administration
Reversal agents and time administered
Intravenous fluids
Procedure site; dressings; concerns

Patient's status
Vital signs
Level of sedation
Adverse events and their treatment

should be stabilized prior to transport. When the care of the patient is transferred from one caregiver to another, adequate communication of the patient's condition is the first consideration. Although the sedation documentation record should reflect the pertinent medical history, the procedural information, medications, and the patient's vital signs and physiologic status (*see* Chapter 10), a brief verbal report from one care provider to the next can serve to highlight critical information such as the patient's risk factors, medication history, and adverse events that may have occurred. Table 1 identifies information that should be included in the verbal report.

Equipment that should be available for sedation emergencies is presented in Chapter 10, Table 4. There are several considerations that help determine the necessary equipment for transportation. If the route from the procedure area to the recovery setting is remote and offers little access to medical help, the transportation team should carry more emergency equipment. Depending upon the patient's depth of sedation, continuous monitoring of oxygen saturation may be appropriate, and equipment to administer oxygen during transport may be necessary. For patients with significant cardiac disease, or for those who have undergone certain cardiac procedures, the transport stretcher should carry an electrocardiograph device, and in some cases, a defibrillator. If the patient remains deeply sedated and is therefore at risk for loss of airway reflexes, it is necessary to have appropriate airway, ventilation, and suctioning devices available.

Frequently, transportation of the sedated patient requires the assistance of more than one care provider. In some cases, unlicensed personnel may be utilized for such assistance, and in others, a physician or registered nurse should be in attendance. For example, patients who have experienced an adverse event or are at increased risk because of their medical history or the nature of the procedure, probably warrant the presence of additional medical staff during transportation. The Joint Committee on the Accreditation of Health Care Organizations (JCAHO) sedation and analgesia guidelines state that sufficient numbers of qualified personnel must be present when patients are moderately or deeply sedated *(7)*. This allows one person to be solely responsible for patient monitoring and care, while the other may attend to other tasks such as pushing the stretcher, procuring an elevator, or seeking medical help if necessary.

Occasionally, an unforeseen event occurs that impedes the smooth transport of sedated patients to the recovery area. Equipment failure is probably the most common of these events. It is important to check the proper functioning of monitoring and/or suctioning devices, including the battery life of such equipment. Furthermore, oxygen tanks should be checked to ensure an adequate supply. Less often, elevator failure or closed corridors may impede transportation. It may therefore be prudent to assess the route of transport prior to moving the patient. Additionally, the care provider should be aware of potential patient-related complications that may occur en route, and be familiar with the location of telephones and emergency crash carts. Finally, high-traffic public hallways should be avoided if possible to ensure efficient and uninterrupted transport of the patient.

3. MONITORING AND ASSESSMENT DURING RECOVERY

National and institutional guidelines specify the physiologic parameters that must be monitored and documented during the postprocedure period *(1,4,5,7–9)*. Generally, these parameters include the patient's ventilatory status, oxygenation, hemodynamic status, and level of consciousness *(1,8)*. The frequency of patient assessment and documentation during the recovery phase is dependent upon the general condition of the patient, the type and length of the procedure, and the types and amounts of medications administered *(1)*. Certain procedures, such as cardiac catheterization, angiography, bone marrow aspiration, and transcutaneous biopsies require regular monitoring of an incision site or dressing. Documentation requirements for ongoing physiologic monitoring are discussed in Chapter 10.

As during transportation, patients who remain moderately or deeply sedated require continuous monitoring of oxygen saturation for early detection of hypoxemia. Continuous observation and monitoring of ventilatory function by observation of respiratory activity or ausculation of breath sounds is also warranted in these patients. There is some evidence that monitoring of end-tidal carbon dioxide (CO_2) via capnography offers an advantage over the pulse oximeter in early detection of ventilatory changes that permits early intervention prior to the occurrence of hypoxemia *(10)*. Thus, certain sedation guidelines have added capnography as "desirable" monitoring for patients who are deeply sedated *(11)*, and others suggest that end-tidal CO_2 monitoring could become standard of practice for sedation monitoring in the near future *(12)*. A complete discussion of pulse oximetry and capnography monitoring is presented in Chapter 8.

Early intervention in response to changes in the patient's respiratory and ventilatory status is critical to the prevention of adverse events or complications. Stimulating the patient to breathe may be all that is required in patients whose depth of sedation has decreased the respiratory drive. The provision of supplemental oxygen will prevent the development of further hypoxemia; however, this may delay the detection of apnea by pulse oximetry. Monitoring of ventilatory status in these patients must therefore continue throughout the recovery period. Airway obstruction may be readily corrected with the head-tilt, chin-lift maneuver in some cases. The placement of oral or nasal airways may become necessary in others. Once placed, these devices should not be removed until it is determined that the patient's airway reflexes have returned.

Appropriate monitoring of cardiovascular status is warranted in high-risk patients to permit early detection of hemodynamic instability and facilitate appropriate intervention. The presence of pre-existing comorbidities and the nature of the diagnostic or medical procedure will determine whether continuous electrocariogram (ECG) monitoring or increased frequency of blood pressure monitoring is warranted. It is recommended that continuous ECG and regular noninvasive blood pressure monitoring (NIBPM) be implemented in patients with hypertension, or a history of significant cardiovascular disease or dysrhythmias *(1)*. Patients who undergo cardiac catheterizations for ablation or diagnostic reasons, electrophysiologic studies or cardioversion, and pacemaker procedures also warrant this level of monitoring. Hypotension is the most common cardiovascular complication that occurs during and following sedation and analgesia. Regular monitoring of the patient's circulatory status, including heart rate, blood pressure, temperature, skin color, and peripheral pulses, will identify problems so that appropriate intervention

Table 2
Suggested Calculation of Fluid Requirements

Weight (kg)	mL/h
<10 kg	4 mL/kg/hr
10–20 kg	40 mL + 2 mL/kg above 10 kg
>20 kg	60 mL + 1 mL/kg above 20 kg

can be implemented. Furthermore, a careful assessment of the patient's fluid status will facilitate appropriate volume replacement. This requires calculation of the patient's volume deficit by determining the duration of fasting and fluid maintenance requirements (*see* Table 2).

Hypothermia is a less common problem that nonetheless warrants monitoring and early intervention. Inadvertent hypothermia occurs more often in the perioperative environment, but can also occur in patients who are sedated for diagnostic and therapeutic procedures (*13*). Sedative agents can alter the threshold temperatures in the thermoregulatory centers in the brain, placing the patient at risk for hypothermia. Additionally, certain patient populations are more vulnerable to thermoregulatory failure, including the elderly and infants. In addition to compromising patient comfort, hypothermia may decrease drug metabolism, resulting in prolonged sedation. Furthermore, hypothermia can impair coagulation, which can lead to complications in some patients, such as those who have undergone angiography or catheterization. It is therefore important to assess the patient's temperature upon arrival to the recovery area, and implement strategies that will preserve normothermia. The use of warm blankets is generally sufficient; however, the use of a convective warmer such as the Bair Hugger® may be needed in some cases.

Pain during diagnostic and therapeutic procedures is generally limited to the procedure itself; however, it may occasionally persist or worsen during the recovery period. Some procedures that are associated with pain include percutaneous nephrostomies, liver biopsies, bone marrow biopsies, and angiography. Additionally, some patients have pre-existing conditions such as osteoarthritis or spasticity that result in pain even during non-painful procedures. Pain can be readily assessed in many patients using self-reported pain scores. The 0–10 number scale (0 = no pain; 10 = worst pain) is the most commonly used pain tool in the clinical setting. For young children, and for those who cannot conceptualize numbers, there are other types of self-report pain tools available that can help to identify the intensity of pain (*14–16*). The FACES scale is the most common of these (Table 3). In patients who cannot self-report pain because of age, cognitive impairment,

Table 3
The FACES Pain Tool for Use in Young Children

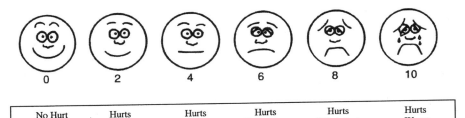

No Hurt	Hurts Little Bit	Hurts Little More	Hurts Even More	Hurts Whole Lot	Hurts Worst

Reprinted with permission from ref. *(35)*, copyrighted by Mosby, Inc., 2001.

or inability to verbalize, behavioral observation techniques are available to provide the caregiver with an objective means to assess pain. The Faces, Legs, Activity, Cry and Consolability (FLACC) scale is an example of one such tool *(17)* (Table 4). Prior to administering analgesics during the recovery period, the care provider must assess the dose(s), timing, and route(s) of administration of previous sedatives, analgesics, and their reversal. Doses of opioid analgesics should take into consideration their synergistic effects with sedatives, with particular attention given to the duration of action of these agents. The pharmacology of sedatives and analgesics is reviewed in detail in Chapters 6 and 7. The use of non-opioid analgesics, including acetaminophen or ibuprofen, may be the drugs of choice for mild to moderate postprocedural discomfort. It is important to differentiate pain that may be caused by a major procedural complication from discomfort that is anticipated as a result of the procedure. Hemmorhage, perforation of a vital organ, or myocardial infarction are rare adverse events, but should be ruled out when pain is present.

Certain sedative and analgesic agents are associated with a high incidence of nausea and vomiting *(18)*. Additionally, pain, obesity, hypovolemia, procedural interventions such as the use of contrast agents, and early resumption of oral intake may contribute to postprocedural nausea and vomiting *(9,19)*. Although administration of antiemetics may be beneficial, virtually all anti-emetics have sedative effects that may prolong the patient's recovery.

4. DISCHARGE CRITERIA

Ongoing monitoring of the patient's condition should continue until the patient has achieved a stable status that is close to baseline, and the

Table 4
FLACC Behavioral Pain Tool *(17)*

		Score
Face	0 = No particular expression or smile	0
	1 = Occasional grimace/frown, withdrawn or disinterested	1
	2 = Frequent/constant quivering chin, clenched jaw	2
Legs	0 = Normal position or relaxed	0
	1 = Uneasy, restless, tense	1
	2 = Kicking, or legs drawn up	2
Activity	0 = Lying quietly, normal position, moves easily	0
	1 = Squirming, shifting back and forth, tense	1
	2 = Arched, rigid or jerking	2
Cry	0 = No cry	0
	1 = Moans or whimpers; occasional complaint	1
	2 = Crying steadily, screams or sobs, frequent complaints	2
Consolability	0 = Content and relaxed	0
	1 = Reassured by occasional touching, hugging, or being talked to. Distractable	1
	2 = Difficult to console or comfort	2
	Total:	

Reprinted from *Pediatric Nursing,* 1997, Volume 23, Number 3, p. 294. Reprinted with permission of the publisher, Jannetti Publications, Inc., East Holly Ave Box 56, Pitman, NJ 08071–0056; phone (856) 256–2300; fax *(856)* 589–7463. For a sample copy of the journal, please contact the publisher.

patient can be safely discharged to an unmonitored setting *(4–7)*. Although there is no consensus on specific discharge criteria, in general, the patient must have achieved a stable respiratory and hemodynamic status, and be awake and alert *(20–23)*. Recent guidelines of the American Society of Anesthesiologists (ASA) state that, "Discharge criteria should be designed to minimize the risk of central nervous system or cardiorespiratory depression after discharge from observation by trained personnel" *(1)*. Furthermore, the JCAHO recommends that sedated patients should be discharged from the post-sedation recovery area by qualified independent practitioners or according to criteria approved by the licensed independent practitioner staff *(7)*. Suggested discharge criteria are presented in Table 5.

Table 5
Suggested Criteria for Discharge
Following Sedation and Analgesia *(1,20–22,34)*

1. Patients should be easily aroused, alert and oriented, or returned to their baseline status (i.e. infants, cognitive impairment).
2. Vital signs should be stable and within acceptable limits
3. Patient is not at risk for resedation (i.e., sufficient time has elapsed since administration of reversal agents)
4. The patient's protective reflexes have returned, and there is no risk for airway obstruction or aspiration
5. Pain is minimal and can be easily controlled in the post-discharge setting
6. Nausea is controlled and can be managed in the post-discharge setting
7. Outpatients should be discharged into the care of a responsible adult
8. Outpatients must be provided with written instructions regarding medications, activity, and emergency phone contacts

When evaluating the patient's readiness for discharge, particular attention should be given to the level of consciousness and alertness. Patients who have received sedative agents are often readily aroused and responsive in busy, stimulating environments, but may become very sedated and unresponsive when left undisturbed *(3,24–27)*. Cases of resedation following discharge have been reported, resulting in return to the emergency department in several cases *(26,27)*. In one of these cases, the scheduled procedure had been aborted because of failed sedation, yet the child became excessively sedated at home *(26)*. This case emphasizes the importance of monitoring all patients who have received a sedative agent, even if the sedative effects are not initially apparent. In another case, a child became resedated en route home, obstructed his airway, and died *(28)*. These cases emphasize the importance of rigorous discharge criteria. The patient should not only be easily aroused, but should be able to maintain wakefulness when left undisturbed.

A recent study suggested that bedside nurses may tend to overestimate the patient's level of alertness at discharge *(29)*. Other investigators have warned against such liberalization of the definition of sedation and discharge readiness *(30)*. Efficiency and the need for rapid patient throughput in the diagnostic setting must not compromise the safety of sedated patients. The caregiver must assure that each patient has stringently met discharge criteria prior to releasing the patient to an unmonitored setting, even if this means extended monitoring or escalation of care.

The requirement that patients be able to retain oral fluids prior to discharge remains controversial. Most discharge criteria do not include a provision for oral intake, and many believe that early resumption of oral intake may increase the likelihood of nausea and vomiting. The decision to feed the patient should be individualized, and should never be attempted until it is certain that the patient has regained protective reflexes. Perhaps more importantly, adequate volume status should be assured by the appropriate replacement with intravenous (iv) fluids.

Previous investigators have demonstrated a significant incidence of delayed adverse events following discharge from the sedation recovery area *(25,27,31,32)*. Of particular concern is the high incidence of agitation and aggressive behavior in children following sedation *(26)*. This effect may be more pronounced in children following administration of chloral hydrate. Furthermore, a high incidence of motor imbalance, that lasts up to 24 h in some cases has been reported *(26)*. Patients and parents should be educated regarding the potential for delayed side effects, so that their occurrence is less distressing and appropriate care can be provided.

Previous investigators have suggested that administration of reversal agents may expedite readiness for discharge (*see* benzodiazepine flumazenil citation). However, the routine use of reversal agents is not advocated, and may result in premature discharge of patients in some cases. In the event that reversal agents have been administered, a sufficient time must elapse after administration to ensure that resedation or renarcotization will not occur. For inpatients, a verbal report must be given to the unit staff prior to transferring their care. The report should include all of the elements discussed in Table 1.

5. DISCHARGE EDUCATION

Plans for discharge should begin with pre-procedure instructions so that appropriate planning can take place. It is important that discharge instructions be provided verbally and in writing to the person who will be responsible for the patient's care following discharge. In this manner, families can refer to the written instructions at home when adverse events may occur. Instructions should be concise, but should include the medications administered, expected behavior and side effects, activity restrictions, resumption of diet, symptoms that warrant follow-up care, procedural instructions, and emergency contact phone numbers *(1,9,33)*. Table 6 presents an example of discharge instructions. A copy of the discharge instructions should be kept in the medical record.

Table 6
Recommended Discharge Instructions for Sedated Patients

1. Sedative and analgesic agents administered
2. Potential adverse effects following discharge
3. Recommended diet post-sedation
4. Recommended supervision of the patient (i.e., close supervision of children who may have motor imbalance)
5. Activity restrictions, including when to resume driving, work, school, and which activities to avoid (i.e., bicycle riding, playground equipment, etc.)
6. Signs and symptoms that require a call to the physician or follow-up care
7. Procedure-related restrictions and care (i.e., dressing change, etc.)

6. SUMMARY

The safety of sedated patients will be optimized by adherence to national and institutional guidelines throughout the sedation episode until the patient is fully recovered. Sedated patients require the same degree of vigilant monitoring by appropriately trained personnel during transport and recovery that is required during the procedure itself. Finally, specific discharge criteria and careful patient/caregiver education regarding the potential for delayed side effects will promote the patient's well-being following discharge.

REFERENCES

1. Practice guidelines for sedation and analgesia by non-anesthesiologists. (1996) A report by the American Society of Anesthesiologists Task Force on Sedation and Analgesia by Non-Anesthesiologists. *Anesthesiology* **84(2),** 459–471.
2. Coté, C. J. (1994) Sedation for the pediatric patient. A review. Pediatr. Clin. N. Am. **41(1),** 31–58.
3. Zeltzer, L. K., Jay, S. M., and Fisher, D. M. (1989) The management of pain associated with pediatric procedures. *Pediatr. Clin. N. Am.* **36(4),** 941–964.
4. American Academy of Pediatrics Committee on Drugs (1992) Guidelines for monitoring and management of pediatric patients during and after sedation for diagnostic and therapeutic procedures. *Pediatrics* **89(6 Pt 1),** 1110–1105.
5. Guidelines for the elective use of conscious sedation, deep sedation and general anesthesia in pediatric dental patients. (1998) *Pediatr. Dent.* **21,** 68–73.
6. Clinical policy for procedural sedation and analgesia in the emergency department. (1998) American College of Emergency Physicians. *Ann. Emerg. Med.* **31(5),** 663–177.
7. Joint Commission on Accreditation of Healthcare Organizations (2001) Comprehensive Accreditation Manual for Hospitals: The Official Handbook, in JCAHO, Oakbrook Terrace, IL: http://www.jcaho.org/standards_frm.html.
8. Dlugose, D. (1997) Risk management considerations in conscious sedation. *Crit. Care Nurs. Clin. N. Am.* **9(3),** 429–440.

9. Zeigler, V. L. and Brown, L. E. (1997) Conscious sedation in the pediatric population. Special considerations. *Crit. Care Nurs. Clin. N. Am.* **9(3)**, 381–394.
10. Croswell, R. J., Dilley, D. C., Lucas, W. J., and Vann, W. F., Jr. (1995) A comparison of conventional versus electronic monitoring of sedated pediatric dental patients. *Pediatr. Dent.* **17(5)**, 332–329.
11. Wilson, S., Creedon, R. L., George, M., and Troutman, K. (1996) A history of sedation guidelines: where we are headed in the future. *Pediatr. Dent.* **18(3)**, 194–199.
12. Yaney, L. L. (1998) Intravenous conscious sedation. Physiologic, pharmacologic, and legal implications for nurses. *J. Intraven. Nurs.* **21(1)**, 9–19.
13. Sessler, D. I. (1994) Temperature Monitoring, in *Anesthesia*, 4th ed. (Cucchiara, R. F., Miller, E. D., Reves, J. G., Roizen, M. F., and Savarese, J. J., eds.), Churchill Livingstone, New York, NY, p. 1363–1382.
14. Beyer, J. E., Denyes, M. J., and Villarruel, A. M. (1992) The creation, validation, and continuing development of the Oucher: a measure of pain intensity in children. *J. Pediatr. Nurs.* **7(5)**, 335–346.
15. Hester, N., Foster, R., and Kristensen K. (1990) Measurement of pain in children: Generalizability and validity of the pain ladder and the poker chip tool, in *Advances in Pain Research Therapy* (Tyler, D. C., and Krane, E. J., eds.), Raven, New York, NY, pp. 79–93.
16. Wong, D. L., Hockenberry-Eaton, M., and Wilson D. (1999) Reaction of Child and Family to Illness and Hospitalization, in *Nursing Care of Infants and Children*, 6th ed. (Whaley, L., and Wong, D. L., eds.), Mosby-Year Book, Inc., St. Louis, MO, p. 1153.
17. Merkel, S. I., Voepel-Lewis, T., Shayevitz, J. R., and Malviya, S. (1997) The FLACC: a behavioral scale for scoring postoperative pain in young children. *Pediatr. Nurs.* **23(3)**, 293–297.
18. Malviya, S., Voepel-Lewis, T., Eldevik, O. P., Rockwell, D. T., Wong, J. H., and Tait, A. R. (2000) Sedation and general anaesthesia in children undergoing MRI and CT: adverse events and outcomes. *Br. J. Anaesth.* **84(6)**, 743–748.
19. Lazear, S. E. (1999) Conscious Sedation. Continuing Education for Michigan Nurses **(1053)**, 29–75.
20. Deady, A. and Gorman, D. (1997) Intravenous conscious sedation in children. *J. Intraven. Nurs.* **20(5)**, 245–252.
21. Somerson, S. J., Husted, C. W., and Sicilia, M. R. (1995) Insights into conscious sedation. *Am. J. Nurs.* **95(6)**, 26–32; quiz 33.
22. Proudfoot, J. (1995) Analgesia, anesthesia, and conscious sedation. *Emerg. Med. Clin. N. Am.* **13(2)**, 357–379.
23. Shaw, C., Weaver, C. S., and Schneider, L. (1996) Conscious sedation: a multidisciplinary team approach. *J. Post. Anesth. Nurs.* **11(1)**, 13–19.
24. Frush, D. P., Bisset, G. S., 3rd, and Hall, S. C. (1996) Pediatric sedation in radiology: the practice of safe sleep. *AJR Am. J. Roentgenol.* **167(6)**, 1381–1387.
25. Coté, C. J., Karl, H. W., Notterman, D. A., Weinberg, J. A., and McCloskey, C. (2000) Adverse sedation events in pediatrics: analysis of medications used for sedation. *Pediatrics* **106(4)**, 633–644.
26. Malviya, S. (2000) Prolonged recovery and delayed side effects of sedation

for diagnostic imaging studies in children. *Pediatrics* **105(3)**, http://www.
pediatrics.org/cgi/content/full/105/3/e42.

27. Malviya, S., Voepel-Lewis, T., and Tait, A. R. (1998) Adverse events and risk
factors associated with the sedation of children by nonanesthesiologists [pub-
lished erratum appears in *Anesth. Analg.* Feb; **86(2)**, 227. *Anesth. Analg.* **85(6)**,
1207–1213.

28. Coté, C. J., Notterman, D. A., Karl, H. W., Weinberg, J. A., and McCloskey, C.
(2000) Adverse sedation events in pediatrics: a critical incident analysis of
contributing factors. *Pediatrics* **105(4 Pt 1)**, 805–814.

29. Malviya, S., Voepel-Lewis, T., Tait, A., Merkel, S., Tremper, K., and
Naughton, (2002) N. Depth of Sedation in Children Undergoing Computerized
Tomography: Validity and Reliability of the University of Michigan Sedation
Scale (UMSS). *Br. J. Anaesth.* 88(2), 241–245.

30. Coté, C. J. (1995) Monitoring guidelines: do they make a difference? *AJR Am.
J. Roentgenol.* **165(4)**, 910–912.

31. Kao, S. C., Adamson, S. D., Tatman, L. H., and Berbaum, K. S. (1999) A
survey of post-discharge side effects of conscious sedation using chloral
hydrate in pediatric CT and MR imaging. *Pediatr. Radiol.* 29(4), 287–290.

32. Slovis, T. L., Parks, C., Reneau, D., Becker, C. J., Hersch, J., Carver, C. D., et al.
(1993) Pediatric sedation: short-term effects. *Pediatr. Radiol.* **23(5)**, 345–348.

33. Algren, C. L. and Algren, J. T. (1997) Pediatric sedation. Essentials for the
perioperative nurse. *Nurs. Clin. N. Am.* **32(1)**, 17–30.

34. Frush, D. P. and Bisset, G. S., 3rd. (1997) Sedation of children for emergency
imaging. *Radiol. Clin. N. Am.* **35(4)**, 789–797.

35. Wong, D. L., Hockenberry-Eaton, M., Wilson, D., Winkelstein, M. L., and
Schwartz, P. (2001) *Wong's Essentials of Pediatric Nursing,* 6th ed., St. Louis,
MO, p. 1301.

12

Quality Assurance and Continuous Quality Improvement in Sedation Analgesia

J. Elizabeth Othman, MS, RN

1. INTRODUCTION

Technological and pharmacological advances have prompted the movement of painful invasive procedures and diagnostics away from traditional operating rooms and the direct purview of the anesthesiologist. The need to assure a higher level of care and consistent quality outcomes in a decentralized environment is particularly challenging. This chapter discusses the application of principles and concepts of Quality Assurance (QA) and Continuous Quality Improvement (CQI) to Sedation Analgesia practice.

2. SEDATION ANALGESIA AND THE JCAHO

Traditionally, the operating room was the standard location for many procedures requiring patient sedation. The operating room offers a highly standardized and predictable environment in which to perform high-risk procedures. In this highly controlled setting, functions and required competencies are well-defined, standardized and monitored. In addition, processes and outcomes are formally monitored and reported. Indeed, largely because of mandates from regulatory agencies such as the Joint Commission on the Accreditation of Healthcare Organizations (JCAHO), the processes are predictable across health care organizations in the United States. Over several decades, the anesthesiology, surgery, and nursing professions have observed, monitored, defined and redefined, researched, and developed safer and more efficient perioperative practices. New anesthetic agents have been developed, and monitoring equipment has become more user-friendly and affordable (1).

In recent years, the double-edged sword of cost control and technological advances has prompted the movement of procedures out of the operating room into hospital and ambulatory care procedure rooms, the patient's bedside' and the physician's office (2). In order to complete the procedure and

From: *Contemporary Clinical Neuroscience: Sedation and Analgesia for Diagnostic and Therapeutic Procedures*
Edited by: S. Malviya, N. N. Naughton, and K. K. Tremper © Humana Press Inc., Totowa, NJ

keep the patient comfortable, sedation and/or analgesia is administered. The aim of sedation analgesia is to minimize patient anxiety, pain, and/or movement in order to safely and efficiently complete a treatment or procedure.

With the higher volume of procedures moving out of the well-controlled operating room environment with its proscribed peri-operative processes, reports of patient problems, injury, and even death began to surface *(3)*. Potent sedating agents that are widely available for use by non-anesthesiologists have been implicated in many cases. In an unregulated environment, many of the regimens so deeply ingrained in safe Operating Room practice had been shelved. Professional organizations and associations attempted to define standards of care for patients undergoing "conscious sedation," but unfortunately, during a period of cost constraints, health care administrators and even practitioners were reluctant to institute practices that would add personnel and equipment costs to an already strained budget.

As it did at the turn of the century, when it began regulating surgical practice, the JCAHO turned its attention to regulating sedation practice by non-anesthesiologists. The most significant early development for the regulation of "conscious sedation" occurred with the publication of the 1994 JCAHO standards of care *(2)*. Health care organizations were now required to implement a single standard of care across the institution—regardless of location or circumstances—whenever patients in any setting received for any purpose, by any route, sedation or analgesia that might reasonably be expected to result in the loss of protective reflexes. These standards required hospitals to define the practice of sedation by non-anesthesiologists to conform to the standards in place for anesthesiologists. The JCAHO now required that institutions practicing "conscious sedation" provide sufficient qualified staff and appropriate equipment for the assessment, monitoring, care, and resuscitation of patients. In addition, the JCAHO mandated that the "conscious sedation" process be monitored for adverse events and patterns *(4)*.

3. THE 2001 SEDATION STANDARDS

In previous editions of the JCAHO Comprehensive Accreditation Manual for Hospitals (CAMH), sedation was not an integral part of the Anesthesia Standards. In 2001, the JCAHO included the sedation standards as part of the Anesthesia Standards *(5)*. Sedation was conceptualized as continuum of increasingly deeper sedation with defined points along this continuum, as depicted in Fig. 1. These defined points serve as a measurable scale of sedation levels from 0 to 4. This change paralleled the American Society of Anesthesiologists (ASA) Committee on Quality Management definition of sedation, as occurring on a continuum from minimal sedation to anesthesia *(6)*.

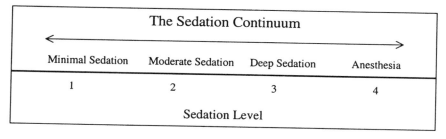

Fig. 1. The sedation continuum.

Thus, references to anesthesia now became sedation and anesthesia. There is now a clear intent that patient care, along the entire sedation continuum, must be of the same standard. These revised standards retained the previous requirements regarding personnel, equipment, assessment, monitoring, and documentation. The term "conscious sedation" was replaced with the term "moderate sedation". The level of sedation beyond moderate, "deep sedation," had now been identified, defined, and recognized as within the purview of the non-anesthesiologist. The adoption of a continuum (Fig. 1) as a framework for managing sedation now mandated that specific requirements be set regarding the capabilities and qualifications of the practitioner ordering and overseeing the sedation.

Because of patient variability and the unpredictable nature of pharmacological response, this continuum is a slippery slope, as shown in Fig. 2, which requires specific practitioner skills in order to maintain the desired level of sedation and to be able to rescue the patient from the next, deeper level of sedation. Since a patient can easily slip into a deeper than desired level of sedation—with the concomitant respiratory, hemodynamic and cardiac risks—it is imperative that a quality improvement mechanism exists for tracking, analyzing, and improving the outcomes of patients who receive moderate and deep sedation. Any patient can be expected to slip into a deeper than desired state of sedation.

As a result, in addition to assessment and monitoring requirements, a clear delineation of specific competencies for non-anesthesiologists who practice moderate and deep sedation is now required *(5)*. The organization is responsible for assuring that only competent individuals participate in sedation analgesia activities and that the competency is current. The 2001 JCAHO standards also strengthened the requirement for quality monitoring for sedation. The requirement specifically states: "Outcomes of patients undergoing moderate and deep sedation are collected and analyzed in the aggregate in order to identify opportunities to improve care" *(5,7)*. A quality improvement

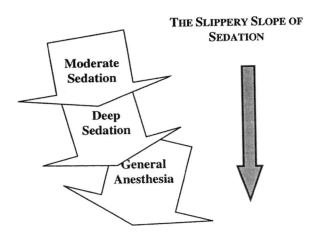

Fig. 2. The slippery slope of sedation.

process must exist for tracking, analyzing, and improving the outcomes of patients who receive moderate and deep sedation. Since sedation has a relatively low occurrence of adverse events but a high risk factor, tracking in the aggregate allows for discernment of low threshold activities and the ability to compare results both internally and externally. Over time, the JCAHO has adopted performance improvement standards that contribute value to the patient and the health care organization, with the goal of improved outcomes and efficiency, which in turn lead to better yet more economical care. The standards specific to quality improvement are found in the Performance Improvement (PI) Section of the JCAHO Standards Manual *(5)*. These general requirements—that data be systematically collected, analyzed and acted upon for the purpose of process improvement—apply in the specific to the practice of sedation. Selected standards are listed in Table 1.

4. THE QUALITY MOVEMENT

Over the years, the conceptualization and measurement of health care quality has undergone considerable maturation. Quality Assurance (QA) is a process of continual monitoring and periodic evaluation of the quality and appropriateness of patient care as defined by regulatory and professional entities *(3,8)*. Traditionally, QA has been a focus of individual services or departments and may include individual case review.

Continuous Quality Improvement (CQI) arises out of the early work of Deming and Juran in the manufacturing sector *(9)*. The concepts underlying CQI include a focus on key processes, trending, and analysis of data leading

Table 1
JCAHO Performance Improvement Standards
Applicable to Sedation Analgesia Practice

JCAHO performance improvement/chapter (reference)	Selected performance improvement standards
PI/3 *(1)*	The organization collects data to monitor its performance
PI/4 *(1)*	Appropriate statistical techniques are used to analyze and display data
PI/4 *(2)*	The organization compares its performance over time and with other sources of information
PI/4 *(3)*	Undesirable patterns or trends in performance and sentinel event are intensively analyzed
PI/4 *(4)*	The organization identifies changes that will lead to improved performance and reduce sentinel events

to improvements that are monitored and sustainable, simplification of work processes, elimination of rework and waste, identification and satisfaction of customers, and teamwork across boundaries *(10)*.

5. DEVELOPMENT OF A QUALITY IMPROVEMENT PROGRAM FOR SEDATION ANALGESIA

In order to achieve a systematic, ongoing Quality Improvement Program for Sedation Analgesia, a systematic multidisciplinary approach to the development of the integral components of the program is essential *(11)*. Such development is best approached by a small team composed of members who are knowledgeable about the process and desired outcomes of sedation. This team should include members from anesthesiology as well as several medical and nursing specialty areas, pharmacy, computer information systems, and the institutional QI committee. Potential objectives for a team are listed in Table 2.

5.1. Development of Quality Indicators

In order to develop quality indicators, an understanding of the conceptualization and language of "quality" is helpful. Avedis Donabedian, a pioneer in the development of quality indicators, recommended that the assessment of health care quality should include the three components of structure, process, and outcomes *(12)*.

5.1.1. Structure Indicators

This aspect of care examines the existing structural component of care and resources that the organization has to work with. Typically, structural

Table 2
Objectives for a Multidisciplinary Sedation Analgesia QI Team

- Development of quality indicators
- Development of the indicator measurements, including operational definitions, and formulas
- Development of standard report format(s) and frequency
- Development of a systematic continuous data collection methodology includ ing other variables of interest
- Development of a process for transforming data into ongoing information using statistics, graphic representations, aggregation and breakdown of the data
- Development of processes for practice evaluation, improvements, and re-evaluation

components of care refer to resources such as numbers, preparation, and qualifications of staff, patient acuity, and number of operating rooms. These measurements often provide the foundation of understanding and describing the process of care.

5.1.2. Process Indicators

Process indicators evaluate how the work of the organization is done. Understanding the way care is actually delivered is critical to the formulation of process indicators. Key events that should be evaluated include decision-making, documentation of care, and the appropriateness and timeliness of care. The examination of process can lead to a heightened awareness of inter-dependencies and areas of variability. These aspects of care are typically measured as counts of inclusion (how often did an appropriate event occur) or counts of exclusion (how many times was an appropriate intervention not instituted). Often what we work with (structure) and how we do our work (process) has a bearing (good or bad) on the outcome of care.

5.1.3. Outcome Indicators

This aspect of care evaluation examines the results of the work done in an organization. Outcomes are often directly linked to the process and are highly influenced by the structure. Although all three aspects are important, early health care quality evaluations focused on structure, and more recently, outcome indicators have taken precedence.

Structure indicators are usually the most obvious and easiest to measure; therefore, initial quality improvement efforts focus on these. As information is gathered and more questions surface, process indicators become more useful. As a fuller understanding of a process is achieved, outcome indicators can be defined and measured. If a process is stable—the resources used and methods employed remain unchanged and constant—outcome indicators are the measurement of choice. Stable processes are those that have outcomes that are consistent and predictable within a very small range of acceptable variability *(13)*. However, in clinical care it is frequently difficult to predict or control the human response, both in the patient and the caregiver. The unpredictability of such responses, coupled with the constant introduction of new technologies and pharmacology, and with management pressures for cost containment, makes it critical to evaluate the structure and process of care as an "early warning system." Changes in the measurements of early warning indicators may foreshadow a change in outcomes. Indeed, if meaningful process indicators are selected, negative trending over time can indicate a risk of deteriorating outcomes. However, unless quality indicators are constantly refined and validated it is possible to have unacceptable outcomes even without activation of the early warning system. Thus, knowledge of the process being evaluated and the interrelationships among its activities is critical in developing indicators.

5.1.4. Quality Indicators

Quality indicators are quantitative measures that can be used as a guide to monitor and evaluate the quality of important clinical activities. As numerical representations of key functions or processes, they represent an evaluation of that activity. Sequential measurements can provide information regarding the stability of the process or activity or the variations therein. This is the essence of the monitoring. The purpose of these measurements is to identify opportunities for improvement, which is the foundation of continuous quality improvement. Thus, the development of appropriate indicators is critical for valid and useful monitoring of important clinical processes *(10,11)*.

5.2. Developing Quality Indicators for Sedation Analgesia

An important first step in developing indicators for sedation analgesia is an understanding of the goals and key activities of the sedation analgesia process. A review of the literature—including clinical guidelines, interviews with practitioners and patients, and the use of quality improvement tools such as flowcharting, cause-and-effect diagrams, and root-cause analyses— is often helpful in identifying the critical elements of the activity *(2,15)*. These critical elements can then be categorized as structure, process, and outcome variables.

A very useful tool in understanding a process is a flow diagram or flowchart. A process flowchart is a symbolic representation of the processes or activities involved in achieving a goal or an end result. An example of a

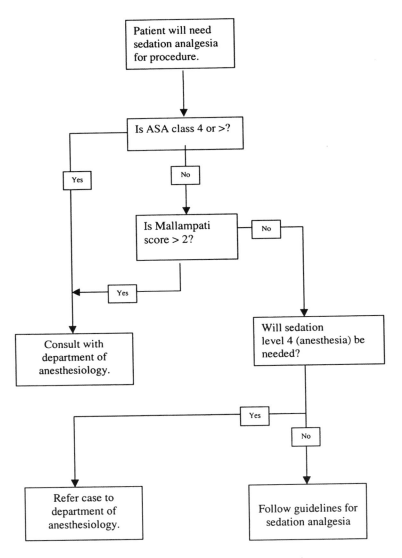

Fig. 3. Sedation decision-making flowchart.

flowchart for a patient undergoing a diagnostic procedure with sedation analgesia is shown in Fig. 3. This flowchart, even at a fairly macro level, reveals
several points for quality monitoring that are listed in Table 3.

Within the sedation process, several preventive measures must be taken
to protect the patient and to minimize the occurrence and the severity of
adverse events such as oxygen desaturation and respiratory arrest. For example,

Table 3
Examples of Monitoring Opportunities Derived from Figure 3

- Appropriate privileging and competencies of physicians targeting moderate or deep sedation
- Documentation of ASA physical status
- Proportion of procedures in which the target level of sedation is achieved
- Frequency of exceeding intended depth of sedation, particularly deep sedation

Table 4
Development of Quality Indicators

Aspect of Care: Maintenance of Respiratory Function

Example of key activities	Possible indicators	Indicator type
Airway assessment	• Airway assessment completed	Process
	• Anesthesia consult for Mallampati Score >2	Process
NPO protocols	• Occurrence of nausea	Process
	• Occurrence of aspiration	Outcome
Supplemental oxygen	• Supplemental oxygen immediately available	Structure
Pulse oximetry	• Compliance with pulse oximetry	Process
	• Occurrence of O_2 desaturation >10%	Outcome
Reversal agents	• Occurrence of use of reversal agent	Outcome
Monitoring protocols	• Compliance with ECG guidelines	Process
Prevention of respiratory arrest	• Occurrence of respiratory arrest	Outcome
	• Occurrence of intubation	Outcome

patients are screened for respiratory disease and airway abnormalities, fasting protocols are followed, oxygen saturation is monitored, and oxygen is readily available, as are reversal agents. Any one or several of these preventive activities could be quantified and used as an indicator. In this example, many structural, process and outcome indicators may be measured. Several possibilities are indicated in Table 4.

Not all indicators are equally predictive or useful. Even with computer-assisted data collection, there is a human resource cost. Numerous and very complex indicators may not necessarily yield the quality monitoring results or quality improvement as anticipated. Thinking economically, it is important to select indicators that are clinically meaningful—those than can act as predicators of patient care, can be linked to a desired outcome of care, and are reflective of activity that is within the realm of the organization's or practitioner's ability to change. For example, quality assessment activities in the early post-implementation phase of sedation guidelines often focus on documentation of particular activities such as consent, airway assessment, and fasting duration. Once the basics are in place, the focus should shift to clinical outcome-related indicators.

Adherence to documentation standards can and should be measured on an ad hoc basis as part of a medical record audit or review *(14)*. For example, completion of an airway assessment is an important step in the sedation process, but does not directly relate to the occurrence of respiratory arrest. However, the measurement via chart audit of noncompliance can, at the very least, speak to noncompliance with documentation standards, and perhaps more meaningfully, as an early warning of high-risk behavior.

Even with careful assessment and monitoring, it is not possible to always maintain a patient's position along the sedation continuum. Patients may have idiosyncratic responses to central nervous system (CNS) depressants, and the synergistic effect of a sedative and opioid is difficult to predict. With any administration of sedatives or combination sedatives and analgesics, patients are at risk for a deeper than targeted level of sedation with concomitant respiratory and cardiovascular compromise. Thus, the most common adverse outcomes relate to oxygenation, circulation, and consciousness. At their most extreme, these outcomes are expressed clinically as respiratory arrest, cardiac arrest, and death *(16,17)*.

Measurement of quality of care provided may be reflected in the incidence of respiratory arrest, cardiac arrest, and death. Since these outcomes are relatively rare, intermediate steps or outcomes that may lead to these adverse events may be defined and tracked. Examples include severely decreased oxygen saturation, aspiration, arrhythmia, and hypotension. Thus, the measurement of an indicator such as oxygen desaturation >10% may be helpful in indicating practice patterns that may lead to the occurrence of a major adverse event.

Other outcome indicators may be patient-related, such as patient satisfaction or pain and comfort scores during the procedure. Management-related indicators, such as the total time needed to do the procedure, may also be useful in the aggregate analysis of the sedation process. Thus, acceptable quality of care may be indicated by successful completion of the procedure in a safe and efficient manner while optimizing patient comfort, avoiding major complications, and minimizing the occurrence of other complications.

Occurrences are expressed as rates. A rate of occurrence or a rate of compliance is a key measurement in Quality Improvement *(8)*. An indicator is measured by the number of occurrences when compared to the number of potential occurrences. In order to be precise, the indicator should be clearly defined or operationalized. Considering the example of oxygen desaturation, the indicator may be defined as: "Occurrence of oxygen desaturation greater than 10% of baseline for more than 30 s as measured by pulse oximetry." The quantifiers of 10% and 30 s can be determined by literature review or clinician consensus. The occurrence of this event must be recorded, counted, and expressed as a rate of occurrence before it can be used as an indicator of clinical practice.

The following formula is used to express the rate of occurrence:

$$\text{Rate of occurrence} = \frac{\text{Number of occurrences (during the specified time period)}}{\text{Number of cases (during the specified time period)}} \times 100$$

The rate of occurrence derived over one specified time period may not, in itself, be useful in describing clinical practice or in identifying an opportunity for improvement. Variables such as a patient population that is not representative of the overall population must be considered. However, when such measurements are collected over time, the data can yield important information. Furthermore, when graphically represented as a trend line, the data may indicate changes in clinical practice that with further study could point to opportunities for improvement. Fig. 4 demonstrates, in a run chart, trends in the rate of oxygen desaturation over time. Certain questions may prompt further data collection and analysis in the search for decreasing the incidence of negative outcomes. The impact of the clinical significance of the event, the seasonal variation, the type of procedures more likely to result in the event, and patient characteristics associated with the event are additional possible considerations.

Traditionally, in health care quality assurance, acceptance levels of problems were usually arbitrarily assigned. Since this type of level of acceptance is usually set up prior to evaluation and not statistically defined, it usually favors a static acceptance of errors and problems *(18)*. In order to move toward a more dynamic model for quality improvement, an understanding of the data regarding unacceptable performance, defect problem, or incident is critical. A threshold rate must be established. The threshold can be considered as a level of tolerance or acceptance of defects or incidents beyond which further investigation is necessary. The threshold can be established

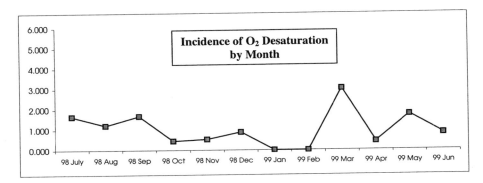

Fig. 4. Example of a run chart.

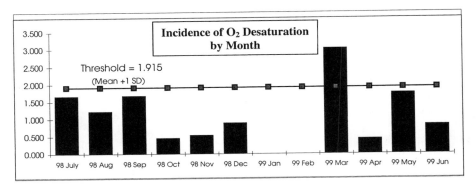

Fig. 5. Example of a control chart: bar graph with threshold.

by the data itself or by benchmarking. Once initial quality improvement data collection has been completed, the data can be used to generate a threshold performance standard. The mean or average occurrence can serve as a threshold. It is important to calculate the weighted average because each measurement is the average of the cases for that time period. Since the volume of activity varies, the effect of each measurement should be in accordance with its proportionate volume *(18)*.

An important concept in threshold development is variation—specifically, the variation around the mean. If the goal is to consistently meet performance standards, the weighted mean average can also serve as the threshold of acceptable performance if a defined level of standard deviation (SD) of the mean is added *(18)*. Fig. 5 demonstrates the resultant threshold obtained by adding one standard deviation to the calculated mean average for the rate

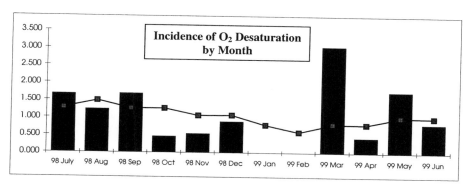

Fig. 6. Example of a control chart: bar graph with rolling mean.

of oxygen desaturation over a 1-year period. If this threshold number is continually recalculated as more data points are collected over time, a rolling mean is obtained that continually drives for improved performance (Fig. 6). This dynamic measurement approach is consistent with the philosophy of continuous quality improvement *(2)*.

The second approach, benchmarking, is a comparison of the published or non-published experience or the results of other similar programs. These could be within the same institution, with other similar institutions, or to a national database. Benchmark data, when compared to institutional data, can identify obvious initial areas for improvement and often allow for identification of practices, which might be used to improve performance. Over time, if used alone, benchmark data tends to result in acceptance of the status quo once the performance matches that of the benchmark.

One nationwide study, The Quality Indicator Project (QI Project) sponsored by The Association of Maryland Hospitals & Health Systems (MHA) began in 1985 as a voluntary pilot project of seven Maryland hospitals *(18)*. The goal of the QI Project is to serve as a tool to assist hospital leadership in overseeing patient care quality and identifying opportunities for improvement. The MHA QI Project now provides clinical performance measurement and national comparative databases for over 1,800 participating hospitals. Quality indicators relating to Sedation Analgesia were added to the database in 1999. The results are available in the aggregate to non-member hospitals and can serve as a beginning source of benchmarking *(19)*. The project reports an overall rate of severe oxygen desaturation during sedation analgesia between 1.5% and 4.2%. Before accepting this range as a benchmark, it is important to note that hospitals of varying sizes participate in the project and that the measurement is for all sedation locations within those institutions. A measurement of interest for one particular location may not reflect the case mix of an entire institution. The project also defines severe desaturation as a drop of 5% or more. At this level of measurement (5%), the result would be a larger number of severe desaturations than if 10% were used as the quantifier for the indicator. Thus, care must be taken in interpreting and using any benchmarking results.

5.3. Quality Monitoring of Sedation Analgesia

Once indicators are chosen for measurement, a methodology for data collection, analysis, and reporting must be defined. Depending on available resources, the data is usually collected by either random sampling of sedation cases or by databasing all sedation cases. Because sedation is a high-risk activity and occurrences of adverse events are relatively rare, it may be advisable to collect data on all cases. Databasing all sedation cases has certain advantages. Low levels of compliance and variation can be better detected. Demographic and clinical information can be readily available to understand the results of the quality indicators. Aspects of sedation practice that are of interest to practitioner credentialing, such as number of cases performed or levels of sedation attained, can be reported.

In order to understand what is being measured, a flow chart of the data process can be helpful. Fig. 7 depicts the methodology used for data collection, analysis and reporting of all sedation cases. Fig. 8 is a replication of the screening tool, the Clinical Quality Indicator Screen, (QI Screen) used at the author's institution. As shown in Fig. 7, the QI Screen is critical to two outputs: the Quarterly Report of activity and quality indicator events including the Case Review Process. The shaded areas indicate possible points of lost information. It can be seen that the denominator for quality indicators is the number of cases for which the QI Screen was completed and databased. Given the particular culture of an organization, lost information could be significant. Thus, an important QA activity would be to occasionally evaluate the proportion of sedation cases for which a screening form is submitted.

5.4. The Quality Improvement Process

Over the years, the management of quality has been intensely studied and conceptualized. Quality assurance has evolved to incorporate sophisticated methodologies and measurements. The development of quality indicators provides a framework within which to objectively and systematically pursue opportunities to improve care and clinical performance. By the early 1990s, hospitals and health care associations across the country had embraced quality improvement, also known as "Continuous Quality Improvement"

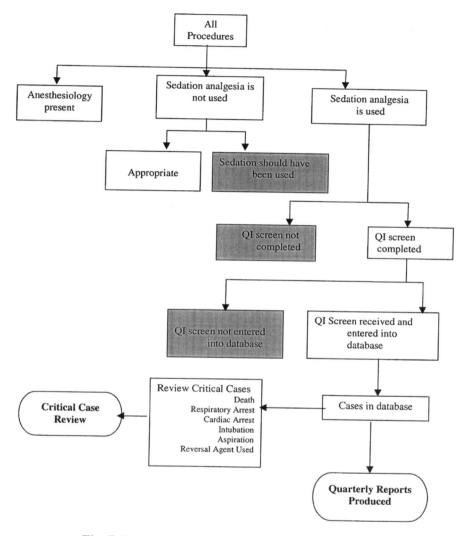

Fig. 7. Sedation analgesia QI methodology flowchart.

(CQI) or "Total Quality Management" (TQM), as an integrated, coordinated approach to systematically review and evaluate clinical performance *(2)*. The broad inclusive concepts of continuous quality improvement today overshadow the traditional department-based QA programs. Indeed, one of the basic tenets of the Quality Movement is that quality is not a department, a technique, or a philosophy. It is a fundamental way of managing organizations as well as the systems, processes, and activities that define its outputs *(20)*.

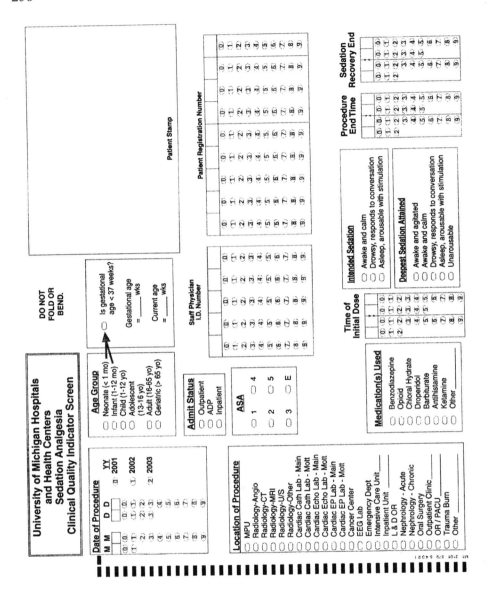

University of Michigan Hospitals
and Health Centers
Sedation Analgesia
Clinical Quality Indicator Screen

Patient Stamp

DO NOT
FOLD OR
BEND.

Date of Procedure

Age Group
Neonate (< 1 mo)
Infant (1-12 mo)
Child (1-12 yo)
Adolescent (13-16 yo)
Adult (16-65 yo)
Geriatric (> 65 yo)

Is gestational age < 37 weeks?

Gestational age = ____ wks
Current age = ____ wks

Admit Status
Outpatient
ADP
Inpatient

ASA
1   4
2   5
3   E

Patient Registration Number

Staff Physician I.D. Number

Location of Procedure
MPU
Radiology-Angio
Radiology-CT
Radiology-MRI
Radiology-U/S
Radiology-Other
Cardiac Cath Lab - Main
Cardiac Cath Lab - Mott
Cardiac Echo Lab - Main
Cardiac Echo Lab - Mott
Cardiac EP Lab - Main
Cardiac EP Lab - Mott
Cancer Center
EEG Lab
Emergency Dept
Intensive Care Unit
Inpatient Unit ____
L & D OR
Nephrology - Acute
Nephrology - Chronic
Oral Surgery
Outpatient Clinic
OR / PACU
Trauma Burn
Other ____

Medication(s) Used
Benzodiazepine
Opioid
Chloral Hydrate
Droperidol
Barbiturate
Antihistamine
Ketamine
Other

Time of Initial Dose

Intended Sedation
Awake and calm
Drowsy, responds to conversation
Asleep, arousable with stimulation

Deepest Sedation Attained
Awake and agitated
Awake and calm
Drowsy, responds to conversation
Asleep, arousable with stimulation
Unarousable

Procedure End Time

Sedation Recovery End

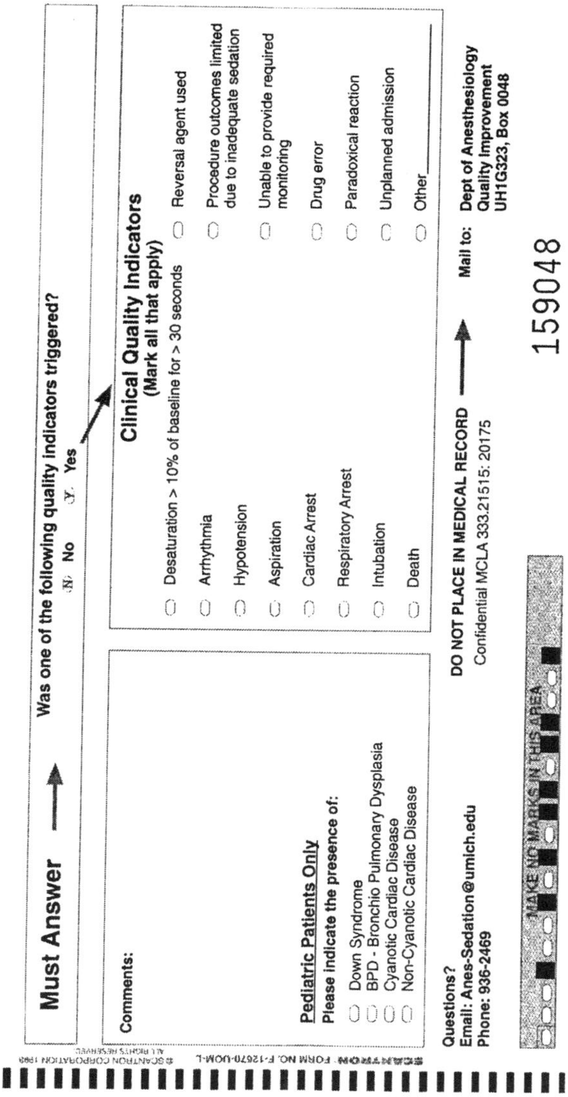

Must Answer → Was one of the following quality indicators triggered?

⊙ N: No ⊙ Y: Yes

Clinical Quality Indicators
(Mark all that apply)

○ Desaturation > 10% of baseline for > 30 seconds   ○ Reversal agent used

○ Arrhythmia   ○ Procedure outcomes limited due to inadequate sedation

○ Hypotension

○ Aspiration   ○ Unable to provide required monitoring

○ Cardiac Arrest   ○ Drug error

○ Respiratory Arrest   ○ Paradoxical reaction

○ Intubation   ○ Unplanned admission

○ Death   ○ Other

Comments:

Pediatric Patients Only
Please indicate the presence of:

○ Down Syndrome
○ BPD - Bronchio Pulmonary Dysplasia
○ Cyanotic Cardiac Disease
○ Non-Cyanotic Cardiac Disease

DO NOT PLACE IN MEDICAL RECORD →
Confidential MCLA 333.21515: 20175

Mail to: Dept of Anesthesiology
Quality Improvement
UH1G323, Box 0048

Questions?
Email: Anes-Sedation@umich.edu
Phone: 936-2469

159048

MAKE NO MARKS IN THIS AREA

Fig. 8. Clinical quality indicator screen.

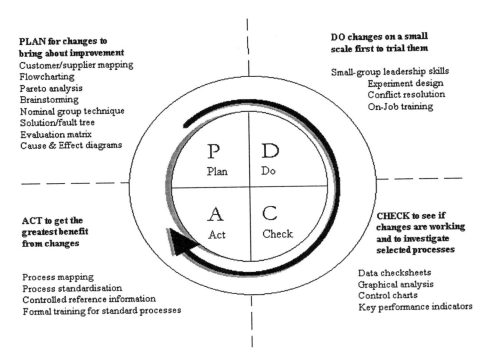

Fig. 9. The PDCA cycle. Reprinted with permission from ref. *(22)*.

Many health systems use the Plan-Do-Check-Act (PDCA) cycle (Fig. 9) or a variation of it, as both a managerial and a quality tool *(21,22)*. The PDCA cycle is a checklist of the four stages which move from understanding a process, evaluating a process, identification of a problem, correcting a problem, and again evaluating the process. This continuous feedback loop as depicted in Fig. 9.

The collection and analysis of QI data is within the check stage of the cycle. This is traditional quality assurance or quality control. Checking is a critical element in the sedation quality improvement process. Since sedation is a high-risk activity, the occurrences of indicators that are determined to be critical or adverse events are reviewed. The critical indicator case review is an important source of information and identification of opportunities for improvement. A sample critical indicator case review process is described as a flowchart in Fig. 10. Quality improvement is practiced when there is a systematic movement from checking to acting, doing, and then re-checking.

The assessment of quality indicators involves determining current levels of performance, stability of the processes over time, comparison to external

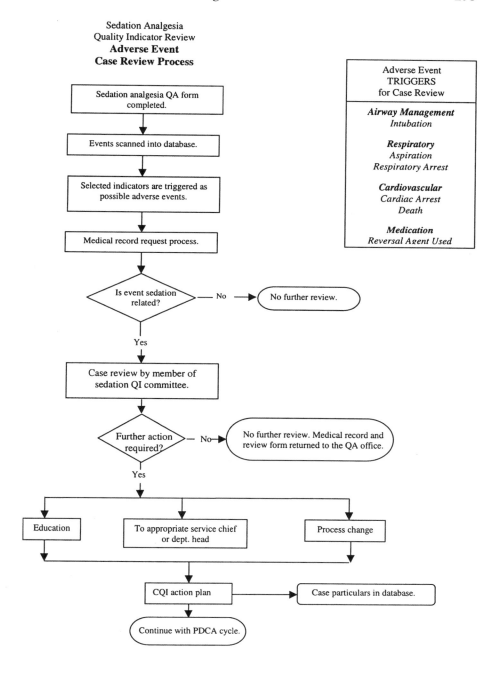

Fig. 10. Case review process flowchart.

benchmarks, identification of areas that can be improved, prioritization of improvement opportunities and development of improvements. The role of an interdisciplinary sedation quality improvement committee is critical in the QI process. A well-functioning sedation QI committee, not only acts as an institutional resource for sedation but allows for the cross pollination of ideas, consensus building, and the development and implementation of sedation practices that are safe, effective, and institutionally acceptable.

6. CONCLUSION

Quality Management is now an integral component of health care management. Although QA remains an important part of high risk clinical practice such as sedation analgesia, CQI, with its concepts of cross departmental problem solving and the understanding and redesigning key processes, is a model for quality improvement in sedation practice. Once sedation is taken out of the sheltered environment of the operating room, interaction with hospital systems and varied personnel can cause unwanted variability in the sedation analgesia process. Only by working within a systematic framework, in partnership with the clinical and support staff responsible for sedation performed by the non-anesthesiologist, can variability be decreased and quality outcomes be attained more consistently.

REFERENCES

1. Mokhashi, M. and Hawes, R. (1998) Struggling Toward Easier Endoscopy. *Gastroint. Endosc.* **48(4)**, 432–440.
2. The American College of Radiology Committee on Quality Assurance. Guide to Continuous Quality Improvement in Medical Imaging. *The American College of Radiology Publications* 1998.
3. Patterson, E. (2000) New Rules impact sedation and anesthesia care, Part 1. *Nursing Management* **31(5)**, 22.
4. Smith, D. F. (1999) Conscious Sedation, Anesthesia and the JCAHO, in *The JCAHO's Anesthesia-Related Standards.* Marblehead, MA: Opus Communication Inc., pp. 59–122.
5. Joint Commission on Accreditation of Healthcare Organizations (2000) Revision to anesthesia care standards. *Comprehensive Accreditation Manual for Hospitals* Effective January 1, 2001; http://www.jcaho.org/standard/aneshap.html.
6. American Society of Anesthesiologists. (October 13, 1999) Continuum of depth of sedation: Definition of General Anesthesia and Levels of Sedation/ Analgesia. *American Society of Anesthesiologists* http://www.asahq.org/ Standards/20.htm.
7. Joint Commission Resources. (2001) Anesthesia and Sedation, in *Topics in Clinical Care Improvement.* Joint Commission on Accreditation of Healthcare Organizations, 41–45.

8. Schroeder, P. (1991) Clinical indicators: development and use. *Journal of Nursing Quality* **6(1)**, 1–87.
9. Deming, W. E. (1986) *Out of the Crisis,* MIT Press, Cambridge, MA.
10. Berwick, D. M. (1989) Continuous Improvement as an Ideal in Health Care. *N. Engl. J. Med.* **320(1)**, 53–56.
11. Sales, A., Moscovice, I., and Lurie, N. (2000) Implementing CQI Projects in Hospitals. *The Joint Commission Journal on Quality Improvement* **26(8)**, 476–487.
12. Donabedian, A. (1980) The Definition of Quality and Approaches to its Assessment. Ann Arbor, MI, Health Administration Press.
13. Laffel, G. and Blumenthal, D. (1989 Nov. 24) The Case for Using Industrial Quality Management Science in Health Care Organizations. *JAMA* **262(20)**, 2869–2873.
14. Ross, P. and Fochtman, D. (1995 July) Conscious sedation: a quality management project. *Journal of Pediatric Oncology Nursing* **12(3)**, 115–121.
15. Brassard, M. and Ritter, D. (1994) The memory Jogger: A pocket guide to tools for continuous improvement and effective planning. GOAL/QPC, Methuen, MA.
16. Foster, F. (2000) Conscious sedation: coming to a unit near you. *Nursing Management* **31(4)**, 45, 48–52.
17. Kost, M. (1999) Conscious sedation: guarding your patient against complications. *Nursing* **20(4)**, 34–38.
18. Matthes, N. and Wood, N. (2001) Developing performance measures for sedation and analgesia: the approach of the quality indicator project. *Journal of Healthcare Quality* **23(4)**, 5–10.
19. The Association of Maryland Hospitals & Health Systems (MHA). (2000) *Quality Indicator Project* http://www.qiproject.org/
20. Thomas, P., Kettrick, R., and Singsen, B. (1992) Quality Assurance and Continuous Quality Improvement: History, Current Practice and Future Directions. *Delaware Medical Journal* **64(8)**, 507–513.
21. Institute for Healthcare Improvement Quality Improvement Resources: A Model for Accelerating Improvement. *National Academy Press* 2001; http://www.ihi.org/resources/qi/
22. HCi, PDCA Cycle: From Problem Faced to Problem Solved. *HCi Toolkits* 2000; http://www.hci.com.au/hcisite2/toolkit/pdcacycl.htm.